Engaged Jainism

SUNY series in Religious Studies

Harold Coward, editor

Engaged Jainism

Critical and Constructive Studies of Jain Social Engagement

Edited by

CHRISTOPHER JAIN MILLER and
COGEN BOHANEC

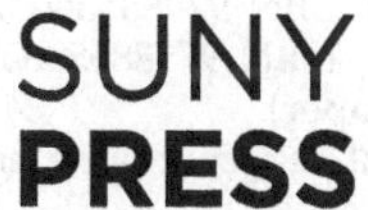

Cover: Clockwise from top right: Mehool Sanghrajka (Institute of Jainology), left, preparing to present Dr. Jasvant Modi (Vardhamana Charitable Foundation), right, with the Ahimsa award at the UK House of Commons (2024); Ruchika Chitrabhanu (The Earthen One) holding a rescued baby goat at an animal sanctuary in India; Pramodabhen Chitrabhanu (PETA India) taking care of a rescued cow at an animal sanctuary in India; Dr. Nitin Shah (right) performs a free eye examination for a patient in need (left) at the Healthfair at Huntington Park, California; Mahersh Shah, Nishma Shah, and Rehma Chandaria (from left to right) speaking with a fellow member of the Jain community about veganism at the Jain Vegans booth in the UK, with special thanks to Sagar Shah at Jain Vegans (jainvegans.org) for providing this photo; Dr. Tushar Mehta (left front with sunglasses) volunteering with Health Education Project Haiti (hephaiti.com/education) in the town of Tiburon for a dental and medical project as well as a family planning program (2018); and Dr. Parveen Jain (CEO and President, Arihanta Institute) giving a keynote speech about Arihanta Institute at the Arihanta Institute Gala in Northern California (2023).

Published by State University of New York Press, Albany

Printed in the United States of America

EU GPSR Authorised Representative:
Logos Europe, 9 rue Nicolas Poussin, 17000, La Rochelle, France
contact@logoseurope.eu

For information, contact State University of New York Press, Albany, NY
www.sunypress.edu

Library of Congress Cataloging-in-Publication Data

Names: Miller, Christopher Patrick, 1981– editor. | Bohanec, Cogen, editor.
Title: Engaged Jainism : critical and constructive studies of Jain social engagement / edited by Christopher Jain Miller and Cogen Bohanec.
Description: Albany : State University of New York Press, [2026]. | Includes bibliographical references.
Identifiers: LCCN 2025034947 | ISBN 9798855805710 (hardcover : alk/ paper) | ISBN 9798855807127 (epub) | ISBN 9798855805734 (PDF) | ISBN 9798855805727 (pbk. : alk. paper)
Subjects: LCSH: Jainism—Social aspects | Jaina ethics | Jaina philosophy | Jainism—Doctrines
Classification: LCC BL1375.S63 E54 2025
LC record available at https://lccn.loc.gov/2025034947

For Parveen Jain

First knowledge of the world, then compassion for it.

—*Daśavaikālika Sūtra* 4.10

Contents

Part V: Interfaith Engagement

Acknowledgments

We would like to express our sincere gratitude to Arihanta Institute for its unwavering support of our research and this volume. Particular thanks goes out to our CEO and president, Dr. Parveen Jain, to whom this volume is dedicated, as well as to our entire team of faculty, staff, volunteers, and supporters, including Jonathan Dickstein, Pramod Patel, Kamlesh Mehta, Kavita Mahendra, Taina Rodriguez-Berardi, Opal Shah, Biren Shah, Umesh Sagar, Sunil Mehta, Bijal Vakil, Shobha Vora, Pramod Khincha, Suman Khincha, Sharvari Dixit, Prem Jain, Narendra Parson, Jasvant Modi, Mohini Jain, Hope Bohanec, Diana Hulet, and Dhanesh Kothari. Special thanks also goes to all of our colleagues at Claremont School of Theology, especially Grant Hagiya, Jeff Kuan, Andrew Dreitcer, Yuki Schwartz, Grace Kao, and Venu Mehta. Christopher Jain Miller would like to personally thank his mentor and PhD advisor Dr. Smriti Srinivas at the University of California, Davis, who introduced him to the concept of engaged Buddhism and engaged religion a decade ago, and Professor Nicolas Martin and the Asien-Orient-Institut at the University of Zürich for their support for his research. He also extends gratitude to the Berlin Wall Foundation (Stiftung Berliner Mauer) for its generous assistance with the images of the East Side Gallery in chapter 4. Cogen Bohanec would like to pay gratitude to Dr. Rita D. Sherma for being an important advisor, a stalwart supporter, and an inspiring mentor in our work, as well as to the esteemed scholars of the Dharma Academy of North America (DANAM), held in conjunction with the Annual Meeting of the American Academy of Religion, for consistently providing a forum for innovative approaches to the study of dharma traditions. An earlier version of chapter 2 was originally published in the *International Journal of Hindu Studies* and has been reprinted in part here with the kind permission of Springer.

We thank all of our authors for their passion and dedication to establishing research in the field of engaged Jain studies, as well as our three anonymous peer reviewers for their feedback and enthusiastic support of this volume.

Finally, we express our deep gratitude to the Uberoi Foundation for their support of Arihanta Institute's research project titled "Compassion in Jainism, Buddhism, Hinduism, and Sikhism," which contributed to the publication of several chapters.

Foreword

PARVEEN JAIN

On Earth Day in April 2023, Arihanta Institute hosted a two-day conference titled Defining Applied Jain Studies to bring together some of the leading Jain scholars from around the world who are researching Jain engagements with various contemporary social, environmental, and animal advocacy concerns. This conference was a preamble to the MA in England Jain Studies program that was initiated in fall 2023 in partnership with Claremont School of Theology. By supplementing the traditional application of Jain principles to societal issues with critical and constructive frameworks from historical, philosophical, and anthropological perspectives of the Jain tradition, the Engaged Jain Studies graduate program is an essential and highly relevant field of study in today's complex world.

Jains have always actively engaged with society to deal with wide-ranging social concerns. The ancient scriptural aphorism, *parasparopagraho jīvānām*, meaning "all life is bound together by mutual support and interdependence," best illustrates the tradition's distinctive nature. Jains have always known that "mutual support" can be possible only through active engagement with everything around us—humans and other living beings, the environment, ecology, etc.

For Jains, the concept of engagement begins with the Tīrthaṅkaras themselves. To facilitate effective engagement between spiritual practitioners and society, Lord Mahāvīra, the last Tīrthaṅkara of the current era, like his predecessors, established a fourfold organization (*caturvidh saṅgha*) constituting female and male mendicants and male and female householders. Both types of mendicants engaged with the general populace to promote nonviolence through teachings, and both types of householders engaged in worldly affairs with an unwavering focus on philanthropy and service. In parallel, all four constituents persevered—while fully engaged with society—with their own internalized practices for self-improvement.

Ahiṃsā, the bedrock of Jain teachings, is paramount and essential to how Jains engage with others. Over 2,550 years ago, Lord Mahāvīra regularly engaged with all levels of society to expose the ill effects of slavery, gender inequality, the caste system, animal sacrifice, and other violent and hurtful customs prevailing at that time. In every instance—and his life involved many inspirational episodes—to facilitate social reform, he engaged and persuaded the rulers, politicians, social leaders, and others with compassion, friendliness, and mutual respect without ever deploying confrontational tactics. One of the many widely documented episodes from Mahāvīra's life that illustrates his endeavors is the episode involving Candanbālā, a princess who underwent many traumatic experiences involving female abuse, slave trading, forced imprisonment, and more. Her plight was brought to light by Mahāvīra through his penance of fasting where he vowed that he would only accept alms from such a princess who was a destitute, starving young lady with shaved head, in shackles, in a small room, with a bowl of roasted chickpeas, and in tears—a set of preconditions that only Candanbālā seemed to fulfill. This episode is an example of Mahāvīra's endeavors to engage society without harshly confronting anyone but instead by making his message clear with self-imposed austerities and penance.

Throughout history, following Mahāvīra, Jains actively engaged with ruling and "elite" classes for the betterment of society. They actively advised and supported rulers but rarely became the rulers themselves. For instance, as noted by Dr. Padmanabh Jaini in his well-known work *The Jaina Path of Purification*, Jain mendicants, such as Hirāvijaya Sūri, convinced the Mughal Emperor Akbar to enact promotion of *amāra* (prohibition of animal sacrifice) in the Muslim kingdoms of northern India on the days considered auspicious by the Jain community (Jaini 1979, 284). Under Hirāvijaya Sūri's influence, Akbar renounced his much-loved hunting, he restricted fishing practice, and subsequently abstained almost wholly from eating meat.

Jains have traditionally engaged in business and trade, but always with an eye on society's welfare. The *Upāsakadaśāṅgasūtra*, a highly revered Jain scripture on the traits of the ideal Jain layman, features Ānanda Śrāvaka, who was involved in massive business deals but restrained himself by taking the vow of limited personal assets and committing his profits to philanthropy for social welfare. For ideal Jain householders, business is not for self-indulgence—it is a vehicle for social service and fulfilling the community's needs. For example, trading was encouraged to meet regional supply and demand by ensuring the wide use of articles produced at one location by moving them to avoid shortages at other places. Even today, on average, the philanthropic contribution of Jains is generally believed to be many times higher than any other community.

In recent times, perhaps one of the most venerable Jain gurus of our times Shrimad Rajcandra played a catalytic role in shaping Mahatma Gandhi's sociopolitical outlook by enlightening him with the power of nonviolence to the point that Gandhi concluded that nonviolence is the weapon of the brave and not of the timid. Shrimad's teachings guided him to craft methods to engage with Indian citizens on the one hand and the British empire on the other, and transformed an ordinary "Mohandas" into the "Mahatma." We all know how Mahatma Gandhi influenced Dr. Martin Luther King Jr., Nelson Mandela, and others, carrying the influence of Jain teachings into the majority of democratic social movements in the twentieth century and beyond.

In 1975, Ācārya Sushil Kumar, a revered Jain monk of India, came to America with the mission to enlighten the world about the importance of *ahiṃsā*. Having successfully organized multiple World Religion Conferences and having interacted with the highest level of political and social leaders like the president and prime minister of India, he knew the profound impact of engaged spirituality on society's cultural, social, and political fabric. He traveled worldwide to inspire the Jain diaspora to organize and engage with communities and institutions around them to familiarize them with Jain values. Ācārya Sushil Kumar established Siddhachalam—the first Jain *tīrtha* outside of India—as the center for disseminating

Jain teachings. He built strong affiliations with the United Nations and many of the leading faith-based organizations, and he worked with a plethora of universities and other institutions. He regularly met with the world's leading religious and political leaders, such as presidents of the US and USSR and the Pope, and frequently delivered talks at the UN and other institutions. He always reminded everyone of the importance of peace and emphasized *ahiṃsā* as the most important and sustainable way for the world to move forward. His vision inspired the founding of many Jain institutions, including Arihanta Institute.

Jains have always understood the importance of staying engaged, but engagement methods have continually changed with time, circumstances, and place—*kāla, bhava,* and *kṣetra*. We know that what worked just a few decades ago may not work today, and what works in India may not work in the Western world. Thus, strategy and engagement methods must evolve, and our Engaged Jain Studies graduate program at Claremont School of Theology, as well as the volume before you, is designed to develop methods for studying Jain engagements with the world.

The publication in your hands is a compilation of articles on *Engaged Jainism: Critical and Constructive Studies of Jain Social Engagement* documenting the research and scholarship of some of the leading experts in the field. As Dr. Christopher Jain Miller states in the introductory chapter, the three methodological tendencies in engaged Jain studies include the "constructive-reproductive," "critical-analytical," and "critical-constructive," which together seek to provide a balanced representation that includes and underscores the shortcomings of Jain engagements as well. Keeping the principle of *anekāntavāda* in mind, it is important to note that an academic volume like this one does not seek to reduce discussions of engaged Jainism to a one-sided overestimation of Jain contributions without simultaneously applying a critical lens, an approach that was established with Arihanta Institute's Defining Applied Jain Studies Conference (2023).

Finally, with escalating human tendencies in thought, speech, and actions to be at war with each other, with everything around them, and, to some extent, with themselves, Jain values based on *ahiṃsā* and *karuṇā* and their optimal engagement are more critically important now than ever before. The featured researchers in this volume, and those who we spotlight at Arihanta Institute, are leading the way in articulating the methods that Jains employ for bringing peace to our turbulent world through social *engagement*.

Parveen Jain, PhD
Founder and CEO, Arihanta Institute

Introduction

Conceptualizing "Engaged" Jainism and the Field of "Engaged" Jain Studies

CHRISTOPHER JAIN MILLER

At the beginning of his introduction to Jainism, *The Jains*, the late Paul Dundas (1952–2023) described "a tendency which has persisted into modern times and would interpret one of the world's oldest religions in a manner so narrow as to be little better than caricature" (Dundas 2002, 2). Dundas was issuing a corrective to the ubiquitous portrayals of the Jain tradition as colorless, austere, and pathologically preoccupied with the practice of nonviolence found not only in modern Orientalist Indological research but also in similar depictions of the Jains found in early classical Hindu literature (ibid., 2–3). These portrayals tended to focus on the ascetic community and ignored the very active householder community, thereby misrepresenting Jains and their tradition in ways that have trickled down to the present. Dundas was therefore offering an important critique toward those who produced these unfair stereotypes of Jains and Jainism as obsessively *disengaged* from the world. Like Dundas, scholarship in the field of Jain studies has clearly shown that Jains—both lay and ascetic—are, in the broadest sense of the word, *engaged* with the world in manifold ways both now and in the recent and distant past. Jains are indeed "Jains in the World" (Cort 2001), and therefore the question as to whether or not Jain traditions are "engaged" is, at this point, irrelevant.

The more important question to ask, then, is what exactly do we mean by "engaged," and why is it urgently necessary to conceptualize a field of "engaged Jain studies" and a corresponding object of study, "engaged Jainism"? In this introduction I seek to answer these questions by considering the multiple forms of engagement Jains and Jainism—as well as those who study and research both—have been implicated in, both in the past and present. I include close consideration of historical issues and methodological tendencies in Jain studies and in doing so propose a reevaluation of both the "field" of Jain studies and the field's object, "Jainism."

Let us begin by considering that since 2010, Jain donors working first with the Jain Education and Research Foundation (JERF) and, since 2015, with the Academic Liaison Committee (ALC) of the Federation of Jain Associations in North America (JAINA) have "established Endowed Chairs, Professorships, Post-Doctoral Fellowships, Lectureships, Adjunct Professorships, Fellowships in Prakrit, Annual Lecture programs etc. in more [than] 30 universities in [the] USA, Canada, Belgium and [the] U.K. and this efforts [*sic*] is continuing" (JAINA 2023). The generosity of these Jain donors, who have donated tens of millions of dollars, continues to exponentially expand viable career paths for Jain scholars in North America and Europe, where careers in the humanities have been otherwise shrinking. It has also made it possible for students in these settings to learn about the Jain tradition.

Also consider that these new research and teaching positions fall under the ALC's mission, "To establish liaison with Academic institutions in North America that are promoting or willing *to promote the study, teaching and research* in the principles, philosophy, culture and history *of Jain Dharma*" (JAINA 2023, emphases added). The primary principles to which the ALC and most any diasporic Jain will refer are nonviolence (*ahiṃsā*) but also often include non-possession (*aparigraha*) and tolerance for perspectives that are different from our own (*anekāntavāda*). Frequently added to these three core A's of *ahiṃsā*, *aparigraha*, and *anekāntavāda* is the oft-quoted Sanskrit phrase *parasparopagraho jīvānām* ("The function of souls is to help one another"), which seeks to convey the notion of the interconnectedness of all souls and our corresponding duty to care for and respect all forms of life. From the Jain perspective, these and other related principles have much to offer our troubled world and the many challenges we collectively face as a global society.

Indeed, the emphases I have added in italics in the previous paragraph are meant to highlight one of the frequent imperatives many Jain scholars filling their newly funded positions in the academy face as they find themselves placed in a role of continuous relational engagement with the North American Jain community who are interested in promoting and "applying" Jain principles to the manifold crises and challenges of contemporary life. Scholars who have trained for years in critical academic fields such as history, the social sciences, philosophy, or philology and who are expected to objectively and critically identify nuance and particularity in religious traditions now find themselves engaging with a diasporic Jain community who regularly seek to "apply" Jain principles to select issues normatively, constructively, and universally to *"promote the study, teaching and research,"* as I have italicized, *"of Jain Dharma"* (JAINA 2023).

In other words, academic imperatives of retaining etic objectivity come into close contact with emic Jain imperatives aimed at applying Jain principles, often leaving scholars in a self-consciously "torn" (Miller et al. 2023) position wherein they confront the obligation to maintain scholarly impartiality while simultaneously remaining sympathetic to the worldviews of Jains and the donor communities subsidizing their academic careers. These recent productive frictions between both of these "engaged universals" (Tsing 2005, 8)—academic and Jain—give rise to an urgent need for the field of Jain studies to conceptualize a field of engaged Jain studies whose central imperative is to study what I have called "engaged Jainism."

Affixing "Engaged" to "Jainism" and "Jain Studies"

I affix the term "engaged" to "Jainism" and "Jain studies" following four very particular and intentional frameworks. These frameworks include the notions of (1) "engaged universals" (Tsing 2005, 8), (2) "engaged scholars" (Broad 2016, 12), (3) "engaged learning" (Miller

2019), and (4) "engaged Buddhism" (e.g., Queen and King 1996; Fuller 2021). These four frameworks are already operating in the field of Jain studies to varying degrees, though I make them explicit here to be able to provide a foundation for us to conceptualize the field of engaged Jain studies and its object, engaged Jainism, in the sections that follow.

Anthropologist Anna Tsing uses the phrase "engaged universals" to refer to the transformative process that occurs when universal epistemes such as neoliberal ideology, science, etc. come into contact and produce frictions with local contexts and alternative cultural logics. Tsing writes, "Cultures are continually co-produced in the interaction I call 'friction': the awkward, unequal, unstable, and creative qualities of interconnection across difference . . . Engaged universals travel across difference and are charged and changed by their travels. Through friction, universals become practically effective . . . Engaged universals must convince us to pay attention to them. All universals are engaged when considered as practical projects accomplished in a heterogeneous world" (Tsing 2005, 4, 8). Tsing's "engaged universals," and in our case diasporic Jainism but also the episteme of the Western academy, are necessarily transformed from the frictions they encounter when they come in contact with one another. Frictions also occur anytime that "universal" Jain principles encounter new cultural terrain wherein Jains attempt to promote and retain their way of life (see Miller and Dickstein 2021a). This has been true for Jains historically as well, as their epistemic systems became entangled with and experienced intellectual friction against rival schools of thought, for example. "Engaged Jainism" accounts for the epistemic frictions Jains have encountered, challenged, and adapted to both past and present, while also taking into consideration the epistemic frictions between sometimes irreconcilable Jain and academic ways of knowing.

Whether they subscribe to or themselves espouse Jain values in their work, many scholars researching and teaching the Jain tradition today are directly engaged with the Jain community in some meaningful way. Some, though certainly not all, of these scholars understand Jain principles to hold promise for the many challenges we face globally and thereby often work as partners with the Jain community to propagate and apply these principles. In doing so, they become "engaged scholars" in a very specific sense, insofar as they are often "participating in everyday struggles for social justice" of some kind (Broad 2016, 12).[1] As Broad, a scholar working with Black communities for food justice explains, an engaged scholar participates in engaged scholarship, which seeks

> to produce scholarly knowledge while simultaneously conducting research that may help research participants advance, facilitate, and reflect upon their own social change efforts. This engaged approach differs from some of the traditional standards in American academia, which has often called for a sharp break between researcher and research subjects. Those who follow this engaged methodology, however, believe that a collaborative research practice is ethically sound and can serve as a foundation for the production of scholarly insights that would be difficult to garner through a more neutral observational approach. (Ibid., 13)

Engaged scholars use the methods of the Western academy to carry out their research, though they do so in collaboration with the communities that they study and take seriously, though not uncritically, those communities' voices, cultural imperatives, and truth claims. In my own collaborative work with the Jain community, for example, I have sought to demonstrate how Jains and those who take Jain principles seriously might significantly reduce their climate impact by considering giving up dairy (Miller 2023).

Similarly, scholars often share their engaged scholarship with students in their graduate and undergraduate classrooms and even bring their students into engagement with their research communities. Here, the transformative pedagogical technique of engaged learning (Miller 2019, 1) and its counterpart, high-impact learning (Kuh et al. 2013), become useful for putting students into direct engagement with the local Jain community. Such engaged educational encounters, as I have written elsewhere regarding my own experience using these techniques, "involve experiential learning experiences that take place within particular communities, collaborative undergraduate projects aimed at addressing real social challenges, and transformative intercultural exchanges intended to expose students to alternative worldviews" (Miller 2019, 5). Through these engaged learning experiences, students are transformed and sometimes themselves become long-term active partners and scholars of Jain traditions. For example, many former International School for Jain Studies (ISJS) students, having engaged with the Jain community in India, now occupy Jain professorships and chairs in North America and Europe.

Finally, scholars of engaged Buddhist studies consider how Buddhists engage (or perhaps even disengage, as we will see) with the world, through social issues past and present, in light of Buddhist principles, as well as how these engagements transform Buddhism and also the broader social landscapes in which Buddhists are engaging. In like manner, engaged Jain studies draws from the methods and debates in engaged Buddhist studies, outlined in the section that follows, to consider the manifold ways that Jains do so, albeit with careful attention to what makes Jains' worldly engagements unique.

Collectively, engaged universals, engaged scholars, engaged learning, and engaged Buddhism help us account for the manifold ways Jains and scholars engage with one another, the way that these engagements can be both culturally and intellectually transformative and productive, and the ways Jain-specific cultural and religious principles are applied to issues of contemporary social and intellectual relevance. As Jain principles and traditions are applied within specific cultural circumstances, the Jain tradition is transformed in particular ways, but so too is the cultural context, including academia itself, with which Jains are engaging. "Jainism" becomes "engaged Jainism," while the academic field of "Jain studies" becomes "engaged Jain studies."

I now turn our attention to a more detailed consideration of the robust field of engaged Buddhist studies, which, having confronted many of the promises and challenges common to Jain studies today, provides a well-formed lotus upon which we will be able to conceptualize the discipline of engaged Jain studies.

Standing on the Shoulders of Giants: Engaged Jain Studies on the Lotus of Engaged Buddhist Studies

In their groundbreaking *Engaged Buddhism: Buddhist Liberation Movements in Asia*, Queen and King observed how the Three

Refuges (Pali: *tisaraṇa;* Sanskrit: *triśaraṇa*) or Three Jewels (Pali: *tiratna;* Sanskrit: *triratna*) of Buddhism, which include the Buddha (leader of the tradition), the Dharma (teachings on liberation), and the Sangha (practicing community), provide a useful framework through which one can understand "important patterns of thought and action" in the various forms of contemporary engaged Buddhism that their volume considered (Queen and King 1996, 6). As they show, leaders of Buddhist traditions have reinterpreted the Three Refuges from ancient texts and teachings, sometimes with the help of scholars, including members of the Theosophical Society in the late nineteenth century (ibid., 22). These Buddhists have re-envisioned liberation as a soteriological goal accomplished not through withdrawal from the world, but through active engagement in particular social struggles. Writing in the mid-1990s, Queen and King observed how these struggles often included "animal liberation, women's liberation, liberation theology, gay liberation, or the liberation of Kuwait," for example (ibid., 9).

Despite these innovative applications of Buddhism, Queen and King argue, "A tradition may be transformed without being betrayed, and heresies may enrich and broaden a cultural heritage while leaving behind those elements—beliefs, practices, institutional forms, public roles—that no longer meet the needs of living communities in a changed world" (ibid., 31). In other words, Buddhist traditions can still be regarded as authoritatively "Buddhist" as they transform to grapple with the particular social contexts with which they are engaged so long as they have, at a minimum, the Three Refuges as a part of their fundamental ideological framework.[2] While such an approach may risk essentializing Buddhism, it helpfully provides a very basic ground upon which one can identify engaged Buddhism as an object of study and as a form of community and practitioner identity.[3]

Because the field of engaged Buddhist studies[4] (e.g., Kraft 2000) has been well-developed over the past three decades, we have much to gain from starting with some of the primary themes and issues in this scholarly work as we conceptualize the field of engaged Jain studies. In doing so, we will gain some useful methodological tools and analytical frameworks while also avoiding potential pitfalls that scholars in engaged Buddhist studies have already become keenly aware of.[5] Though I will address some critical differences, the structural similarities between engaged forms of Buddhism and Jainism are striking. The similarities we will see here arise no doubt on account of the fact that proponents of Buddhism and Jainism share not only origins in South Asia's ancient renouncer cultures (*śramaṇa*, "strivers" for liberation) from the early centuries BCE, but even more so because both traditions have been forced to address many of the same social challenges over the past century and a half in light of colonialism, imperialism, modernization, and globalization through the lenses of their particular traditions.

Like Jains, many Buddhists have been actively concerned with and engaged with the world since the time of the Buddha, applying Buddhist principles such as karma, causality, dependent origination, interdependence, the Four Noble Truths, compassion, loving kindness, giving, and the five precepts, including, like their Jain counterparts, *nonviolence* to issues of contemporary relevance (King 2009, 13–14, 22, 24). Buddhist scholars nevertheless tend to identify "engaged Buddhism" as a very particular type of engagement among Buddhists that began in Asia in the nineteenth century, the likes of which has become entangled with particular contemporary social justice initiatives and liberation movements around the globe concerned with addressing not only individual but also collective suffering (*duḥkha*).

Though the socially engaged Buddhist Thich Nhat Hanh (1926–2022) is credited with coining the phrase "engaged Buddhism" in 1964 in light of the anti-Buddhist violence taking place in Vietnam (Fuller 2021, 5, 178), Chinese Master Taixu (1890–1947) is considered the preeminent modern reformer of Buddhism who provided a template for engaged Buddhism in Asia in light of the social challenges wrought by imperialism and modernization in the early twentieth century (DeVido 2009, 413–414). Taixu used Buddhism's Three Jewels of the Buddha, the Dharma, and the Sangha to promote a "world-engaging Buddhism that ' . . . reforms society, helps humankind to progress, and improves the whole world' " (Shi Taixu 1933, as cited in DeVido 2009, 417). Many engaged Buddhists throughout Asia and beyond, including most prominently Thich Nhat Hanh, would build upon Taixu's blueprint in the generations that followed (DeVido 2009, 425).

Even before Thich Nhat Hanh, however, other reformers were already engaging Buddhism as a means to achieve radical social transformation in South Asia. Bhimrao Ramji Ambedkar (1891–1956) has served as the paramount exemplar of engaged Buddhism in India. Along with millions of his fellow Dalits, Ambedkar publicly converted to Buddhism in 1956 as a symbolic rejection of the caste discrimination[6] he experienced from within his native Hindu tradition (Queen and King 1996, 2–3). In Sri Lanka, Ahangamage Tudor Ariyaratne founded the Sarvodaya Shramadana Movement in 1958. Combining with Gandhian ideals, Ariyaratne's revival movement united the Buddhist quest for individual liberation with the goal of social liberation in a struggling, impoverished, postcolonial Sri Lanka (Bond 1996, 121–122). Around the same time, the fourteenth Dalai Lama fled Tibet in 1959 to Dharamshala in India, a base from which he would disseminate Buddhism globally even as he nonviolently advocated for the independence of the Tibetan people (Cabezón 1996).

Meanwhile, Buddhism was being engaged beyond Asia. In America, Gary Snyder wrote his manifesto titled "Buddhist Anarchism" in 1961, attempting to fuse what would become the growing Western countercultural concern for social revolution and environmentalism with the teachings of Buddhism (Snyder 1961). Engaged forms of Buddhism have indeed spread globally since, as Buddhist traditions have attempted to confront a plethora of global challenges including climate change, animal rights, structural racism, sexism, capitalism, and other social injustices (see Capper 2022; Vesely-Flad 2017; King 2009). To address these and other issues, some engaged Buddhists have recognized that "the principles and even some of the techniques of an engaged Buddhism have been latent in pre-modern Asian settings" but "can now be actualized through Buddhism's exposure to the West, where ethical sensitivity, social activism, and egalitarianism are emphasized" (Kraft, as cited in Eppsteiner 1988, xiii; see Queen and King 1996, 33).[7] In scenarios such as these, scholars' engagement with practitioners and practicing communities produces novel applications of Buddhism whose message and teachings are entangled with, and amplified by, scientific and academic knowledge (see Simmer-Brown 2020).[8] Some "engaged Buddhists," as Gleig more recently explained, "explicitly identify alternative systems of knowledge that have influenced their reading of Buddhist doctrines, such as feminism or systems theory" (Gleig 2021, 11–12), although not without controversy insofar as these movements can sometimes reinforce an "Orientalist binary of a mystical/passive East and a rational/active West and a 'Western savior' model in which modernity rescues Buddhism from its supposed apolitical, asocial slumber" (ibid., 18). For this reason, other scholars have critiqued the field of engaged Buddhist studies altogether, with Hsu recently naming it "Academic Engaged Buddhism," which is a predominantly white, baby boomer, and "hegemonic . . . Western Buddhist practitioner-facing anthological project of Euro-American scholars with potentially powerful but unevenly distributed effects on Buddhist thought and practice from around the world" (Hsu 2022, 17, 22). Some forms of engaged Jain studies, as we shall see, seek to avoid these hegemonic pitfalls through their collaborative approaches with the global Jain community.

Here I have so far provided examples of well-known forms of engaged Buddhism advocating for social justice whose leaders are men. Women have also, however, taken a significant lead toward shaping engaged forms of Buddhism in the past and the present, in Asia and beyond (Storch 2020; Tsomo 2009). As Simmer-Brown has recently shown, for example, Pema Chodron has been engaged in anti-racism dialogue critiquing white privilege in the United States (though not without controversy; see Simmer-Brown 2020). Tsomo has demonstrated how the relocation of women-led forms of engaged Buddhism from Taiwan to other particular global locations has presented unique sets of social challenges and new opportunities. While prominent nuns including Bhiksuni Cheng Yen, Bhiksuni Chao Hwei, and Bhiksuni Shig Hiu Wan have been able to engage Buddhism with issues pertaining to social service, women's rights, animal rights, art, and education in Taiwan, for example, Tsomo also shows how other Taiwanese nuns' engaged Buddhism has become constrained and transformed as it has moved from Taiwan to North America to serve a predominantly Chinese immigrant diaspora (Tsomo 2009).

It is also important to note here that although the field of engaged Buddhist studies at first only considered "consistent advocates and activists for world peace" (Queen and King 1996, 5), not all Buddhist teachers, lineages, or practitioners have adhered to or promoted the values of contemporary social justice movements. Cases such as those at Shambhala, an institution that Pema Chodron has since left in response to the organization's legacy of sexual abuse, remind us of the potentially catastrophic consequences of romanticizing any religious tradition as a solution to global social justice and other challenges. Myanmar's (Burma's) Aung San Suu Kyi provides an even more apt case in point: Following her early "striking example of Buddhist nonviolent resistance" (Queen and King 1996, 2) against her country's ruling military junta that earned her a Nobel Peace Prize in 1991, she has "received widespread criticism for her silence on the Rohingya issue" (Rosenthal 2018) from both within and outside of the global Buddhist community. As a result of this and other cases where Buddhists are not acting as "consistent advocates and activists for world peace" (Queen and King 1996, 5), some scholars of engaged Buddhism have encouraged that the breadth of the field be expanded to include the complexity and messiness of engaged forms of Buddhism worldwide as Buddhism intersects with all forms of political, ethnic, nationalist, and other seemingly less attractive expressions both today and in the past (Main and Lai 2013, 3; see also Fuller 2021; Brown 2023).[9]

Finally, we also need to recognize that not all Buddhists throughout history have found it necessary, worthwhile, or even plausible to practice engaged forms of Buddhism. There are in fact traditions of "Disengaged Buddhists" who "reject involvement with social and political issues as unfruitful and even harmful" and whose doctrines, focusing on the pursuit of wisdom, comprise "a coherent, thoughtful position to be found across a variety of at least classical Indian Buddhist texts" (Lele 2019, 241–242). Regarding the social justice initiatives that engaged Buddhists are involved in, Jeffreys has also argued that "ascribing rights to persons requires that we revise Buddhist ontology" since "ontologically, the self does not exist" (Jeffreys 2003, 271). Such philosophical positions stand counter to many contemporary projects of engaged Buddhists, whether they are advocating for or against social justice and violence.

This overview of key concerns and methodological approaches in the field of engaged Buddhist studies provides the lotus upon which engaged Jain studies sits. From their lotus seats, however, the Jinas disseminated teachings that, though sharing many practical and theoretical foundations with Buddhism, were often in direct conflict with the teachings and practices of the Buddha since the fifth century BCE—and remain so today. Thus in the next section I draw from engaged Buddhist studies while nevertheless highlighting the particular historical, philosophical, and cultural circumstances that require engaged Jain studies to depart from engaged Buddhist studies in important ways.

The Jina on the Lotus: Key Features of Engaged Jain Studies

The Jain tradition possesses its own "Three Jewels" (*ratna-traya*), which are nevertheless quite different from their aforementioned Buddhist counterparts. These are correct worldview (*samyag-darśana*), correct knowledge (*samyag-jñāna*), and correct conduct (*samyak-cāritra*), which, along with a firm commitment to the teachings of their tradition's twenty-four liberated teachers known as the Jinas ("conquerors"), form the basis of Jain identity. As Paul Dundas explains, "The Jains are *at the most basic level* those who credit [the Jinas] with total authority and act according to their teaching of the Three Jewels" (2002, 3, emphasis added). Various interpretations of the elements comprising each of these Three Jewels provide the basic prism through which self-identifying Jains "engage" with the world, and like their Buddhist counterparts, provide a way for us to identify and study various forms of engaged Jainism.

The First Jewel, correct worldview (*samyag-darśana*), assumes that a person subscribes to and "sees" (*darśana*, from √*dṛś*, "to see") and accepts the operations of karma through their personal experience or through the study of Jain scriptures, as well as understands how their individual karma keeps them bound to the world of suffering.[10] The Second Jewel, correct knowledge (*samyag-jñāna*), includes five classical forms of acceptable knowledge (*jñāna*, from √*jñā*, "to know") including empirical knowledge (*mati-jñāna*), scriptural knowledge (*śruta-jñāna*), knowledge from clairvoyance (*avadhi-jñāna*), knowledge from mind-reading (*manaḥparyāya*), and, as a final goal, omniscience (*kevala-jñāna*) (see Tatia 2011 [1994], 5–16; *Tattvārtha Sūtra* 1.1–1.15). Lay Jains typically only have access to empirical (sensory) knowledge and scriptural knowledge (Jain texts), while Jain ascetics can potentially access the final three, and more "direct" (*pratyakṣa*) forms of spiritual knowledge beyond the senses. Finally, the Third Jewel, correct conduct (*samyak-cāritra*), refers to the ways that Jains, possessing as they do an understanding of the operations of karma (*samyag-darśana*) and a concomitant commitment to acquiring correct knowledge (*samyag-jñāna*), must behave correctly (*cāritra*, from √*car*, "to act or conduct one's self") in the world in order to eliminate their karma, access the most direct levels of knowledge, and, eventually, lead their soul (*jīva*) to eternal liberation (*mokṣa*) from suffering.

While Jain scriptures require, in a limited sense, that one intervene when witnessing violence around them,[11] the process of eliminating karma outlined by the Three Jewels in Jain scriptures is highly individualistic and bears minimal references to the necessity to avoid what we would today consider structural violence. Jains instead emphasize the paramount ethic of nonviolence (*ahiṃsā*) and its manifold accompanying ethical restraints, or vows (*vrata*, from √*vṛ*, "to cover, choose"), as *individual choices* applied in quotidian life to avoid the accumulation of individual unmeritorious karma (*pāpa*), to maximize the accrual of individual auspicious karma (*puṇya*), and, ultimately, to eliminate one's individual karma altogether. This does not mean that Jains are disengaged from the world, but that they make habitual choices to avoid unnecessary individual harm while remaining as fully engaged as possible. This is why, first and foremost, most Jains are vegetarian and some are transitioning to becoming vegan, for example (Miller and Dickstein 2021a).

As a religious minority whose population today counts somewhere between five to seven million adherents worldwide (with the vast majority still in India), the Jains' well-known ethical system and generosity in philanthropy has, over the past several centuries, allowed the community to garner prestige and respectable business reputations (Persian: *ābrū*; Sanskrit: *pratiṣṭhā*) (Dundas 2002, 196) as they have participated in "cautious integration" (Jaini 1979, 287) with societies in the Indian Ocean region and now globally. The dearth of collective social justice activism within the global Jain community is likely a reflection of their tradition's wealthy minority status as well as their particular understanding of karma focusing on individual choice and action. This helps explain why Jains will routinely donate generously for social causes, though they typically avoid activism that speaks out against social injustice and in many ways benefit from their place within hierarchical caste, class, and gender systems, which their scriptures and discourses ascribe to individual karma.[12] All of these facets of Jain tradition efficiently merge with neoliberal capitalism and its concomitant predisposition of neoliberal subjectivity, which champions individual "self-discipline and self-mastery" (Godrej 2016, 783)[13] and thereby limits the possibilities for radical activism by the community in any manner resembling what we might encounter in some forms of engaged Buddhism.

The way Jains "engage" with society is thus shaped by their very particular practical social circumstances and ideological commitments. It is also important to recognize that they do not seek converts (as many forms of contemporary Buddhism do), but rather seek to disseminate and proselytize (Qvarnström and Birch 2012) their values and the "Jain Way of Life" at the level of civic society and not at the level of politics within the context of post–World War II Westphalian internationalism (Ikenberry 2020). Jain tradition and philosophy has thus been less likely to be coopted by those not born into the tradition or to be used to engage in radical political activism, as one would expect to encounter in many forms of engaged Buddhism, though there are people not born into the Jain tradition who have adopted a commitment to Jain principles and what is often conveyed as the "Jain Way of Life" by emic community standards.

This is not to say that Jains are apolitical, however, as they have remained engaged in and have influenced politics for thousands of years. As Banks observes, though "Jains and their apologists have always been at pains to stress the secular nature of Jain social organization in view of the fact that Jainism aims to liberate the individual from this world and its concerns, and is therefore not concerned with how society should operate," there is nevertheless "ample evidence that Jains have been involved in large-scale political activity, both in a personal capacity, and in the name of Jainism" (Banks 1986, 455). Not only have Jains been directly involved in political activity, including in the work of the Jain freedom fighter Lala Lajpat Rai, for example, but they have also directly influenced the nonviolent political activism of Gandhi as well as, consequently, those directly influenced by Gandhi including Martin Luther King, Jr. and Nelson Mandela. Jain political activity continues into the present, where Jains can be found in many countries on all levels of the political spectrum, including as advocates for LGBTQ+ rights in the UK (PinkNews 2023), for example, but also even as ascetics serving as allies in support of anti-Muslim Hindu nationalism in India (Organiser 2015) or scholars whose theological work reinforces the continued exploitation of animals (Jain 2014).

As this volume seeks to highlight, we indeed find Jains engaging with society in very compelling ways, and some even in the form of activism. Engaged Jain studies therefore follows engaged Buddhist studies in its pursuit to document these various engagements that religious practitioners and institutions have and continue to make within society, for better or for worse, in what we call "engaged Jainism." In many cases, we will even see scholars of the Jain tradition become engaged in various social, animal advocacy, and environmental justice issues through their own engagement with, and advocacy of, particular Jain principles.

The engagements considered in this volume and in engaged Jain studies more broadly are not necessarily limited to justice initiatives, but to *all* initiatives including, but not limited to, those engagements that may seem to be counter to modern conceptions of social justice as well as those more conservative Jains who do not see social engagement as even necessary or advisable. Like developments in engaged Buddhist studies, which have begun to consider non-justice-oriented material into the field's corpus, engaged Jain studies benefits from being as inclusive as possible. This is not to say that scholars of engaged Jain studies necessarily condone movements counter to social justice, but that they seek, with as much scholarly impartiality as possible, to engage, understand, deconstruct, and analyze these engaged Jain practices, worldviews, and discourses, rather than ignore them altogether.

Engaged Jain studies could, and in many ways already does in extant scholarship, include critical studies of key Jain figures and organizations as diverse as, but not limited to, the world ambassador Virchand Gandhi, spiritual leader Shrimad Rajchandra, Indian nationalist Lala Lajpat Rai, Mahatma Gandhi and other social justice leaders he has inspired, Anuvrat's Acharya Tulsi (see Bothra in this volume), Acharya Mahaprajna and Acharya Mahashramana, Siddhachalam's Acharya Sushil Kumar, Chitrabhanu and Pramoda Chitrabhanu, Veerayatan's Acharya Chandanaji, the Adani Group's billionaire Gautam Adani, Digambar monk Tarun Sagar, Shrimad Rajchandra Mission's Rakeshbhai, and Digambar Jain Trilok Sodh Sansthan's Aryika Jnanamati, as well as movements and institutions such as JAINA and their committees including the ALC and the Ahimsak Eco-Vegan Committee, the Jain International Trade Organization (JITO), the Jain Education and Research Foundation (JERF), the Global Jain Network, the Jain Vegan Initiative, Young Jains of America, and Young Jain Professionals. These are but a few of the understudied Jains and their institutional endeavors that have or continue to engage the world in particularly captivating—and very different—ways. There are also Jains in precolonial and colonial India and lesser known Jains who have nevertheless played important roles in shaping Jainism and Jain studies and also deserve closer attention (see Cort et al. 2020). Like engaged Buddhism, these and other manifestations of engaged Jainism have roots in South Asia but are now global. They engage in manifold social, cultural, economic, educational, and political activities. And they are led by lay and ascetic Jains, including both men and women.

Like their counterparts in engaged Buddhism, Jain women indeed play central roles in various forms of engaged Jainism. Not only are women playing important roles within the Jain community (Kelting 2009), but they are also making impacts on society at large. Consider the diverse impacts of the following Jain women. Grounded in a commitment to compassion inspired by her reinterpretation of Jain tradition, Acharya Chandanaji's Veerayatan seeks to provide medical treatment, education, and other forms of support in Bihar and now globally (Vallely 2020). Nirva Patel, a Jain lawyer and animal law advocate from Boston, is the executive director of Harvard's Animal Law and Policy Program as well as executive producer of the influential and highly acclaimed film *Game Changers*, advocating for the health benefits of a plant-based diet through the stories of famous vegan athletes from around the world (Patel 2023). The Global Jain Network's Jain Vegan Initiative also includes notable women taking leadership roles, such as Ruchika Chitrabhanu (related to Chitrabhanu and Pramoda Chitrabhanu), who actively educates the public on intersectional issues relating to animal welfare, diet, human health, climate change, environmentalism, and consumption (Chitrabhanu 2023a; 2023b). Finally, Aryika Jnanamati continues to advocate and convince others that the Earth is flat according to Jain scriptures at the Digambar Jain Trilok Sodh Sansthan in Hastinapur (Auckland 2016). These are but a few of the countless engagements Jain women are making in global society, all of which deserve scholarly attention.

With these parameters regarding what makes engaged Jainism unique in mind, there are three primary models within which engaged Jain studies can be undertaken, broadly categorized in the sections that follow as the constructive-reproductive, the critical-analytical, and the critical-constructive models. These three models are meant to be as accommodating and interdisciplinary as possible; they sometimes overlap and in many ways reflect the aspirations and methods of scholarly work already being undertaken in the academy. The summary that follows organizes these particular methodological approaches and makes them explicit to demonstrate the possible approaches for undertaking research in engaged Jain studies. One will undoubtedly observe that as we proceed from one model to the next, the level of methodological sophistication necessarily increases. These models have particular strengths and weaknesses as well as risks and rewards, which should become apparent as one reads through each.

The Constructive-Reproductive Model of Engaged Jain Studies

The constructive-reproductive model of engaged Jain studies *constructively reproduces* emic Jain discourse, teachings from Jain texts, Jain philosophy, and other Jain cultural and historical phenomena in a normative, universal, and constructive manner. Scholars embracing this model are, to varying degrees, seriously committed to the principles of the Jain tradition and do not attempt to bring their commitment or the data they are presenting into any particular critical-analytical framework. Instead they adopt something akin to what Cort has described as the "internal model *for* the Jains" (Cort 1990, 55). The constructive-reproductive model often reproduces approaches to the study of the Jain tradition initiated by romantic Orientalist European and American scholars of the nineteenth century, who, working with Jain interlocutors, were searching for universal, ancient wisdom that they understood to have applications for the many challenges facing modern society.

We find the origins of the constructive-reproductive model of engaged Jain studies in organizations such as the Theosophical Society who perceived an increasingly disenchanted, modern Western society that could only be redeemed by India's scriptural "treasures." Consider, for example, this 1891 methodological directive from Irish American Theosophist William Quan Judge:

> There are *men* in India today who are qualified and willing to aid in translating works hitherto untranslated, in collecting that which shall enable us to disseminate and popularize true doctrines of *man's life and destiny* . . . Let us then get ready to use the material in the *ancient storehouse of India, treasures that no man can be called a thief for taking,* since the truths acquired by the mind respecting *man's* life, conduct, constitution, and destiny are the *common property* of the human race, a *treasure* that is lost by monopoly and *expanded by dissemination.* (Judge 1891, 346, emphases added)

Quan's directive here reflects an ethos found in romantic Orientalist studies of India wherein European and American scholars, who were often, though not always, men (cf. Foxen 2020), understood themselves to be recovering and disseminating—rather than "taking"—India's "treasures" as found and translated from sacred, often Sanskrit, texts for the benefit of "the human race."

A number of subsequent "Jain Theosophists" (Flügel 2005, 8) adopted this approach and applied it toward the study of Jain scriptures. Herbert Warren's *Jainism in Western Garb, as a Solution to Life's Great Problems* is a shining example, though what makes Warren's case particularly special is the fact that he was collaborating with Virchand Gandhi, the famous Jain barrister who had traveled to the Parliament of the World's Religions in 1893 under the direction of Acharya Vijayanandasuri (Atmaramji) to share Jain teachings alongside the Hindu representative Swami Vivekananda and the Buddhist Anagarika Dharmapala (Warren 1912). Warren was the honorary secretary of the Jaina Literature Society in London, and had compiled his book based explicitly on his "notes of Talks and Lectures by Virchand R. Gandhi," the Jain teachings of whom Warren was quite fond of (ibid., front matter). In the preface to his work, Warren wrote, "I have been asked to write a manual of Jain doctrine; this I am not competent to do, but I make the request a very welcome opportunity for trying to present to the world that which Mr. Gandhi gave me, and which I hold in the very highest esteem as being of priceless value" (ibid., vi). Following Warren's preface, German Indologist Hermann Jacobi congratulated Warren for his achievement, adding, "Your book brings it home to the reader that Jainism is an ethical religion which is calculated to morally improve those who earnestly and intelligently obey its commands" (ibid., vii). Members of the Jain community also congratulated Warren, including Lalan, who acknowledged, "As far as my present knowledge of my own religion goes, and as far as my humble practice of its noble and convincing principles is concerned, I venture to say that I have never come across in the whole range of my English reading on Jainism such a faithful and correct representation of it and of its principles . . . The reader will find the truths of Jainism put into western garb without any change or even slight modification of the Jain principles" (ibid., viii–ix). By the beginning of the twentieth century, what we might call "engaged Jain studies" had already become a transnational collaborative endeavor wherein educated Western writers were working with prominent and highly educated Jains to apply Jain teachings in "Western garb" as potential solutions "to Life's Great Problems" (Warren 1912).

A number of other collaborative initiatives followed Warren's work, including the formation of the Mahavira Brotherhood or Universal Fraternity (est. 1913), the Rishabh Jain Lending Library in London (est. 1930), and the World Jaina Mission in London (est. 1949) (Flügel 2005, 7–8). As Flügel observes, these societies "resembled the Theosophical Societies and it would not be out of place to call their members 'Jain Theosophists.' They were educated professionals, vegetarians, and greatly influenced by the international peace movement" (ibid.).

While there was an apparent hiatus in collaborative, constructive work between Jains and non-Jains from the mid-1950s onward (ibid., 8), North American Jains have since the establishment of JAINA (est. 1981) gradually increased such endeavors within the North American and European academies, resulting in JAINA's current initiative to endow Jain studies positions in universities therein.

An example of the constructive-reproductive model of engaged Jain studies that has recently emerged can be found in Chapple's *Living Landscapes: Meditations on the Five Elements in Hindu, Buddhist, and Jain Yogas* (2020, 2), which reflects something akin to Hsu's aforementioned Academic Engaged Buddhism (Hsu 2022). This book considers the "treasure trove of resources that find enduring application" in various Indic traditions, including those of the Jain tradition (ibid., 2). In the introduction to this monograph, which includes translations of Jain scriptures relating to yoga, Chapple writes,

> The methodology employed in this study of Yoga in relationship to elemental concentrations does not fit into a strictly Indological category, though it includes textual analysis and translation. Nor does this book offer a sociological descriptive approach or analysis of the practice of Yoga, though it does describe Yoga practices and many field experiences. Rather, in keeping with my own disciplinary training and prior research projects, *this book is a work of constructive theology*. It seeks to explore how various Yoga texts and practices and social realities regard the intersection between the human being and nature as expressed through the five elements and animals. (ibid., xxiii, emphasis added)

Here, Chapple explicitly acknowledges his work as "constructive theology," and the contents of the book itself primarily focus on the translation and dissemination of Jain primary sources alongside those from Buddhist and Hindu traditions, or the "treasure trove of resources that find enduring application" (ibid., 2), which, as he suggests, can help humanity produce a renewed relationship with the natural world in light of our collective environmental challenges.

Other notable examples of the constructive-reproductive model come in the work of Rankin's *Jainism and Environmental Philosophy: Karma and the Web of Life* (2018) and *Jainism and Environmental Politics* (2020), as well as in Shah and Rankin's *Jainism and Ethical Finance: A Timeless Business Model* (2017). A number of chapters in Shugan Jain's edited volume *Social Consciousness in Jainism* (2013) and several chapters in Chapple's earlier edited volume *Jainism and Ecology: Nonviolence in the Web of Life* (2002) also belong to this model of engaged Jain studies. We should likewise consider that a number of scholarly voices from within the Jain community are contributing to the constructive-reproductive model, including, as already mentioned, Atul K. Shah and Shugan Jain, but also Parveen Jain's (see foreword to this volume) *An Introduction to Jain Philosophy* (2020).

Jain Vishvabharati in Ladnun as well as Shugan Jain's International School for Jain Studies (ISJS) in India have institutionalized the constructive-reproductive model through a process Auckland identifies as "academization" (Auckland 2016, 200). ISJS continues to produce a number of publications within this framework in its journal *Transactions* (ISJS 2022) as well as in other recent publications including *Social Consciousness in Jainism* (Jain and Jain 2014), *Jain Business Engagement and Ethics: An Overview* (Jain et al. 2023), and its edited volume *Applications of Anekāntavāda: Jain Pluralism* (Jain and Jain 2025).

Following early Theosophical impulses, each of these works engages Jain scriptural principles and Jain ways of living past and present sincerely as approaches and potential solutions to a number of contemporary ecological, social, animal advocacy, and economic issues (see Shah in this volume), albeit without using critical-analytical frameworks, and thereby constitute what I have called the constructive-reproductive model of engaged Jain studies. Contrary to this methodological tendency, we also have the critical-analytical model of engaged Jain studies.

The Critical-Analytical Model of Engaged Jain Studies

The constructive-reproductive model has as its contrary the critical-analytical model of engaged Jain studies. As the name suggests, the critical-analytical model *critically analyzes* emic Jain discourse, teachings from Jain texts, Jain philosophy, and other Jain cultural and historical engagements using etic, interdisciplinary frameworks. Though often engaged with the Jain community, scholars embracing this model maintain a commitment to objectivity and to the empirical methods of the post-Enlightenment Western academy and thereby subscribe to something akin to what Cort has described as the "scholarly model *of* the Jains" (Cort 1990, 55). Scholars embracing the critical-analytical model study Jain engagements with the world using interdisciplinary tools, including critical-historical, anthropological, philological, and philosophical methods and frameworks. Nevertheless, these scholars do not themselves actively engage with contemporary issues by applying Jain principles to issues of contemporary relevance. If those embracing the constructive-reproductive model are Jain Theosophists (Flügel 2005, 8), those using the critical-analytical model might be considered Jain Orientalists.

Like the constructive-reproductive model, the critical-analytical model of engaged Jain studies also finds its origins in nineteenth century studies of the Jain tradition initiated by Orientalist Euro-American scholars in dialogue with Jain interlocutors who were again often, though not always, men. Unlike the Theosophists, however, these scholars' motivations blended colonial, missionary, theological, anthropological, philological, and/or Indological impetuses and were not concerned, nor did they believe, that the Jain tradition necessarily had any "treasure" to plunder (cf. Chapple 2020, 2).

A particularly revealing place to start in order to understand the aspirations of the critical-analytical approach are found in the opening pages to the *Monier-Williams Sanskrit-English Dictionary*, first published in 1851 following decades of work by Orientalists at the Asiatic Society in India. Sir Monier Monier-Williams dedicated his dictionary to ease the burdens of "all those zealous *men* who have devoted themselves to the social, religious, and intellectual improvement of the natives of our Indian Empire" (Monier-Williams 1899 [1851], x, emphasis added). To these "zealous men" he counted "missionaries, and other philanthropists and scholars, whose aim has been to communicate scriptural and scientific truth to the learned natives" (ibid., x). Monier-Williams's motivations were driven by colonial and missionary translation imperatives, which sought to translate religious scriptures, law books, and other texts to identify, objectify, subordinate, and dominate Indian cultures and their religious and legal frameworks in order to support the imperialist goals of the British Empire. Quite interestingly, the 1899 edition is printed by Narendra Prakash Jain at Shri Jainendra Press, demonstrating just one of the manifold types of worldly engagements Jains have had with those in power in their recent past. Jain engagements with colonial, Indological, and missionary projects were indeed complex and widespread in the eighteenth, nineteenth, and first half of the twentieth century (Cort et al. 2020; Premchand 2020).

Prior to Monier-Williams's systematic rendering of Sanskrit vocabulary, British imperialists from the Asiatic Society had already been engaged with Jains in colonial India for quite some time. The chapters contained in the volume *Asiatic Researches; or, Transactions of the Society Institute in Bengal, for Inquiring into the History and Antiquities, the Arts, Sciences, and Literature of Asia* present an early example of the critical-analytical model applied anthropologically in this colonial context (Asiatic Society 1809). The chapters titled "Account of the Jains, Collected from a Priest of this Sect at Mudgeri" and "Particulars of the Jains" present detailed ethnographic accounts of Major C. Mackenzie's and Doctor F. Buchanan's engagements with unnamed Jain "priests" who apparently shared basic information with them about Jain universal history, philosophy, beliefs, and cultural customs, though the chapters reflect a general assumption that Jains were a subsect of Hinduism widely held (though not universally; see Orr 2020; Luithle-Hardenberg 2020) among British colonial administrators at the time (Mackenzie 1809, 244, 279). Also in this volume are Henry Thomas Colebrooke's "Observations on the Sect of Jains," the conclusions of which are quite critical and condescending, suggesting, for example, that the Jains "precaution to avoid injuring any being is a practice inculcated in the orthodox religion, but which has been carried by them to a ludicrous extreme" (Colebrooke 1809, 290).

Alongside and even prior to the work of Colebrooke and other colonial Orientalists in Calcutta, a number of other missionaries and colonial intellectuals using the critical-analytical model were in dialogue with self-identifying Jains. Together these Jains and Europeans were effectively establishing Jainism as a distinct religious tradition (see Cort et al. 2020). The early studies that emerged from these engagements would lead to definite changes in the ways that Jains perceived themselves within the context of what the Western world understood as the world's great religions. In South India, the Madras School of Orientalism identified the Jains as a unique tradition from records kept by earlier missionaries who had interacted with Jains there as early as the seventeenth and eighteenth centuries (Orr 2020). During the first decade of the nineteenth century in Baroda, the East India company's Scottish officer Alexander Walker demonstrated that Jain religious tenets were different from those religious doctrines of other traditions with which the Jains were socially integrated (Luithle-Hardenberg 2020). In the decade that followed, Lieutenant-Colonel James Tod identified and wrote about the Jains in dialogue with a Jain ascetic as his reliable associate (Babb 2020). In 1848, Reverend John Stevenson, one of a number of Scottish missionaries in Bombay, translated the *Kalpa Sūtra*, which marked the first time that someone from Europe would attempt to translate a Jain text. The work of Stevenson and the missionaries he worked with demonstrated that Jains already had at least a semi-formed notion of what the category of "Jainism" meant before it was mediated to them in their engagements with missionaries and colonial Orientalists (Numark 2020).

As Schubring notes, critical approaches to the study of the Jain tradition saw "the beginning of a philological and creative epoch" (Schubring and Beurlen 1962 [1935], 3) in Europe in the later work of Albrecht Weber from 1865 to 1867, who eventually published his work in his book titled *The Sacred Literature of the Jains* (*Über die heiligen Schriften der Jaina*) (Weber and Smyth 1893). Europeans were not working alone on many of these translation projects, supplied as they sometimes were by Jain manuscript brokers in India (Balbir 2020). Writing about this particular time period in Jain studies, Flügel has argued,

> Because no textual evidence was presented by the Jains in public, "Jainism/Jinism" was not recognised as an independent "religion" until 1879 when Hermann Jacobi in the introduction of his edition of the *Kalpasūtra of Bhadrabāhu* furnished for the first time textual proof that the ancient Hindu and Buddhist scriptures already depicted the *nigganthas* as a separate "heretical" (*tīrthyā*) group. With this, Jaina Studies was established as an independent field of academic research. Before Jacobi, the Jains were regarded either as "Buddhists" or as a "Hindu sect." After Jacobi's publication, Jainism became

> gradually recognized as a universal or "world religion." (Flügel 2005, 2)

Following the aforementioned new evidence presented in Cort et al., Flügel's dating of the establishment of Jainism as a world religion and the origins of Jain studies as a Western field of study here has since been challenged and dated much earlier to the eighteenth and nineteenth centuries (Cort et al. 2020). Nevertheless, Flügel's earlier conclusions remain highly relevant: Europeans' elite Jain counterparts in India recognized, as he writes, "The political value of the academic study of Jainism" and, as a result, "the educated Jain elite . . . for some time demanded the public recognition of 'Jainism' and the 'Jainas' from the colonial government and in the courts" (Flügel 2005, 2–3; see also Orr 2009).

While Jain traditions certainly existed prior to the colonial period,[14] it is critical to recognize that a very particular and novel Jain identity formed as a result of colonial Orientalist, missionary, and Indological engagements, an identity that would become the basis for today's diasporic Jainism, which seeks to overcome sectarian differences to instead purvey a "universal Jainism" around the world (Banks 2003, 81–82; see also Cort 2020a, 262). In their colonial encounters, self-identifying Jains recognized an opportunity for cross-cultural communication of their tradition's principles in light of the colonial situation in which they found themselves. Where European Indological and Orientalist "objectivity" waved its wand, the Jains were quick to capitalize, creating opportunities for Jains such as, as we have already seen, Virchand Gandhi and his interlocutor Herbert Warren to later disseminate Jain teachings for the betterment of society, for example.

Critical approaches to Jain studies continued to take new directions in the early twentieth century. Working with Jains, Helen M. Johnson, Maurice Bloomfield, and W. Norman created "The First 'School' of Jain Studies in the U.S." by exploiting the availability of Jain texts from India, which had been facilitated by India's colonization (Cort 2020b, 479). Meanwhile in Ireland, and shortly after Warren had published his *Jainism in Western Garb* (1912), Margaret Stevenson wrote a critique of the Jain tradition titled *The Heart of Jainism* (1915) apparently instigated by the "deep impression" that the "pathos" and "sadness" of a Jain ritual she had witnessed years before in a temple in Ahmedabad had imprinted upon her (Taylor, in Stevenson 1915, xvii). As the introductory chapter written by Dr. G. P. Taylor tells us, Stevenson's "kindly sympathies have won her many friends in the Jaina community, and have even procured her a welcome entree into the seclusion of a Jaina nunnery. Time and again she has been present by invitation at Jaina functions seldom witnessed by any foreigner" (ibid., xvii–xviii). Stevenson indeed worked closely with, gained the trust of, and was quite grateful for her many Jain interlocutors in India. Reflecting on her ongoing engagements with the Jain community, she herself wrote, "Whatever language they spoke, every one whom the writer asked showed the same readiness to help; indeed almost every fact recorded in this book owes its presence there to the courtesy of some Jaina friend, and every page seems to the writer water-marked with someone's kindness" (Stevenson 1915, x). Stevenson's critical study was, nevertheless, not concerned with discovering what the Jain Theosophists would have considered "treasures," but rather argued in its concluding pages, "The more one studies Jainism, the more one is struck with the pathos of its empty heart" (ibid., 289). As a Christian writing primarily for missionaries, she invited her Jain interlocutors to a "personal friendship with the Incarnate Son of God which is the great gift that Christianity has to offer to the Jaina" (ibid.). On the basis of an alleged objectivity, which she frames as her effort to "try reverently and sympathetically to grasp the inner meaning of an Indian faith" (ibid., 1), Stevenson's critical study, which places the Jain tradition in dialogue with what she perceived as her own superior and unquestionable universal Christian framework, betrayed the apparent trust and hospitality she had garnered in her years of ethnographic research with the Indian Jain community.

Further critical-analytical studies of the Jain tradition emerged as the twentieth century advanced that were more self-conscious and far more neutral toward Jain traditions than Stevenson's had been. Schubring's more sophisticated *The Doctrine of the Jainas: Described After the Old Sources* (*Die Lehre der Jainas, nach den alten Quellen dargestellt*), originally published in German (1962 [1935]), provided a basic overview of Jain history and Śvetāmbara and Digambara textual teachings in a hope to contribute to what he perceived as work by "Western scholars—including many Germans" that had been to date aimed toward making "the world acquainted with one of the finest products of the Indian mind," by which he meant Jainism (Schubring and Beurlen 1962 [1935], iv).

As the field of Jainology emerged in the mid-nineteenth century (Flügel 2005, 6), Jain and non-Jain scholars from South Asia have also since engaged the critical-analytical model in historical, philosophical, and philological studies. A. B. Dhruva, H. R. Kapadia, and B. K. Matilal produced widely-read philosophical scholarship pertaining to the popular topic of *anekāntavāda*, for example (Cort 2000; Matilal 1981). In 1979, Padmanabh S. Jaini published *The Jaina Path of Purification*, a highly reliable resource explaining Jain history, philosophy, and culture that is still widely used in Jain studies today (Jaini 1979).

During the decades that have followed, a robust and now global network of Jain scholars committed to the critical-analytical model comprises the majority of the work in the field of Jain studies. These scholars use etic, interdisciplinary approaches that have become increasingly sophisticated, much more nuanced, and far more inclined to observe and study specific ways that Jains engage with their social, economic, political, textual, ritual, and intellectual environments (see Zhang in this volume; see also Cort 1990; Banks 1992; Laidlaw 1996; Dundas 2002; Kelting 2009). Recent scholarship illustrative of this approach, for example, is Andrea Jain's consideration of Acharya Mahaprajna's engagement with the discourses and practice of transnational postural yoga in the creation of his eclectic *prekṣā dhyāna* yoga system (Jain 2015, 56). Shalin Jain's *Identity, Community, and State: The Jains Under the Mughals* (2017), wherein Jain focuses on Jain ideological engagements with the Mughals, is another notable example, as is Vose's *Reimagining Jainism in Islamic India: Jain Intellectual Culture in the Delhi Sultanate* (Forthcoming; see also Vose 2022).[15] More recently and no less significant is Gregory Clines's *Jain Rāmāyaṇa Narratives: Moral Vision and Literary Innovation* (2022), which considers how Jain writers engaged with and adapted premodern *Rāmāyaṇa* narratives to shape their own Jain models of what it meant to be a moral person.

Along with the constructive-reproductive model, this overview of the development of the critical-analytical model of engaged Jain studies is not intended to be exhaustive. Rather, it is intended to illustrate a methodological tendency that focuses on increased precision, analytical distance, and a historically locatable pursuit of etic objectivity and impartiality typical of the Western academy that has now become global and can be productively used to study various forms of "engaged Jainism."

It is crucial to recognize that methodologically, the objectivity of the field of religious studies (and by extension other colonial-era Orientalist studies) was shaped through particular historical processes during the European enlightenment, where "religion was thought of . . . as an objective reality—rather like natural objects . . . that could be explored, compared, and classified through scientific enquiry. A religion was 'a system' with shape and boundaries—one religion being clearly divided from another" (Oddie 2016, 8). The notion of academic objectivity in the study of religion is thus a historically constructed project with origins in self-interested European and American undertakings, and the claim that objectivity alone is methodologically superior is indeed anything but objective. As we have seen, those involved in these projects were often driven by particular motivations to establish racial and religious superiority, and the translation and identification of Indian religions remained a core part of their endeavors. All of this is to say that while scholars using the critical-analytical model of engaged Jain studies are committed to maintaining scholarly objectivity, it is important to take into account the colonial, Orientalist, missionary, theological, and Indological legacy within which their presumedly impartial and objective methodological framework was developed. As recent studies demonstrate, Jain scholars have begun to use the critical-analytical model self-reflexively, pointing their methodological frameworks onto the discipline of Jain studies itself, where they have started to discover the fascinating ways that historical engagements between colonial, Orientalist, missionary, theological, Indological, and Jain actors have shaped their current approaches to the study of Jainism (see Cort et al. 2020).

The Critical-Constructive Model of Engaged Jain Studies

The critical-constructive model draws from both the critical-analytical and constructive-reproductive models of engaged Jain studies, creatively blending emic and etic perspectives in research and teaching. Inheriting both the romantic Orientalist impulse and the colonial Orientalist and Indological legacies that created the binary that distinguishes etic/outsider from emic/insider, this third model is both "of" *and* "for" the Jains (Cort 1990, 55), engages the etic *with* the emic, and in the process remains open to the transformation of both. Because those scholars embracing the critical-constructive model walk a fine line between these perspectives, they must be particularly vigilant in all dimensions of research and teaching.

Scholars who participate in this model of engaged Jain studies are committed to maintaining academic objectivity, following the ethos of the empirical methods of the post-Enlightenment Western academy to which they are committed. This does not mean, however, that scholars cannot take seriously the principles and ethical commitments of many Jains who wish to apply Jain principles in light of contemporary global issues and challenges. Scholars might therefore espouse Jain values critically, observing what emerges when the "engaged universals" (Tsing 2005, 8) of their respective academic disciplines encounter frictions when they come into contact with Jain ways of knowing. In doing so, scholars using the critical-constructive model acknowledge the historical provenance of scholarly "objectivity" and become something akin to Broad's "engaged scholar" (Broad 2016, 12). Both scholars and Jains alike have much to gain by embracing the methods of the critical-constructive model's "engaged scholarship" (ibid., 13). Together, both can help provoke questions of enduring relevance for society, Jains can engage with scholars to respond to these questions, and in doing so, Jains can also learn how to reduce their own violence in the world.

The critical-constructive model of engaged Jain studies shares origins with our two previous models, though its particular provenance emerges from the more recent frictions that have taken place between academic commitments to impartiality and objectivity and the JAINA ALC's mission to endow Jain studies positions in North American and European universities to spread the study, teaching, and research of Jainism intended to promote Jain Dharma. Not referring to the JAINA ALC's mission explicitly, Auckland has referred to this process of institutionalizing Jain studies in the university as "academization" (Auckland 2016, 200).[16]

Flügel had presaged the JAINA ALC's mission and the current "academization" in which many Jain scholars are now intimately entangled in 2005 when he wrote:

> It may well be that we are presently witnessing the uncoupling of the doctrines of Jainism from the traditional institutional bedrock of the Jain communities and the establishment of a universal religion of non-violence (*ahiṃsā*) embodied in a set of texts which, after their release from the vaults of the *bhaṇḍāras* and the monopoly of interpretation of the *ācāryas*, gained a life on their own in the form of printed or electronic texts which are freely available to anyone anywhere. "Jainism" as a disembodied text-based set of ideologies or dogmas from which one can pick and chose [*sic*] can be individually interpreted and applied in manifold ways without fear of social or supernatural sanctions. The consequences of the ongoing transformation of Jain lay religiosity from ritual to reflection for the future of the Jain tradition have [yet] to be seen. (Flügel 2005, 9–10)

There were of course precursors to the phenomenon of a universal Jainism about which Flügel writes. Śrīmad Rajcandra had already developed a form of Jainism detached from ascetic authority in Gujarat that would eventually make its way into the diaspora where it still thrives today. Virchand Gandhi had already shared Jain teachings at the Parliament of the World's Religions in the United States in 1893. Acharya Tulsi's Anuvrat Movement, founded in the mid-twentieth century following World War II, to improve individuals and society by espousing Jain values had already created a traveling order of ascetics (*samaṇīs* and *samaṇs*) for global outreach (see Bothra in this volume; see also Reading 2020). Chitrabhanu and Acharya Sushil Kumar had already broken traditional Jain ascetic vows to travel to Europe and North America to teach universal Jain principles. Finally, Acharya Chandanaji had already reinterpreted fundamental Jain principles and founded Veerayatan to provide education and healthcare globally (Cort 2020a, 257–259).

Nevertheless, since the establishment of the first endowed Jain professorship in Jain studies at Florida International University in 2010 (FIU 2010), we have been witnessing an explosion of the outcome of Flügel's earlier speculations regarding the creation of a transnational, universal Jain religion fundamentally detached from ascetic authority. The historical developments outlined in this chapter and the current activities in Jain studies show us how the roots of JAINA's project to "establish liaison with Academic institutions . . . to promote the study, teaching and research . . . of Jain Dharma" (JAINA 2023) find their provenance in the late nineteenth century and in the work of pioneering Jains, both lay and ascetic, since then. From a scholarly perspective, it is urgent that these newly emerging trends in global Jainism be studied carefully and in a spirit of interdisciplinarity in order to understand the historical, cultural, and philosophical entanglements that continue to emerge as a result of global Jain engagements with society and the scholarly community, as well as *who*, in particular, receives the authority to define and construct what "Jainism" is and how it ought to be practiced.

Furthermore, it is critical that scholars embracing the critical-constructive model also recognize their own particular historical inheritance and social location that produced Jain studies in the first place. As we have seen, the academic field of Jain studies and Jainism are not self-evident, a priori entities, but rather culturally co-constructed projects now internalized by both scholars and Jains alike. Both bear identifiable colonial, Orientalist, theological, and Indological origins that result from the engagements and frictions between newly self-identifying Jains and their European interlocutors in the nineteenth century. Members of the academy have since made careers out of studying the historically locatable object of "Jainism" produced in these encounters, while self-identifying Jains continue to receive much-sought-after acknowledgment of the existence and ongoing significance of their tradition worldwide.

Scholars embracing the critical-constructive model therefore work closely with Jains to disseminate the findings involved in their academic research widely and for the benefit of the Jain community and society at large. Following similar trends in some forms of engaged Buddhist studies (e.g., Gleig 2021, 11–12), the critical-constructive model of engaged Jain studies requires that those Jains engaging the scholarly community fulfill a coinciding obligation to accommodate and take seriously the findings and frameworks of peer-reviewed, data-supported scholarship that seeks to support the Jain community's endeavors to apply Jain principles in light of the many issues we face as a globalized society. While it may seem unnecessary to make this point, some Jains' rejection of science and empirical research often places Jain scholars in a difficult position as they attempt to share thoroughly researched and yet sometimes unsettling scientific, historical, philosophical, or anthropological findings that conflict with Jain belief, praxis, doctrine, self-image, and personal beliefs (see Vekemans and Beltz in this volume). For example, in a recent meeting in Zürich between scholars and members of the diasporic Jain community, the topic of Jain implications in the category of caste in India according to ethnographic and historical scholarly research emerged during our conversation.[17] While one Jain suggested that Jains are against caste altogether, I was taken by surprise when another member of the community immediately became defensive and, rather than denying Jain caste issues, tried to justify casteism within the framework of alleged "scientific" evidence supporting the necessity of caste (see Auckland 2016).[18] In another scenario a decade before, while I was visiting the Digambar Jain Trilok Sodh Sansthan in Hastinapur in 2012, many in my fellow graduate student cohort, several professors, and other Jain researchers were perplexed when we were taught, following Jain scriptures, that the Earth is actually flat, not round (Cort 2020a, 261–262; Auckland 2016, 220).

As research partners, scholars in the field of engaged Jain studies oblige the Jains with whom they are collaborating and who make such claims to perhaps more fully embrace the episteme of reliable, international, peer-reviewed science and scholarship. As I argue elsewhere, Jains already have the space within their own epistemic systems in their empirical viewpoint (*vyavahāra-naya*) contained within their doctrine of viewpoints (*naya-vāda*; see Balcerowicz 2020, 850) as well as in their tradition's more general tendency to accept empirical knowledge (*mati-jñāna*) so as to be able to accommodate contemporary materialist epistemologies, including empirical scientific methods (Miller 2023). Auckland has also suggested that those who take into account the findings of scholarly resources as I am suggesting here might then appreciate "a variety of resources with which people explore, reformulate, and express their religion" and may therefore also "be inclined to hand over some ontological queries to the natural sciences or adopt a more reified or historical understanding of their religion" (Auckland 2016, 223). With some degree of "epistemic flexibility" (Donaldson 2020, 190), Jains can indeed admit academic knowledge into their own knowledge systems and in doing so discover many opportunities for how to apply the Jain principles they are asking scholars to help them disseminate. This may require, of course, that Jains be willing to revise, demythologize, or bracket aspects of their tradition that are not scientifically verifiable or tenable, and will involve a process of ongoing dialectical engagement with the scholarly community with whom they are engaged.

As Jonathan Dickstein and I have noted in our research concerning Jain forms of veganism, Jains of all ages are indeed embracing empirical scientific findings from their academic interlocutors. And as public doctors and intellectuals, including Tushar Mehta, Pratik Bhansali, Jonathan Dickstein, and myself, continue to present publicly available science to Jains demonstrating the environmental, animal, social, and human health harms of dairy, for example, more Jains are giving up their centuries-old habit of consuming dairy in light of their commitments to nonviolence (*ahiṃsā*), compassion (*karuṇā*), and the elimination of their karma (Mehta 2021; Vegan Jains 2019; Bhansali 2023; Miller and Dickstein 2021b; Miller 2023; Miller, forthcoming 2026).

More recent scholarly research continues to do the kind of critical-constructive work I have described here, while a number of Jains and Jain organizations are also already acting as dependable collaborators and research partners. We find an early analogue in the work of Nathmal Tatia, for example, who translated the *Tattvārtha Sūtra* for a primarily diasporic Jain readership who continue to reference the text today as the source text of their tradition (Tatia 2011 [1994]; see also Jain and Jain 2023). More recently, Donaldson and Bajželʼs *Insistent Life: Principles for Bioethics in the Jain Tradition* (2021), is "a book on Jainism in relation to contemporary bioethical issues" whose "dual approach of excavating foundational principles and deducing principles of application" seeks to "make a meaningful contribution to future scholarship and clinical analysis in Jainism and bioethics" (1). Donaldson and Bajžel both occupy positions endowed by JAINA's ALC in the positions of Shri Parshvanath Presidential Chair at UC Irvine and Shrimad Rajchandra Chair at UC Riverside, respectively. Their well-known research, which has been celebrated by the Jain community, maintains high academic standards of precision and objectivity and yet applies the results of such meticulous research to difficult and relevant questions we collectively face as a global society, whether we are Jain or not. Other recent creative examples of the critical-constructive model have been put on display—quite literally—at the Museum Rietberg's *Being Jain* exhibition in Zürich, Switzerland (Beltz et al. 2023) and at the Fowler Museum at UCLA's *Visualizing Devotion: Jain Embroidered Shrine Hangings* in Los Angeles, California (Fowler 2023). In both of these exhibitions held from 2022 to 2023, Jain scholars, Jain community members, and museum professionals collaborated, though not without frictions (see Beltz in this volume) to showcase Jain objects, films, history, the Jain way of life, and Jain culture in ways that were both academically rigorous and sympathetic to the possibilities that the Jain tradition offers in light of our shared global challenges (Fowler 2022; Arihanta Institute 2022).

Most recently, Arihanta Institute, a Jain-founded nonprofit online educational organization, was established to advance "education, scholarship, critical research, and public dissemination of real-world application of the Jain principles of nonviolence (*ahiṃsā*) and compassion (*karuṇā*) . . . to empower individuals with knowledge to embrace and apply these principles as a force for positive change, addressing the most pressing issues of our time with courage and compassion" (Arihanta Institute 2023a).[19] Most significantly, the institute's faculty teach for Claremont School of Theology's accredited master's degree program, Engaged Jain Studies: South Asian and Global Perspectives (CST 2023). The Engaged Jain Studies graduate program, where both editors of this volume are faculty members and which has now expanded to include a fully online PhD program, is Jain-supported and engages scholars and Jain community members from around the world embracing all three of the models outlined in this introductory chapter to support research in engaged Jain studies. Arihanta Institute's faculty and the graduate students they serve regularly interact with the global Jain community, forge partnerships with them, and work in a collaborative spirit to study and practice various forms of engaged Jainism. The volume before you in fact emerges from Arihanta Institute's annual Engaged Jain Studies conference titled "Defining Applied Jain Studies" that I organized in 2023. Here, in partnership with Claremont School of Theology, the Graduate Theological Union, and JAINA, academics and community members came together virtually for two days to deliberate what it means to apply Jain principles in everyday life (Arihanta Institute 2023b).

In sum, the critical-constructive model acknowledges the interdependent, dialectical, relational, and sometimes divergent circumstances and objectives of the academic and Jain communities both historically and in the present. Scholars following this model are "engaged scholars" (Broad 2016, 12) and their students participate in "engaged learning" (Miller 2019), partnering with Jains and Jain institutions to study the ways Jains can, or do already, apply and disseminate Jain principles as they engage with specific concerns and challenges pertaining to environmental justice, animal advocacy (see Bridges, Dickstein, Bohanec, and Tuminello in this volume), social justice (see Vose in this volume), interreligious dialogue (see Long in this volume), political, economic, corporate (see Zenk in this volume), and other issues Jains find to be of pressing concern. Scholars embracing the critical-constructive model may themselves participate with Jains in performing and/or disseminating research that seeks to understand the most effective ways Jain principles might be applied to these specific issues.

Though engaging with the Jain community in their research, scholars must nevertheless endeavor to maintain objectivity, and must not feel obliged to limit their research to what is considered "good" in the moral sense, but to explore all forms of Jain engagement (and disengagement) with the world. Therefore, when critical-constructive scholars encounter activities and discourses that they consider to be counter to social justice or human flourishing within the Jain communities that they research, they are obliged to consider, with a critical lens, the particular worldviews and discourses they are encountering and to reflect these phenomena back to the academic community as well as the Jain community supporting their research (see Vose in this volume).

Reading This Volume

This volume is organized thematically to demonstrate interdisciplinary approaches in engaged Jain studies that employ, to varying degrees, the three primary methodological tendencies outlined in this chapter (some authors explicitly state which model they are using, while others have chosen to let the reader decide). We invite our readers to read our entire volume, to focus on thematic sections, or to use individual chapters to teach and/or research possible approaches to engaged Jain studies.

It is worth noting here that six authors currently occupy JAINA ALC–funded university positions, three others belong to Arihanta Institute (two of whom formerly occupied JAINA ALC positions), two were born Jain, and all of the others have had degrees of direct or indirect engagement teaching or performing research in JAINA and Arihanta Institute initiatives. Though we reached out to a number of nonwhite, non-male scholars to contribute, we acknowledge that many, though not all chapters, are written by white scholars and that many, though not all of these scholars, are men. We aim to continue to diversify engaged Jain studies, to bring as many diverse perspectives into the conversation as possible, as these perspectives will undoubtedly continue to reshape the discipline for the better.

The volume is divided into five parts around topics of ongoing relevance and interest in the field of Jain studies as well as within the Jain community itself. Each of the five parts were carefully chosen to organize the topics of research each scholar had presented at the 2023 Engaged Jain Studies Conference at Arihanta Institute, and were therefore determined based upon the available scholarship and scholars researching in their respective areas of expertise and interest. We welcome the addition of further categories of engaged Jainism as the field of engaged Jain studies continues to expand.

In part I, "Critical Issues in 'Engaged Jain Studies,'" Steven Vose and Tine Vekemans more closely interrogate JAINA's diasporic identitarian narrative (Vose) and the engagements between emic Jain mantra healing discourses and etic academic ways of knowing and medical knowledge (Vekemans).

In part II, "Social Engagement in the Diaspora," Johannes Beltz, Yifan Zhang, and I consider engaged forms of Jainism in both India and the diaspora, as Jain art is curated in a major interactive exhibition at Museum Rietberg in Switzerland in collaboration with the Swiss Jain community (Beltz), while a Jain-inspired mural is painted on the Berlin Wall (Miller), and while Jains perform "Jainness" when they engage their social environment in Southeast Asia (Zhang).

Next, in part III, "Engaging with Business and Economy," Benjamin Zenk and Atul K. Shah engage Jain philosophical ideas with questions that regularly arise in business ethics education (Zenk) and corporate sustainability discourses (Shah).

Part IV then includes a topic of utmost relevance to engaged Jainism, "Engaging to Protect Animals and the Environment," with chapters by Cogen Bohanec and Andrew Bridges that productively engage Jain virtue ethics (Bohanec) and the Jain concept of *anekāntavāda* (Bridges) with contemporary considerations in animal advocacy. Jonathan Dickstein and Joey Tuminello then use ethnographic and philosophical approaches to help us understand Jain social engagements with the Western animal sanctuary movement (Dickstein) and the ethical concerns of faux meat (Tuminello). The section then concludes with another chapter that follows a historically important topic pertaining to engaged Jainism by helping us to conceive of a Jain "ecotheology" by engaging thought from the broader field of ecopsychology with Jain philosophy concerned with the environment (Bohanec).

Finally, part V, "Interfaith Engagement," includes five chapters from Alba Rodríguez Juan, Christopher Key Chapple, Corinna May Lhoir, Shivani Bothra, and Jeffery D. Long, which guide us through Jain intellectual engagements with other religious traditions, including the Jain *bhāvana*s, which are shared with the Buddhist and brahmanical *brahmavihāra*s (Rodríguez Juan); early Jain engagement with religious difference in the work of Haribhadra (Chapple); the Jain medieval texts *Yogapradīpa* and *Yogasāra* in dialogue with extant yoga systems (Lhoir); the socially engaged Anuvrat Movement of Acharya Tulsi (Bothra); and *anekāntavāda* in dialogue with modern Vedānta (Long).

This volume is the first of its kind, and though it covers, or at a minimum mentions, many of the key figures and institutions who participate in engaged Jainism, there are innumerable further studies that still need to be undertaken. Our book provides, therefore, a thematic foundation to initiate the discipline of engaged Jain studies while also serving as an invitation to our colleagues to join with us to continue to develop new methodologies, models, and approaches to understand the quickly developing relationships between Jains, scholars, and/or the communities with whom they work.

The future of Jain studies is engaged.

Notes

1. Food studies scholar Garret Broad (2016, 12) is particularly concerned, as are many vegan Jains, with addressing intersectional social justice issues as they pertain to the food system. Broad's study focuses on social justice issues surrounding food in Black communities in the United States, though his concern and methods can be extended to a variety of circumstances wherein scholars working with local communities can advocate for social justice across a range of issues.

2. Queen and King elaborate, "The refuge formula, expressing homage to Buddha, Dharma, and Sangha, offers a standard for regarding a thinker or movement as 'Buddhist,' regardless of the presence of non-Buddhist cultural elements, and regardless of the absence of other traditional teachings" (1996, 32).

3. This is not of course to say that a tradition that actively seeks to change or leave behind one of the refuges could not also be studied as a new Buddhist movement. The particular reasons as to why one would leave behind one of the refuges would need to be carefully considered, however. As Queen and King note, even Ambedkar had misgivings about the third refuge, though ultimately accepted it (Queen and King 1996, 32).

4. I use the phrase "engaged Buddhist studies" here to describe the field of study that takes as its object "engaged Buddhism."

5. The following summary of work in the field of engaged Buddhist studies is by no means intended to be comprehensive. I instead intend to bring out some of the core themes and issues scholars have faced over the past three decades. For a more robust overview of the field of engaged Buddhism, one would do well to read *An Introduction to Engaged Buddhism* (Fuller 2021), "Engaged Buddhism" (Gleig 2021), *Socially Engaged Buddhism* (King 2009), and/or *Action Dharma: New Studies in Engaged Buddhism* (Queen et al. 2003).

6. It is worthwhile to note here that Ambedkar did not choose to convert to the Jain tradition, which though in its earliest textual sources rejected brahminical casteism (as had Buddhism) was in fact "forced to accept it eventually" (Banks 1986, 451). With a minimal number of

adherents in modern India, Buddhism provided a more apt tradition onto which Ambedkar could write his anti-caste aspirations without fear of Buddhists' dissent.

7. I first encountered this quote by Kenneth Kraft from Fred Eppsteiner's *The Path of Compassion: Writings on Socially Engaged Buddhism* (1988) while reading the introduction to Queen and King's *Engaged Buddhism* (1996).

8. Simmer-Brown (2020) describes this dynamic quite well in her chapter "Opening the Heart in Anti-Racism Activism: Pema Chodron and the Lojon Teachings." Here, Pema Chodron's approach to Buddhism is gradually transformed through her engaged dialogue with public concerns over structural racism raised in the Black Lives Matter movement and various insights born from critical race theory.

9. Main and Lai (2013, 3) write, for example, "Our revised definition is an attempt to move away from two problems that affect scholarly analyses of this topic, namely the use of 'socially engaged' as a term of moral praise and one restricted to nonviolent groups founded in the postwar period." This is not to say that scholars condone the alternative forms of engaged Buddhism about which Main and Lai speak, but they also do not ignore them.

10. As Tatia (2011 [1994], 6) elaborates, *samyag-darśana* is a particular "outlook or way of seeing, a conviction backed by reason."

11. See, for example, *Tattvārtha Sūtra* 6.9, wherein simply approving (*anumata*) "someone else's initiative in acting" is understood to be one of the sources of "long-term karmic inflow and bondage" (Tatia 2011 [1994], 154). According to this teaching, when someone witnesses violence around them, they are required to intervene to avoid "approving" (*anumata*) the violence they are witnessing. This teaching, which one could extend to include the structural violence in society today, is rarely, if ever, emphasized in the contemporary Jain community, and has only recently come into focus in Jain ethical practices (see Miller and Dickstein 2021a).

12. See, for example, the canonical *Tattvārtha Sūtra*'s teaching that the three genders (*liṅga*) of male, female, and hermaphrodite emerge based on one's individual conduct-deluding and body-making karma (verse 2.6), wherein males have the clear advantage over females, while both males and females have an advantage over hermaphrodites. Also consider the text's distinction between non-Aryan, outcaste, foreign humans (*mleccha*), and noble humans (*ārya*), wherein the latter to which Jains belong are clearly karmically superior.

13. Here I cite the work of Farah Godrej (2016), who, though writing about the practice of modern yoga, provides an excellent detailed account of the disposition and imperatives of neoliberal subjectivity.

14. It should also be noted here that Flügel later writes, "When exactly the vernacular word 'Jain' was introduced as a self-designation is still an open question" (Flügel 2005, 3).

15. One might also consider scholarship that does not center Jain scholarship and yet demonstrates Jains' historical engagements with other cultural, political, and religious influences, such as *Culture of Encounters: Sanskrit at the Mughal Court* (Truschke 2016).

16. As Auckland (2016, 200) writes, "Academization is linked to the soft sciences and the academic enterprise in general, and might lead to publications of critical editions of sacred texts and conferences on theological subjects . . . whose functions, implications, and effects vary according to context."

17. During this meeting, I had in mind, among other things, Cort's research regarding "Jains and Caste in Patan," where Cort (2001, 57) observes that "references to caste are found at the earliest levels of evidence of Jainism, and it is unlikely that the Jains have ever been less caste-organized than the surrounding population."

18. Auckland (2016) refers to this Jain practice broadly as "scientization," which considers the ways Jains and members of religious traditions make selective use of "science" to buttress their own religious traditions.

19. Arihanta Institute's vision further elaborates, "Arihanta Institute envisions a world where the timeless principles of non-violence (*ahiṃsā*) and compassion (*karuṇā*) inspire global transformation. As a leader in Engaged Jain Studies, we aim to bridge theory and practice, creating inclusive, accessible online education that empowers individuals and communities to apply ancient wisdom to modern challenges, fostering a more peaceful and compassionate future for all" (Arihanta Institute 2023a).

References

Arihanta Institute. 2022. "Jains in Society: Interviews with Jains from Around the Globe." https://www.arihantainstitute.org/jains-in-society.

———. 2023a. "Vision." https://www.arihantainstitute.org/vision.

———. 2023b. "Defining Applied Jain Studies." https://conf.arihantainstitute.org/agenda.

Asiatic Society. 1809. *Asiatic Researches; or, Transactions of the Society Institute in Bengal, for inquiring into the History and Antiquities, the Arts, Sciences, and Literature of Asia*. Vol. 9. Asiatic Society.

Auckland, Knut. 2016. "The Scientization and Academization of Jainism." *Journal of the American Academy of Religion* 84 (1): 192–233.

Babb, Lawrence. 2020. "James Tod and the Jains." In *Cooperation, Contribution, and Contestation: The Jain Community, Colonialism and Jainological Scholarship*. Studies in Asian Art and Culture. Vol. 6, edited by John E. Cort, Andrea Luithle-Hardenberg, and Leslie C. Orr. EB Verlag.

Balbir, Nalini. 2020. "Owners, Suppliers, Scholars: Jains and Europeans in the Nineteenth Century Search for Manuscripts in Eastern India and Bombay Presidency." In Cort, Luithle-Hardenberg, and Orr, eds., *Cooperation, Contribution, and Contestation*.

Balcerowicz, Piotr. 2020. "Jain Epistemology." In *Brill's Encyclopedia of Jaiṇism*, edited by John E. Cort, Paul Dundas, Knut A. Jacobsen, and Kristi L. Wiley. Brill.

Banks, Marcus J. 1986. "Defining Division: An Historical Overview of Jain Social Organization." *Modern Asian Studies* 20 (3): 447–460.

———. 1992. *Organizing Jainism in England and India*. Clarendon.

———. 2003. "Indian Jainism as Social Practice at the End of the Twentieth Century." In *Jainism and Early Buddhism: Essays in Honor of Padmanath S. Jaini*, edited by Ollie Qvarnström. Asian Humanities Press.

Beltz, Johannes, Michaela Blaser, Marion Frenger, Patrick Felix Krüger, and Harsha Vinay, eds. 2023. *Being Jain: Art and Culture of an Indian Religion*. Hatje Cantz.

Bhansali, Pratik. 2023. "Climate and Environment: A Conversation Rooted in Justice." Presentation at Defining Applied Jain Studies Conference, April 22, 2023. Arihanta Institute. https://conf.arihantainstitute.org/agenda.

Bond, George D. 1996. "A. T. Ariyaratne and the Sarvodaya Shramadana Movement in Sri Lanka." In *Engaged Buddhism: Buddhist Liberation Movements in Asia*, edited by Christopher S. Queen and Sallie B. King. State University of New York Press.

Broad, Garret. 2016. *More Than Just Food: Food Justice and Community Change, California Studies in Food and Culture*. University of California Press.

Brown, Donna Lynn. 2023. "Beyond Queen and King: Democratizing 'Engaged Buddhism.'" *Journal of Buddhist Ethics* 30:7–58.

Cabezón, Jose Ignacio. 1996. "Buddhist Principles in the Tibetan Liberation Movement." In Queen and King, eds., *Engaged Buddhism*.

Capper, Daniel. 2022. *Roaming Free Like a Deer: Buddhism and the Natural World*. Cornell University Press.

Chapple, Christopher Key. 2020. *Living Landscapes: Meditations on the Five Elements in Hindu, Buddhist, and Jain Yogas*. State University of New York Press.

———, ed. 2002. *Jainism and Ecology: Nonviolence in the Web of Life*. Center for the Study of World Religions, Harvard University Press.

Chitrabhanu, Ruchika. 2023a. "Jain Roundtable: Applying Jain Principles in Everyday Life." Panel held at Arihanta Institute's Defining Applied Jain Studies Conference, April 23, 2023. https://conf.arihantainstitute.org/agenda?day=23-04-2023.

———. 2023b. "Facets of Veganism in Jainism." Keynote talk at Ahimsa Vegan Conference: Jain Voices in Animal Advocacy. Sponsored by Arihanta Institute, August 27, 2023.

Clines, Gregory M. 2022. *Jain Rāmāyaṇa Narratives: Moral Vision and Literary Innovation*. Routledge Advances in Jaina Studies. Routledge.

Colebrooke, Henry Thomas. 1809. "Observations on the Sect of Jains." In *Asiatic Researches; or, Transactions of the Society Institute in Bengal, for Inquiring into the History and Antiquities, the Arts, Sciences, and Literature of Asia*. Vol. 9. Asiatic Society.

Cort, John E. 1990. "Models of and for the Study of the Jains." *Method & Theory in the Study of Religion* 2 (1): 42–71.

———. 2000. "'Intellectual Ahiṃsā' Revisited: Jain Tolerance and Intolerance of Others." *Philosophy East and West* 50 (3): 324–347.

———. 2001. *Jains in the World: Religious Values and Ideology in India*. Oxford University Press.

———. 2020a. "Jain Society: 1947–2018." In Cort, Dundas, Jacobsen, and Wiley, eds., *Brill's Encyclopedia of Jainism*.

———. 2020b. "In Search of 'Hindu Fiction': The First 'School' of Jain Studies in the U.S." In Cort, Luithle-Hardenberg, and Orr, eds., *Cooperation, Contribution, and Contestation*.

Cort, John E., Andrea Luithle-Hardenberg, and Leslie C. Orr. 2020. "Cooperation, Contribution, and Contestation: The Jain Community, Colonialism and Jainological Scholarship." In *Studies in Asian Art and Culture*. Vol. 6. EB Verlag.

CST. 2023. "Engaged Jain Studies: South Asian and Global Perspectives." https://cst.edu/degree-programs/ma/engaged-jain-studies-south-asian-and-global-perspectives/.

DeVido, Elise A. 2009. "The Influence of Chinese Master Taixu on Buddhism in Vietnam." *Journal of Global Buddhism* 10:413–458.

Donaldson, Brianne. 2020. "Jainism and Darwin: Evolution Beyond Orthodoxy." In *Asian Religious Responses to Darwinism: Evolutionary Theories in Middle Eastern, South Asian, and East Asian Cultural Contexts*, edited by C. Mackenzie Brown. Springer.

Donaldson, Brianne, and Ana Bajželj. 2021. *Insistent Life: Principles for Bioethics in the Jain Tradition*. University of California Press.

Dundas, Paul. 2002. *The Jains*. 2nd ed. Routledge.

Eppsteiner, Fred, ed. 1988. *The Path of Compassion: Writings on Socially Engaged Buddhism*. Parallax Press.

FIU. 2010. "The Bhagwan Mahavir Professorship in Jain Studies." https://jainstudies.fiu.edu/about-us/professorship/professorshiphistory.pdf.

Flügel, Peter. 2005. "The Invention of Jainism: A Short History of Jaina Studies." *International Journal of Jain Studies* 1 (1): 1–14.

Fowler. 2022. "Vital Matters: Applied Jain Ethics for Earth Day." https://fowler.ucla.edu/events/vital-matters-applied-jain-ethics-for-earth-day/.

———. 2023. "Visualizing Devotion: Jain Embroidered Shrine Hangings." https://fowler.ucla.edu/exhibitions/visualizing-devotion/.

Foxen, Anya P. 2020. *Inhaling Spirit: Harmonialism, Orientalism, and the Western Roots of Modern Yoga.* Oxford University Press.

Fuller, Paul. 2021. *An Introduction to Engaged Buddhism.* Bloomsbury.

Gleig, Ann. 2021. "Engaged Buddhism." In *Oxford Research Encyclopedia of Religion*. https://oxfordre.com/religion/view/10.1093/acrefore/9780199340378.001.0001/acrefore-9780199340378-e-755.

Godrej, Farah. 2016. "The Neoliberal Yogi and the Politics of Yoga." *Political Theory* 45 (6): 772–800.

Hsu, Alexander O. 2022. "Coming to Terms with 'Engaged Buddhism': Periodizing, Provincializing, and Politicizing the Concept." *Journal of Global Buddhism* 23 (1): 17–31.

Ikenberry, John G. 2020. "Liberal Internationalism and Cultural Diversity." In *Culture and Order in World Politics*, edited by Andrew Phillips and Christian Reus-Smit. Cambridge University Press.

ISJS. 2022. *Transactions: A Quarterly Refereed Online Research Journal on Jainism* 6 (3 and 4). https://www.isjs.in/july-december-2022/.

———. Forthcoming. *Applications of Anekantavada.* Publisher unknown.

Jain, Andrea. 2015. *Selling Yoga: From Counterculture to Pop Culture.* Oxford University Press.

Jain, Pankaj. 2014. "Bovine Dharma: Nonhuman Animals and the Swadhyaya Parivar. In *Asian Perspectives on Animal Ethics: Rethinking the Nonhuman,* edited by Neil Dalal and Chloë Taylor. Routledge.

Jain, Parveen. 2020. *An Introduction to Jain Philosophy: Based on Writings and Discourses by Ācārya Sushil Kumar.* D. K. Printworld.

Jain, Manoj, and Yogendra Jain. 2023. "Jain Path to Jain Way of Living." Arihanta Institute. https://www.arihantainstitute.org/course/103-jain-path-to-jain-way-of-living.

Jain, Shalin. 2017. *Identity, Community, and State: The Jains under the Mughals.* Primus Books.

Jain, Shugan C., and Prakash C. Jain, eds. 2014. *Social Consciousness in Jainism.* International School for Jain Studies and New Bharatiya Book Corporation.

Jain, Shugan C., and Preeti Rani Jain, eds. 2025. *Applications of Anekāntavāda: Jain Pluralism*. Motilal Banarsidass.

Jain, Shugan, Prakash C. Jain, and Malay R. Patel. 2023. *Jain Business Engagement and Ethics: An Overview*. D. K. Printworld.

JAINA. 2023."Academic Liaison." https://www.jaina.org/page/Academic Liasion.

Jaini, P. S. 1979. *The Jaina Path of Purification*. University of California Press.

Jeffreys, Derek S. 2003. "Does Buddhism Need Human Rights?" In *Action Dharma: New Studies in Engaged Buddhism*, edited by Christopher S. Queen, Charles S. Prebish, and Damien Keown. Routledge.

Judge, William Quan. 1891. *The Path: Vol. 5; 1890–91*. Theosophical Society.

Kelting, Mary Whitney. 2009. *Heroic Wives: Rituals, Stories, and the Virtues of Jain Wifehood*. Oxford University Press.

King, Sallie B. 2009. *Socially Engaged Buddhism, Dimensions of Asian Spirituality*. University of Hawaii Press.

Kraft, Kenneth. 2000. "New Voices in Engaged Buddhist Studies." In *Engaged Buddhism in the West*, edited by Christopher S. Queen. Wisdom Publications.

Kuh, George D., Ken O'Donnell, and Sally Reed. 2013. *Ensuring Quality & Taking High-Impact Practices to Scale*. AAC&U.

Laidlaw, James. 1996. *Riches and Renunciation: Religion, Economy and Society Among the Jains*. Clarendon Press.

Lele, Amod. 2019. "Disengaged Buddhism." *Journal of Buddhist Ethics* 26:240–89.

Luithle-Hardenberg, Andrea. 2020. "Alexander Walker of Bowland's 'Account of the Jeyn': A Starting Point for British Encounters with the Jain Community in Gujarat." In Cort, Luithle-Hardenberg, and Orr, eds., *Cooperation, Contribution, and Contestation*.

Mackenzie, Major C. 1809. "Account of the Jains, Collected from a Priest of this Sect; at Medgeri: Translated by Cavelly Boria, Brahmen." In *Asiatic Researches; or, Transactions of the Society Institute in Bengal, for Inquiring into the History and Antiquities, the Arts, Sciences, and Literature of Asia*. Vol. 9. Asiatic Society.

Main, Jessica L., and Rongdao Lai. 2013. "Introduction: Reformulating 'Socially Engaged Buddhism' as an Analytical Category." *The Eastern Buddhist* 44 (2): 1–34.

Matilal, Bimal Krishna. 1981. *The Central Philosophy of Jainism (Anekānta-vāda)*. L. D. Institute of Indology.

Mehta, Tushar. 2021. "Dismantling 'Regenerative' Animal Agriculture with Dr. Tushar Mehta." *Hope for the Animals Podcast*. Compassionate Living, December 4. https://youtu.be/me8mxaQrRks.

Miller, Christopher Jain. 2023. "Jain Responses to Climate Change." Presentation at Arihanta Institute's Defining Applied Jain Studies Conference, April 22, 2023. https://conf.arihantainstitute.org/agenda.

———. Forthcoming 2026. "Interpreting: Jain Veganism in Dialogue with Jain Vegetarianism: Instrumentalizing Jain Scriptures in Global Debates." In *The Bloomsbury Handbook of Religion and Food*, edited by Yudit Greenberg and Ben Zeller. Bloomsbury.

Miller, Christopher Jain, and Jonathan Dickstein. 2021a. "Jain Veganism: Ancient Wisdom, New Opportunities." *Religions* 12 (7): 512. https://doi.org/10.3390/rel12070512.

———. 2021b. "Revisiting Veganism and the 'Ahiṃsā Crisis': Raising Consciousness according to Karma and Science." Presentation delivered at the Second International Conference on Science and Jain Philosophy, Florida International University, March 22, 2021.

Miller, Christopher Jain, Steven Vose, and Tine Vekemans. 2023. "Theorizing Applied Jain Studies." Panel held at Defining Applied Jain Studies Conference, April 23, 2023. Arihanta Institute. https://conf.arihantainstitute.org/agenda?day=23-04-2023.

Miller, Christopher Patrick. 2019. "Jainism, Yoga, and Ecology: A Course in Contemplative Practice for a World in Pain." *Religions* 10 (4): 232. https://doi.org/10.3390/rel10040232.

Monier-Williams, Monier, Ernst Leumann, and Carl Cappeller. 1899 [1851]. *A Sanskrit-English Dictionary Etymologically and Philologically Arranged with Special Reference to Cognate Indo-European Languages*. Clarendon Press.

Numark, Mitch. 2020. "The British 'Discovery' of Jainism in the Nineteenth Century: Scottish Missionaries, the 'Jain Religion' and the Jains of Bombay." In Cort, Luithle-Hardenberg, and Orr, eds., *Cooperation, Contribution, and Contestation*.

Oddie, Geoffrey A. 2016. "The Emergence and Significance of the Term 'Hinduism.'" In *Hinduism in India: Modern and Contemporary Movements*, edited by Will Sweetman and Aditya Malik. Sage.

Organiser. 2015. "News Roundup: Love Jihad Is a Conspiracy Against Non-Muslims: Tarun Sagar Maharaj." https://organiser.org/2015/03/10/62625/general/ra4dfb98c/.

Orr, Leslie. 2009. "Orientalists, Missionaries, and Jains: The South Indian Story." In *The Madras School of Orientalism: Producing Knowledge in Colonial South India*, edited by Thomas R. Trautmann. Oxford University Press.

———. 2020. "European Imaginings of Jainism in Colonial Madras: Tales of the Coromandel Coast." In Cort, Luithle-Hardenberg, and Orr, eds., *Cooperation, Contribution, and Contestation*.

Patel, Nirva. 2023. "Journeys of a Jain Vegan: From Vegetarian to Vegan, From Engineer to Engaged Animal Advocate." Keynote talk at the Ahimsa Vegan Conference: Jain Voices in Animal Advocacy. Arihanta Institute, August 26, 2023.

PinkNews. 2023. "As an LGBTQ+ Jain, I Felt Completely Invisible Growing Up. Now, I Want to Give Back." https://www.thepinknews.com/2023/02/03/jainism-lgbt-jain-coming-out-just-like-us/.

Premchand, Sushil K. 2020. "The Life of Premchand Roychand (1831–1906): 'Wisdom Above Riches.'" In Cort, Luithle-Hardenberg, and Orr, eds., *Cooperation, Contribution, and Contestation*.

Queen, Christopher S., and Sallie B. King, eds. 1996. *Engaged Buddhism: Buddhist Liberation Movements in Asia*. State University of New York Press.

Queen, Christopher S., Charles S. Prebish, and Damien Keown, eds. 2003. *Action Dharma: New Studies in Engaged Buddhism*. Routledge.

Qvarnström, Olle, and Jason Birch. 2012. "Universalist and Missionary Jainism: Jain Yoga and the Terāpanthī Tradition." In *Yoga in Practice*, edited by David Gordon White. Princeton University Press.

Rankin, Aidan. 2018. *Jainism and Environmental Philosophy: Karma and the Web of Life*. Routledge Focus on Environment and Sustainability. Routledge.

———. 2020. *Jainism and Environmental Politics*. Routledge, Taylor & Francis Group.

Reading, Michael. 2020 "Acharya Sri Tulsi, Anuvrat, and Eco-conscious Living." In *Beacons of Dharma: Spiritual Exemplars for the Modern Age*, edited by Christopher Patrick Miller, Jeffery D. Long, and Michael Reading. Explorations in Indic Traditions: Theological, Ethical, and Philosophical, series editor Jeffery D. Long. Lexington Books.

Rosenthal, Randy. 2018. "What's the Connection Between Buddhism and Ethnic Cleansing in Myanmar?" Lionsroar.com. https://www.lionsroar.com/what-does-buddhism-have-to-do-with-the-ethnic-cleansing-in-myanmar/.

Schubring, Walther, and Wolfgang Beurlen, trans. 1962 [1935]. *The Doctrine of the Jainas: Described After the Old Sources*. Motilal Baṇarsidass.

Shah, Atul K., and Aidan Rankin. 2017. *Jainism and Ethical Finance: A Timeless Business Model*. Routledge, Taylor & Francis Group.

Simmer-Brown, Judith. 2020. "Opening the Heart in Anti-Racism Activism: Pema Chodron and the Lojong Teachings." In Miller, Long, and Reading, eds., *Beacons of Dharma*.

Snyder, Gary. 1961. "Buddhist Anarchism." *Journal for the Protection of All Beings* 1.

Stevenson, Margaret. 1915. *The Heart of Jainism.* Humphrey Milford, Oxford University Press.

Storch, Tanya. 2020. "Beacons of Dharma from the *Biquini zhuan.*" In Miller, Long, and Reading, eds., *Beacons of Dharma.*

Tatia, Nathmal, translator. 2011 [1994]. That Which Is: A Classic Jain Manual for Understanding the True Nature of Reality. Translated from the Tattvārtha Sūtra of Umāsvāti/Umāsvāmi. Yale University Press.

Truschke, Audrey. 2016. *Culture of Encounters: Sanskrit at the Mughal Court.* Columbia University Press.

Tsing, Anna Lowenhaupt. 2005. *Friction: An Ethnography of Global Connection.* Princeton University Press.

Tsomo, Karma Lekshe. 2009. "Socially Engaged Buddhist Nuns: Activism in Taiwan and North America." *Journal of Global Buddhism* 10:459–485.

Vallely, Anne. 2020. "Tai Maharaj, Rebel with a Cause: Acharya Chandanaji's Life of Compassion in Action." In Miller, Long, and Reading, eds., *Beacons of Dharma.*

Vegan Jains. 2019. "Jain Declaration on the Climate Crisis." Accessed June 4, 2023. https://veganjains.com/jain-declaration-on-the-climate-crisis-oct-2019/.

Vesely-Flad, Rima. 2017. "Black Buddhists and the Body: New Approaches to Socially Engaged Buddhism." *Religions* 8 (11): 239. https://doi.org/10.3390/rel8110239.

Vose, Steven M. Forthcoming. *Reimagining Jainism in Islamic India: Jain Intellectual Culture in the Delhi Sultanate.* Routledge.

———. 2022. "Jain Memory of the Tughluq Sultans: Alternative Sources for the Historiography of Sultanate India." *JRAS Series 3* 32 (1): 115–139.

Warren, Herbert. 1912. *Jainism in Western Garb, as a Solution to Life's Great Problems; Chiefly From Notes of Talks & Lectures by Virchand R. Gandhi.* Bibliotheka Jainica.

Weber, Albrecht, and Herbert Weir Smyth. 1893. *Weber's Sacred Literature of the Jains.* Printed at the Education Society's Steam Press.

Part I

Critical Issues in "Engaged Jain Studies"

1

Applied to What? For Whose Benefit?

A Critique of "Applied Jain Ethics"

STEVEN M. VOSE

Scholars have noted as early as the 2002 *Jainism and Ecology* (Chapple 2002) volume that Jains living in the European and North American diaspora have considered Jainism's soteriology—that is, the liberation of the soul from the bonds of karma through rigorous asceticism marked by a thoroughgoing commitment to avoiding harm to even the subtlest forms of life—to be an ethos ill-suited to modern life outside of India. In her contribution to that volume, pointedly titled "From Liberation to Ecology," Anne Vallely writes,

> The geographical and cultural distance from India has led to changes in the beliefs and practices of what constitutes Jainism in North America. Traditional orthodox Jain ethics are renunciatory and individualistic, and their central ethic of *ahiṃsā* [non-harm, nonviolence] reflects this ascetic orientation. However, within a growing segment of the diaspora community, Jain ethics no longer reflect the ascetic ideal. Rather than through the idiom of self-realization or the purification of the soul, ethics are being

> expressed through a discourse of environmentalism and animal rights. (2002, 193)

As Vallely asserts here, Jains who have made their homes abroad have translated the constituent pieces of the soteriological path into an ethical basis for engaging with issues of pressing global concern. As the aim of that volume was to ascertain, from both academic and emic perspectives, just what it means to claim that Jainism is itself ecological or environmentalist, a debate emerged in its essays between the credulous (both scholars and Jains) and skeptics (mainly scholars) that led to both assertive claims of Jainism's inherent environmentalism and critical appraisals of such a possibility, generally rooted in the widely differing historical contexts in which the body of Jain teachings and modern environmentalist thought each arose.

None of the essays in that volume took up the question of why environmentalism and animal rights had become the exclusive avenues in which Jains had chosen to apply their newly developed ethics of engagement. Further, on neither side of the debate in that volume is there an assessment of what effects the assertions of Jainism's inherent environmentalism would have on the very idea of what it means to be a Jain—outside of India or in it—in the late twentieth and early twenty-first centuries, an era increasingly shaped by globalization and transnationalism as much as by the resurgence of ethnonationalist politics and hostility toward multiculturalism in democratic states (India and the US, especially). Rather, Vallely's remarks here reflect a general trend in the volume, and in subsequent scholarship on diaspora Jain communities, which tends to focus on the environmentalism claims as markers of what is distinctive about diaspora perspectives while tacitly or explicitly treating orthodoxy as indicative of "Indian" Jainism.[1] The Jains asserting Jainism's inherent environmentalism are rarely described in specific detail; they are instead characterized with vague language as above—"a growing segment"—or simply as "many." There has been little attempt to assess their specific positions within diaspora communities or to quantify their relative levels of authority in deliberative bodies, such as the Federation of Jain Associations in North America (JAINA), which publish and disseminate these views to diaspora communities in the form of both periodicals (such as *Jain Digest*) and pedagogical materials for use in religious education classes (*pāṭhśālā*). Similarly, the class, caste, and sectarian affiliations of these ideologues have yet to be interrogated such that we might understand the channels of influence their views may have, both within diaspora communities and in India. In short, we have yet to assess *which* Jains are putting forth this message or to understand what the effects, intended or otherwise, may be of steering the conversation of what it means to be Jain into this set of concerns—environmentalism and animal rights—and not into others. The questions of who is being served, and who is silenced, by making (and repeating) such assertions have yet to be asked. And yet there are places where we can see the saturation of this messaging having the effect of hampering efforts made by younger Jains to have other kinds of conversations, especially about Jainism's ability to address human rights, two contrasting examples of which I will discuss in the final section of this chapter.

While this chapter will not be able to offer specific answers to these questions, it delineates them as a program for the future critical study of transnational Jain communities and discusses the implications of what such research may reveal. Additionally, it examines the academy as a newly arisen site for the production of efforts to give, in Clifford Geertz's (1973, 90) terms, an "aura of factuality" to the idea that Jainism's ascetic ethics are indeed "applicable" to address some of the major global problems of our time.[2] That is, the charter documents for endowed chairs in Jain Studies, produced in conversations between Jain donors and university administrators (always before the scholar is hired at the university), present a choice to scholars whether to engage as critical analysts and interpretive descriptors of the body of works and practices in the Jain "cumulative traditions" (what Miller proposes as the critical-analytical model of engaged Jain studies; see the introduction to this volume) or to become de facto constructive theologians (see Miller's constructive-reproductive model) who do the work of making the Jain ascetic ethos into an applied ethics (Smith 1991 [1961], 156ff.). I close by urging attention to the responsibility that scholars have to engage critically with the claims that Jains make about Jainism while balancing their own desires to engage in activism via constructive theology (see Miller's critical-constructive model).

The AAA of Jainism: "Core Jain Values" as Identitarian Discourse

Leaders of diaspora Jain communities today often invoke *ahiṃsā* (non-harm, nonviolence), *anekāntavāda* (doctrine of many-sidedness), and *aparigraha* (non-possession) to describe the "core values" of Jainism when talking to Jains and non-Jains alike. This AAA of Jainism is as likely to be invoked in temples and community centers as it is in universities and other public spaces, in classrooms in Jain temples, and when speakers are invited to give talks that connect Jainism's ethics to issues of global concern. The biennial JAINA conventions customarily include a host of speakers whose talks overwhelmingly focus on these three "values" as they apply to major issues. That this collection of two of the five Great Vows (*mahāvratas*), *ahiṃsā* and *aparigraha*, and a key philosophical principle, *anekāntavāda*, has come to stand in for the core values of Jainism can be traced historically. Indeed, the seeming arbitrariness of why these three items out of the many other readily deployable vows and concepts came to be identified as the essence of Jainism demands a historical reckoning.

It is usually taken as a truism that Jainism is the religion of *ahiṃsā*. However, this statement is only possible to make in a modern episteme, thinkable only when Jainism is coined and thought of as a religion, both epistemological inventions of the eighteenth and nineteenth centuries (Cort et al. 2020; Flügel 2005, 2, 2n5). Further, these terms had to be interpreted and deployed not only by foreign scholars and colonial administrators but also by those who recognized their connection to Jainism as a religion and thereby "became Jains" in this modern mode. This was, to be sure, an uneven historical process among those who considered the teachings (*śāsana*, *dharma*) of the Jinas the basis of their moral code, their ethical and ritual praxis, and, to some extent, their community. The political, social, and cultural upheavals of the colonial and postcolonial eras demanded (as in other, prior periods of historical rupture) the rearticulation of what it meant to be Jain.[3] This was certainly the case as Jains moved from hinterlands and Mughal-era cities into colonial cities such as Bombay in the nineteenth century, where they encountered Scottish missionaries and others who thought about religion in quite different ways from how Jains had been accustomed to thinking about the parameters of one's dharma (Numark 2013). Translating "Jina-dharma" (or "Jaina-dharma") into "Jainism" was a process that included early adopters (who may or may not fall under the category of "progressive" in all their views) and those who resisted the epistemic shift (who, likewise, cannot all be labeled "conservative" in all matters).[4] Those who were first to adopt technologies such as the printing press were able to disseminate their views more widely through pamphlets, periodicals, and the publication of canonical texts, collections of hymns, liturgical manuals, and other popular works. Through print, they were able to shape the contours of this emerging Jain religious identity that partially managed to supersede other identities, such as caste, that had previously been more salient to the lives of those people who also happened to support Jain mendicants, build Jain temples, and to practice Jain rituals.

This was no less the case for Jains who migrated to the US, Canada, and the UK starting in the mid-to-late twentieth century. Those who organized and joined collective bodies such as JAINA, founded in 1981, were able to influence Jains at affiliated centers through the publication of *Jain Digest* and the creation of teaching materials for use in *pāṭhśālā* classes.[5] As they thought about how to communicate Jainism's essential features in a North American or British context, so that they might find ways of connecting their ethos to the conversations and concerns they saw around them, they had two points of reference. One was the nonviolent resistance to colonial rule conceived and enacted by Mohandas K. (Mahatma) Gandhi (1869–1948), which brought "ahimsa" into the English lexicon. The other were the lectures on Jainism given by Virchand Gandhi (1864–1901) at the 1893 World's Parliament of Religions in Chicago. Although overshadowed by Swami Vivekananda's representations of Hinduism in the American *imaginaire*, Virchand Gandhi's presence there, and return to the United States to lecture further in 1896, created some small ripples that fostered connections with American and British vegetarians and animal welfare activists and gave a platform for translating *ahiṃsā* into the basis of a social ethic of engagement (Long 2024).

Jainism's association with a positive, outward-looking commitment to nonviolence toward the planet and our animal brethren has been reiterated in numerous books, articles, and other media in European languages since the 1970s. This grew out of several earlier efforts to draw these connections, an early example of which is Herbert Warren's 1912 *Jainism in Western Garb, as a Solution to Life's Great Problems,* written "Chiefly from notes of Talks and Lectures by Virchand R. Gandhi" (Warren 1916 [1912], i). Although focused largely on the Jain account of the universe and its ascetic path of self-purification, we can see in its pages the association of Jainism with its first vow, *ahiṃsā,* and begin to see its development as an ethical principle as much as an ascetic commitment, refigured as a code of self-discipline for managing life in the modern world. Indeed, on the page before the preface appears an early translation of the axiomatic declaration, *ahiṃsā paramo dharmaḥ,* found in many recent Jain publications in English, rendered by Warren as "Non-injury is the highest religion." Directly below it, a corollary: "Non-injury means the cessation of evil" (Warren 1916 [1912], iv).

Many Jain organizations adopted the phrase, *ahiṃsā paramo dharmaḥ,* as the "official Jain credo" after a 1975 conference between Digambara and Śvetāmbara mendicants in India. Held to commemorate the 2,500th anniversary (more or less) of Mahāvīra's liberation (*mokṣa*), the conference attempted reconciliation between Digambara and Śvetāmbara understandings of Jainism.[6] This effort to find common ground likely gave a fillip to diaspora communities who were themselves looking for a basis for thinking about Jainism apart from the sectarian and caste-based practices and identities that had historically modulated it, largely due to the fact that there were not enough Jains of any one denomination in any metropolitan area to build their own temples. With this new spirit of sectarian reconciliation in place, diaspora Jains increasingly put their efforts into translating the path to liberation into principles of a social ethic. However, that it took roughly a century after scholars and even lay Jain leaders had begun to articulate the nature of Jainism for Jain mendicants to attempt a consensus on the matter shows how unevenly impactful the modern idea of "Jainism" had been for different Jain communities.[7]

Still, in none of these efforts to encapsulate Jainism as "the religion of *ahiṃsā*" was it a foregone conclusion that the ethic of nonviolence would be deployed exclusively in the realms of environmentalism and animal rights. Indeed, taking credit for

Gandhi's use of nonviolence would seem to suggest that Jains would readily translate *ahiṃsā* into political activism on behalf of colonized and oppressed peoples around the world, which has rarely been the case.

Avoiding harm to all forms of life, as subtle as the constituent elements of the physical world—earth, air, fire, and water—is a central tenet of the ascetic path and has been regarded for centuries as the basis of the lay ethics of avoiding overt forms of harm through vegetarianism and through livelihoods that avoid dealing in animal flesh or hides. The animal shelters (*pañjarāpoḷs*, *gauśālās*), birdfeeders, and other forms of care for animals found in Jain community spaces across India translated into a Jain assertion of animal welfare and environmentalism in the late twentieth century, as environmentalist and animal rights discourses became increasingly popular in the West (see Dickstein's chapter in this volume). Jains saw an easy connection between the two. Human rights, however, did not enter the popular Jain *imaginaire* as they thought about the sites where nonviolence should be practiced, despite their efforts to take credit for Mahatma Gandhi's ethic of nonviolence, as it had become part of the left's discourse of activism, especially in the US, through the Civil Rights–era protests and tactics of such figures as Martin Luther King, Jr., Jains had themselves roundly criticized Gandhi in India; their reclamation of Gandhi was also a way to find connections with the West's admiration of Gandhi in circles that would be inclined to be inclusive and welcoming of new Jain immigrants.

While it is certainly true that Jains have long regarded *ahiṃsā* as more than a monastic vow, most commonly understood as a demand for lay Jains to adopt a vegetarian diet and to serve as a justification for engaging in certain occupations adhering to principles of upholding non-harm to other beings, the notion that nonviolence was more than a matter of soteriological concern is not evident even in such seemingly compassionate practices as animal shelters (*pañjarāpoḷs*). Or rather, it has gone without explanation for decades why it is that when Jains assert Jainism's commitment to *ahiṃsā*, we understand that to mean that its application in the fields of environmentalism and animal rights is foregone.

And so Jainism's persona in the West remained as the "religion of ahimsa" until the 1990s, when the discourse of religious pluralism began to gain popular currency. Finding another analogue in their intellectual repertoire, Jains connected the philosophical stance of *anekāntavāda* to pluralism as a platform for accepting the (partial) truths contained in other religious and philosophical traditions. And with the publication of another edited volume, *Ahimsa, Anekanta, and Jainism* (Sethia 2004), Jainism's persona had been successfully modified into being the religion of the AA, of *ahiṃsā* and *anekāntavāda*.

Shortly after I began working at Florida International University in January 2013, a new marketing brochure arrived that included the third A, *aparigraha*, as a "core principle" of Jainism. As many upper-class Jains had come out ahead in India's engagements with global capitalism and began manifesting their wealth in the form of conspicuous consumption, several Jain ideologues, including several prominent Śvetāmbara monks, became increasingly concerned with the personal and environmental effects of unchecked consumerism and began to tout another of its main ascetic vows as an ethical principle for dealing with consumerism in late-stage capitalism. With this, Jainism became the religion of the AAA—*ahiṃsā, anekāntavāda,* and *aparigraha*—two ascetic vows and a philosophical stance. It should be noted that *aparigraha* was contained within the interpretive framework of limited consumerism, never a critique of capitalism itself or its constituent parts: private property ownership, exploitation of labor, wealth hoarding, capital accumulation, etc. This was no endorsement of Marxism or its critiques of capitalism.

It is in this context that the endowment of professorships at universities had a ready discourse in place to identify "core Jain values" and to facilitate the application of them toward solving the world's most pressing problems. With these areas of concern identified and repeated in numerous talks, publications, and other forms of public discourse, the horizon of thought of what Jainism could mean to the world became defined, delineated, and circumscribed to these areas. It is these values and realms of application that were touted to students on the International Summer School for Jain Studies (ISSJS) study abroad program, which began in the summer of 2006. An entry point for many students to discover Jainism that inspired them to pursue academic careers in Jain studies, those who found a home in the study of Jainism increasingly became those who were already committed to veganism, animal rights, and environmentalism. Human rights, for example, never made any headway among Jains or the scholars who committed to Jain studies and the application of Jain ethics. And without a cadre of young Jain intellectuals to put forth alternative discourses to those coming out of JAINA and from other, mostly elderly male Jains, the Jain educational scene was saturated with a form of Jain ethics primarily encapsulating only these few things and not others. The remaining vows—non-stealing (*asteya, acaurya*), truth-telling (*satya*), and celibacy (*brahmacarya*)—hardly made any appearances in public discourses.

Professorships and the Marketing of Jainism's Ethics via Constructive Theology

With the endowment of a series of professorships in Jain studies across North America and Europe, the academy has become the most significant new site to emerge for the development of an "applied" or "engaged" Jain ethics since the publication of *Jainism and Ecology* (Chapple 2002). This process began with the establishment of the Centre of Jaina Studies at the School of Oriental and African Studies (SOAS) in London in 2004, then proceeded in earnest with the endowment of a professorship at Florida International University in 2010. There are now roughly thirty academic positions[8] at universities around the US, most of which are public, with additional new chairs in the UK, Canada, Belgium, South Africa, and Israel.[9]

Many of these chairs, endowed by consortia of Jains residing mainly in the US and UK, have in their founding charters or gift agreements certain stipulations to include programming or to encourage research and teaching that applies Jain "ethical principles" or "values" to issues of pressing global concern, either as part of the professor's research or teaching agenda or through programming put on by the university, such as lecture series and workshops. While universities often differ in their missions and approaches to solving the issues of our time, which may or may not be at odds with a faculty member's own research agenda—and given the fact that all but two professorships are endowed at public research universities—the goodwill of the researchers and the university administration toward their donors has meant that they have tried to implement some efforts to see that "applied Jain ethics" are part of their Jain studies programs.

The effect of these efforts has been to foster a body of work—scholarship, activism, and public discourse—on a number of topics that connect with the delineated areas of interest that donors have seen as relevant to Jain ethics. The scholars who hold these chairs may or may not conduct research on ethics or even agree that there is academic merit to supporting these programs. These scholars often conduct programming that fits the mold with what they know will resonate with donors. For those scholars who do direct work in the field of ethics and even in applied ethics, their ability to be hired in such positions depended on their research agenda's conformity to the selected areas of application of these engaged ethics. Their work may best be characterized as "constructive theology," as they are doing the intellectual work of dredging the Jain canon and intellectual history for ways of bolstering the intellectual basis on which such applications fit with Jain ethics. In short, if Jain ethics are to be applied outside the Jain soteriological framework, as many Jains today wish to assert, the reasons for doing so *as Jains* become the main intellectual imperative of the project. This is work that Jain intellectuals have partially done themselves; they are also creating a platform through these endowed chairs for some non-Jain scholars to aid them in this project. For other scholars whose research agendas are historical, anthropological, analytical, and descriptive, these constructive efforts present a new opportunity to describe and analyze the ongoing development, growth, and historical change happening in Jain communities. Any such scholar's anthropological interest in "engaged Jain ethics," however, sits uncomfortably alongside their job requirements to conduct programming and teach courses that are themselves contributing to the very constructive discourses that constitute the growing archive of material which gives any putative engaged ethics their reality.

For scholars on both the descriptive and the constructive side of things, the words "unease" and "discomfort" have frequently appeared in their evaluations of their roles in building a constructive Jain theology on behalf of Jains, each for different reasons. In this chapter, I am in a way interrogating my own role and experience as a professor of Jain studies at two institutions in the US, one of which had a significant programming component in "applied Jain ethics," and the other of which has a mandate to teach courses on topics that connect with these Jain ethics. I have done so in light of the broader developments of these Jain studies professorships across the Euro-American academy (and now, beyond). Some issues that bear further inquiry are: Whose agenda are we serving by furthering "applied" or "engaged" Jain ethics? How is the institution of the university contributing to the legitimation of this project and what responsibility do scholars have to engage this development critically? What do these efforts do to support other kinds of intra-Jain and intra–South Asian politics? What does a lack of critical attention forestall in terms of other kinds of developments and applications of Jain ethics? What other forms of Jain praxis and thought are being marginalized through our complicity in this project? And what kind of pushback on this is possible?

This chapter has sought to ask specifically *who* is putting forth this vision of Jainism and Jain identity and what other agendas beyond those openly declared are being served by the creation of an "engaged" Jain ethics and the delimitation of areas in which those "engaged" ethics may be "applied." As we can see, at least at a minimum, Jain leaders have outsourced the work of doing this constructive theology to scholars.

In the section that follows, I discuss the group Jains for Justice, founded in the wake of the demonstrations following the police murder of George Floyd in 2020, and the work it did to (1) put forth a Jainism-grounded politics of racial engagement in the US and (2) conduct a survey among Jains in the US about their understanding of, and engagements with, American white supremacist racism. I close by urging attention to the responsibility that scholars have to engage critically with the claims that Jains make about Jainism while balancing their own desires to engage in activism via constructive theology.

So What? Jains for Justice, the Save Shikharji Campaign, and Jain Engagements with Human Rights Issues

In *Jainism and Ecology* (2002), individual essays by Cort and Dundas questioned the very possibility of Jain ethics being considered environmentalist or ecological because of the nature of Jain ethics as soteriologically oriented. Ultimately, as both point out, there is plenty in the vast Jain scriptural and literary corpuses for Jains to explore in order to begin to do the constructive theology of establishing a robust Jain environmentalist ethic (see Bohanec's chapter "Jain Ecotheology Engaging with Ecopsychology" in this volume). Instead, what they were confronted with at the time were insistences and declarations coming from certain members of the Jain community who wished that Jainism were known as, at its heart, an environmentalist ethos. The chief criticisms of these insistences at the time were (1) that Jains had not yet done the work of making a serious engagement with modern philosophical and ethical discourses that had given rise to the conservation and environmentalist movements in Europe and the Americas, (2) that the Jains asserting Jainism's claim to being environmentalist seemed more concerned with Jainism being given universal credit for being the "first ever environmentalist religion" without demanding that Jains themselves adjust widespread current practices to align with these values, (3) a lack of historical understanding of what sparked the environmentalist movement in Europe and North America, (4) the will of Jains to actually influence environmentalist policies in India or other places where they live, and (5) a refusal to engage the differences among human populations regarding who are environmental stewards and who are actually causing the greatest environmental degradation, or their alliances with those most likely to support government policies and economic practices that would lead to massive environmental harm.

If there is a sixth point to add to this, it is a refusal to care for those peoples most subject to massive environmental harm. For Jains, environmentalism has meant harm to nonhuman animals and plants and specifically almost never includes humans. What has seemed to be a mere oversight or blind spot has since become an open hostility. Jains' refusal to engage with human rights was made most starkly apparent in the Save Shikharji campaign, as Jains vilified the tribal communities seeking an economic opportunity, the same communities that have been subject to illegal mining operations in Jharkhand, where Sammet Shikhar sits in the southern part of the state in an area with over 30% of its population labeled as "Scheduled Tribe." Jains' widespread support for the Bharatiya

Janata Party (BJP) government has meant that they have themselves refused to see the issue from multiple perspectives and instead have thrown their support behind a party widely cited (e.g., Drèze and Sen 2013) for having allowed mining companies to operate without permits, and, more troublingly, use private armies to run local tribal communities off their land. The BJP government has labeled tribal resistance as "Naxalite," with claims they are part of a vast, coordinated conspiracy to overthrow the Indian government, thereby placing universal blame on all tribal peoples and distracting the public from any effort to rein in mining companies' violence.

Jains wished to see Sammet Shikhar deemed as a protected sacred site, thereby preventing a tribal community from building a resort nearby. However, despite Jains' own touting of their ethics of seeing issues from multiple perspectives, there have been exactly *no* discussions about the reasons why the community wanted to build the resort in the first place, let alone any alternative plan or aid offered to them to provide an alternative economic opportunity—this, despite Jains' also self-touted business acumen. Given Jains' publicly touted ethics, it seems to defy understanding that they would not attempt to see the issue from the side of those wishing to build the resort and instead engaged in a campaign of fearmongering to other Jains (for which, several scholars, including myself, were approached to offer support) about the environmental degradation and social evils that would be allowed to run amok near their holy site if the resort were allowed to be built there.

The peril here for the Jain leaders involved with this campaign and other attempts to define which causes engaged Jain ethics ought to be applied is that they shut out and forestall the wider application of Jain ethics of non-harm to other areas in which other Jains think they ought to be applied. This is seen most clearly in the abortive effort made by a handful of young Jains to support the Black Lives Matter movement in the US. I say "abortive" because the group, Jains for Justice, has not regularly updated its social media accounts since August 2021; its website, jains4justice.org, is no longer extant.[10] The group conducted research among Jains in North America, surveying them on their understanding of social justice issues facing Black racialized populations in the US as well as on their willingness to discuss these issues within their families and communities.[11] The report's chief finding is that respondents indicated that they found it most difficult to talk with their families (among friends, co-workers, and neighbors) about matters of race, caste, and religion. The two most significant reasons they cited for this difficulty were "differing values" and "respect" (Bhalani et al. n.d., 10–11). Representative qualitative responses indicated that discussing such matters with family was not a preferred conversation topic or was seen as "divisive"; one respondent stated that it was difficult to convince their parents that such matters were "relevant" due to a lack of "interact[ion] with people of other races and religion [*sic*] outside of a business setting" (ibid., 14).

This data speaks to a headwind anticipated in Jains for Justice's open letter to the Jain community on Black Lives Matter (Jain and Mehta n.d.). The letter, which appears to have been released in 2020 before the survey was conducted, is an impassioned plea for Jains to regard racial justice in the United States as a matter for them to engage with as a principle of upholding not only *ahiṃsā* but also other vows and values. The five-page letter makes several statements that appear to anticipate a strong reaction from within the Jain community and speaks to the survey findings of the difficulty in speaking to elders due to norms of respect and differences in values. For example, the opening paragraph closes with "In advance, Micchami Dukkadam" (1). This Prakrit phrase is invoked most commonly during the annual Jain period of atonement, Paryūṣaṇa, to seek forgiveness for wrongs committed throughout the year, "knowingly or unknowingly." I have also observed it being used in common speech among Jains in India and the US today to apologize and seek forgiveness for interpersonal matters, equivalent to "I'm sorry" or "Please forgive me." By using this phrase, the authors of this letter show that they thought it would cause a strong negative reaction among its Jain readers. After the letter's closing, an additional statement of apology appears. I quote it here in its entirety: "If we have written anything which has hurt or upset you in any way, or which goes against the teachings of Mahavir Swami [the last Jina and founder of the Jain community, ca. sixth–fifth c. BCE], we humbly ask for your forgiveness. From the bottom of our hearts, we thank you for reading with an open mind. Once again, Michhami Dukkadam."

After a quick history of slavery, Jim Crow, and anti-Black racism in the US, and statistical data showing the police and carceral violence that Black Americans face today, the letter makes a case for understanding "Ahimsa" as admonishing against racism in thought, speech, and deed. Further, and perhaps following the logic of active engagement with animal protection, they write, "We should take the step to be actively anti-racist, rather than remaining silent" (2). They further invoke three other vows, beginning with *satya* (truth), which they claim "asks us to speak the harmless truth"; they ask readers to consider how to "acknowledge and expose racism in our country, and declare that black lives matter" (3). They then invoke *asteya* (non-stealing), asking readers to think about how Black labor has been "stolen" on a daily basis (3). In a pointed critique of the Jain community in the US, their discussion of *aparigraha,* which they define as "non-attachment," asks readers to consider how the American Jain community's relative prosperity has been attributed to personal and community success and, seemingly, not to structural advantages. They ask readers, "If it is non-attachment we care about, why is it that we seem to care so strongly about businesses being demolished while paying minimal attention to centuries of Black lives being taken?" (3). Finally, they invoke *anekāntavāda* to urge readers to think about the world from a Black perspective by seeking out resources; they also admonish Jains against their condemnations of "looting" by stating that "we cannot tell another group what the 'right way' to protest is" (3). They base their entire discussion in this section on a reading of the now-famous line from the *Tattvārtha Sūtra* (5.21), *parasparopagraho jīvānām,* and translate it as "living beings render service to one another" (2).[12] The authors interpret it to mean, "We must use our voices in service of our fellow humans in their struggle to be accepted as equals. Caring for all life includes all races" (2).

The following section expands on this invocation of sympathy, as they appeal to Jains as Indian immigrants who have themselves been historically subject to racism in the forms of everyday discrimination and racist immigration laws. Here, they show how the Civil Rights Movement helped to replace the Asian Exclusion Act of 1927 with the new laws and policies that made immigration to the US possible for Indians after 1965. Additionally, they take head-on two discourses apparently commonly deployed among Jains in the US.[13] The first is a version of the "model minority" myth; they write, "Some may use our [i.e., Jain community members'] success as an argument to 'prove' that America is not racist" (4). The authors redirect this sentiment to ask readers to consider the differences between the day-to-day racism that they face as South Asians and the systemic racism that Black Americans have suffered. The other is a rebuttal to the obscurantist "all lives matter" phrase that, apparently, was also being invoked among Jains alongside the many white Americans who deployed it. They used the commonly invoked analogy of the burning house requiring our attention in this moment of crisis.

Powerfully, the letter closes with a summation that draws upon all these sources of Jain ethics to both assert a more comprehensive reading of what Jain values are and deflect criticism of property destruction as a form of violence that had apparently allowed many Jains to dismiss the Black Lives Matter protests: "It is our duty to speak the truth, to fight for a world in which violence is unnecessary to bring attention to the plight of oppressed people" (4).

In the failure, or refusal, to engage in social justice and human rights issues by those elder leaders of Jain communities, one wonders if it is not mere oversight to see or hear what other Jains have asserted that Jainism must also engage. Instead, it rings as a concerted effort to control the messaging of what it means to be Jain. Engaging with environmentalism and animal rights allows Jain leaders to limit their activism to causes that are widely supported, minimally controversial, and may be, as the case of the Save Shikharji campaign shows, conveniently self-serving. The unwillingness to engage with pressing social justice issues, where speaking the truth would lead to reducing harm and upholding one of the less-touted of the five *mahāvratas*—*satya,* or truth-telling—has meant its alienation from the Jain public consciousness, limiting younger Jains wishing to uphold social and racial justice from being able to do so *as Jains*.

~

For Paul

Notes

1. Rather than distinguish between "diaspora" and "Indian" forms of Jainism, in several conference presentations (e.g., SOAS Jaina Studies Workshop, 2007) and keynote addresses (e.g., Florida International University, 2014), Peter Flügel has delineated a fivefold typology of modes of engagement that Jains have taken, and continue to take, toward "Jainism" since the nineteenth century. These modes include "canonical," "classical," "mystical," "Protestant," and "modern." The last of these categories is marked by an interest in translating Jain ascetic ethics into an engaged ethics to address global issues, particularly focused on the environment and animal welfare. While avoiding the problematic distinction between the diaspora and Indian Jain communities, the typology has yet to take full account of the transnational nature of Jain communities or to assess specific class, caste, or sectarian dynamics that tend to correlate certain Jains with one or another of these modes of engagement. See Mehta (2015 [2007]).

2. To clarify, my claim here is not that Jain ethics do not translate into social ethics; rather, it is to call attention to the process of making certain ascetic vows and philosophical ideas into ethics that are deployed generally in some areas of activist interest and not others. Paying attention to the process reveals the historical choices of which commitments were considered commensurate with Jain values and which were not so considered.

3. For examples of previous efforts by Jain leaders to rearticulate the meaning of Jain identity and of the nature of the tradition itself, see Vose (forthcoming), focusing on the Delhi Sultanate (thirteenth–fourteenth century) and Truschke (2015), on the early Mughal era (sixteenth–seventeenth century).

4. The most fulsome historical examination of this history can be found in Cort et al. 2020, especially chs. 7–9.

5. Studies of pedagogical materials and curriculum in US-based Jain centers has been the subject of a recent PhD thesis by Shivani Bothra (Victoria University of Wellington, 2017) and an MA thesis by Venu Mehta (Florida International University, 2017). Mehta's thesis focuses on "sectarian negotiations" in the spaces of a Jain center and points out that American Jain temples tend to be multi-sectarian in their ritual spaces and nonsectarian in their classrooms. That is, they seek to teach commonly held beliefs, ideas, and practices. I have also observed that when major intellectuals—such as Hemacandra, Haribhadra, and Kundakunda—are read or discussed in *pāṭhśālā* classes, they tend to do so without mentioning

their sectarian identities. Avoiding sectarianism has been a major point of pride for many leaders of JAINA and local centers; some have even gone so far as to say that this is characteristic of a unique "American Jainism" or even that they are the better Jains for avoiding sectarian strife.

6. This conference also led to the creation of the *Samaṇa-sutta*, a Prakrit rendering of verses from canonical texts of both communities that found mutual agreement. This text is still often taught in *pāṭhśālā*s and to (mostly) non-Jain students who attend the International Summer School for Jain Studies study abroad programs.

7. The watershed moment in Western scholarship for the study of Jains and Jainism is often traced to the publication of Hermann Jacobi's 1876 edition of the *Kalpa Sūtra* published in Leipzig. In the introduction to that volume, Jacobi settles, once and for all, the independence of Jainism as a tradition separate from Hinduism or Buddhism (Flügel 2005, 2). Jains themselves began to try to codify the parameters of Jainism shortly thereafter. One early example is Nahar and Ghosh's 1917 *Epitome of Jainism*, which set out to correct some errors and misconceptions they identified in several works of Western scholarship on the tradition.

8. These positions include tenure-line research professorships, lectureships, and postdoctoral fellowships.

9. The founding of the Arihanta Institute by Parveen Jain in 2021 brought a new institutional avenue for research and teaching in applied or engaged Jain ethics. The institute emulates the structure of institutions of higher education while avoiding many of the bureaucratic and legal constraints typical of universities that can make offering courses or publishing research in these areas difficult. The editors of the present volume inform me that it has established standards for retention and promotion for its faculty and is seeking accreditation. Since its founding, it has become the main advocate for the "engaged" Jainism model by promoting courses and seminars on veganism, climate change, religious pluralism, and yoga, including hosting the conference Engaged Jainism, which was the impetus for this chapter (see the introduction to this volume). It currently partners with the Claremont School of Theology to offer a Master of Arts in Engaged Jain Studies (Arihanta Institute n.d.).

10. The last post on any major social media platform is a January 2022 post on Instagram, which came over five months after their previous post.

11. The jains4justice.org website was last viewably archived on the Wayback Machine of the Internet Archive in January 2024. I was able to download the .pdf of the results of their survey before the website was taken down. See Bhalani et al. (n.d.) for the report citation.

12. Cf. Tatia's translation, "Souls render service to one another" (Umāsvatī 1994, 131). To note the importance of this verse for Anglophone Jains, Tatia includes it as an epigram on p. v of this edition.

13. For a history of anti-Black racism in Indian immigrant communities in the US, see Prashad (2001, ch. 9).

References

Arihanta Institute. n.d. "About Us." https://www.arihantainstitute.org/about. Accessed July 17, 2024.

Bhalani, Mitesh et al. n.d. "Results from the Jains for Justice Community Needs Survey." Jains for Justice, jains4justice.org [website now defunct]. Accessed April 22, 2023.

Chapple, Christopher Key, ed. 2002. *Jainism and Ecology: Nonviolence in the Web of Life.* Center for the Study of World Religions, Harvard University Press.

Cort, John E., Andrea Luithle-Hardenberg, and Leslie C. Orr, eds. 2020. *Cooperation, Contribution and Contestation: The Jain Community, Colonialism, and Jainological Scholarship, 1800–1950.* EB Verlag.

Drèze, Jean, and Amartya Sen. 2013. *An Uncertain Glory: India and Its Contradictions.* Penguin/Viking.

Flügel, Peter. 2005. "The Invention of Jainism: A Short History of Jaina Studies." *International Journal of Jaina Studies (Online)* 1 (1): 1–14.

Geertz, Clifford. 1973. "Religion as a Cultural System." In *The Interpretation of Cultures.* Basic Books.

Jain, Sara, and Sahana Mehta. n.d. "Black Lives Matter: An Open Letter to the Jain Community." Edited by Umang Lathia and Pranay Patni. Jains for Justice, jains4justice.org [website now defunct]. Accessed October 2, 2022.

Long, Jeffery D. 2024. "Emissary of Nonviolence: Virchand Gandhi and the Chicago World's Parliament of Religions, 1893." In *Empire, Religion, and Identity: Modern South Asia the Global Circulation of Ideas,* edited by Soumen Mukherjee. Brill.

Mehta, Manish. 2015 [2007]. "9th Jaina Studies Workshop–Jainism and Modernity–A Manish Mehta Report." HereNow4U. July 30. https://www.herenow4u.net/index.php?id=1512. Originally published May 9, 2007.

Nahar, Puran Chand, and Krishnachandra Ghosh. 1917. *An Epitome of Jainism.* H. Duby Gulab Karnar Library.

Numark, Mitch. 2013. "The Scottish 'Discovery' of Jainism in Nineteenth-Century Bombay." *Journal of Scottish Historical Studies* 33 (1): 20–51.

Prashad, Vijay. 2001. *The Karma of Brown Folk*. University of Minnesota Press.

Sethia, Tara, ed. 2004. *Ahiṃsā, Anekānta and Jainism*. Motilal Banarsidass.

Smith, Wilfred Cantwell. 1991 [1961]. *The Meaning and End of Religion*. Fortress Press.

Truschke, Audrey. 2015. "Dangerous Debates: Jain Responses to Theological Challenges at the Mughal Court." *Modern Asian Studies* 49 (5): 1311–1344.

Umāsvatī. 1994. *That Which Is:* Tattvārtha Sūtra. Translated by Nathmal Tatia. HarperCollins.

Vallely, Anne. 2002. "From Liberation to Ecology: Ethical Discourses Among Orthodox and Diaspora Jains." In Chapple, ed., *Jainism and Ecology*.

Vose, Steven M. Forthcoming. *Reimagining Jainism in Islamic India: Jain Intellectual Culture in the Delhi Sultanate*. Routledge.

Warren, Herbert. 1912. *Jainism in Western Garb, as a Solution to Life's Great Problems*. Central Jaina Publishing House.

2

Jain Mantra Healing

Opportunities and Challenges of Engaged / Applied Jain Studies

TINE VEKEMANS

Throughout history, Jains have sought to find elements—concepts, ways of doing things, exemplary figures, texts, interpretations—in their tradition that allowed them to better cope and even thrive in the context they inhabited.[1] The proliferation of mendicant and lay engagement with global challenges that is often perceived as a recent phenomenon is thus not, in essence, fundamentally new. Rather, it is scholarly research on Jainism that has developed in the direction of the study of Jains and their socioreligious practice after a long period that paid almost exclusive attention to Jainism as a doctrine (Cort 1990). Considering how Jainism is applied in specific temporal and geographical contexts allows scholars to look into, for example, Jain (1) campaigns and organizations for the promotion of animal rights, veganism, and social equality, or focusing on environmentalism and climate change, (2) charity organizations providing medical and educational relief, seeking to alleviate poverty or enabling academic research and teaching on Jain values, and (3) systems promoting mental and physical health.

Factors such as environmental degradation, societal and professional pressures, and the COVID-19 pandemic have contributed to a growing global preoccupation with mental and physical health. Jains have sought and developed curative practices within their own tradition. One such modern curative practice, Bhaktamar Mantra Healing (henceforth referred to as BMH) is a spiritual healing system—or as one healer likes to refer to it, a technology—based on a popular devotional poem called the *Bhaktāmar Stotra*. BMH is an example of a relatively recent practice that builds on but at the same time radically transforms elements derived from the Jain tradition (the text, mantra, *yantra*) and operationalizes them to allay contemporary physical and mental health concerns.[2]

The main part of this chapter is a partial and slightly amended reproduction of a longer paper that was published in 2022 in a special issue on tantra in the *International Journal of Hindu Studies*.[3] I refer to that original paper for the detailed discussion on tantra in Jainism as well as the analysis of differences in the prevailing narratives in various digital resources and social media accounts related to BMH, which I will forego here (Vekemans 2022). This chapter will introduce, historicize, and examine the putative beneficial effects of this Jain mode of healing and demonstrate how this analysis of BMH practices would serve well to start thinking through the deontological difficulties and methodological exigencies of the emerging field of engaged Jain studies. Rather than reproduce the original article's conclusions, this chapter will conclude by indicating where the productive and cordial collaboration between scholars of engaged Jain studies and engaged Jains can give rise to frictions and propose some possible ways in which engaged Jains and engaged Jain studies scholars can foster a robust mutual understanding and respectful collaborative relationship.

Historicizing and Contextualizing Bhaktamar Mantra Healing

The Rich and Multilayered Bhaktāmar Tradition

BMH is the newest layer in a complex textual and devotional tradition that grew from a sixth-century CE devotional poem, the *Bhaktāmar Stotra*. This highly popular text was composed as a devotional hymn to the first Tīrthaṅkara Ṛṣabhadeva (alternatively called Ādinātha) and is attributed to the author Mānatuṅga, who is claimed by both *Śvetāmbara* and *Digambara* Jains (Balbir n.d.). Not much is known for certain regarding the author or the context within which he worked, but a recent study in Hindi by Dhanki and Shah identifies Mānatuṅga as a presumably *Śvetāmbara* Jain author who lived in the second half of the sixth century CE, and the study proposes that the original text probably consisted of forty-four verses, to which four verses were added in a later *Digambara* version (Dhanki and Shah 1999; Cort 2000a; 2005, 94).[4] The German Indologist Hermann Jacobi was the first to publish a scholarly edition of the text with a translation in 1876, and different editions and translations have since followed (see figure 2.1 for chronology).[5]

The hymn subsequently spawned a number of commentaries from the fourteenth century CE onward (for an overview, see Cort 2001, 189). The earliest surviving commentary by Guṇākara (1370 CE) transposes the figurative language of each of the original verses into longer miracle narratives and adds a mantra to each verse (Balbir n.d.). The stories relate how the goddess Cakra (or Cakreśvarī) uses her powers to enable devotees who meditate upon

Figure 2.1. Chronological development of the *Bhaktāmar Stotra*. *Source:* Created by the author.

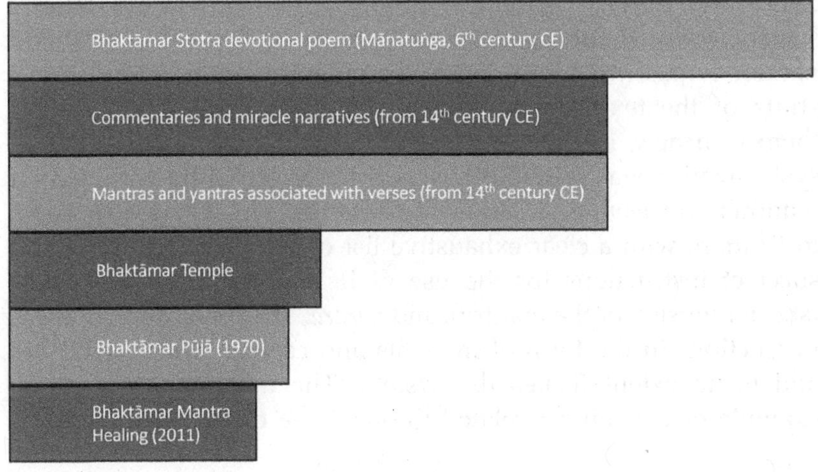

the verses of *Bhaktāmar Stotra* to overcome their problems (Kapashi 2007, 105). These narratives thus translate the aesthetic poem of spiritual devotion into a more mundane transactional process that touches upon the tantric (Lefeber 1995, 426–427; Granoff 1998, 219). In addition to these miracle narratives found in the commentary texts, each of the *ślokas* became connected to its own mantra and *yantra*. In a further transformation, the text itself became a focus of devotion, with temples being devoted to it (e.g., in Sanganer and Bharuch) and a ritual being designed around it (Balbir n.d.; Cort 2005, 107–108; for a detailed description of *Bhaktāmar pūjā*, see Kapashi 2007, 153–155).

BMH is here conceptualized as the most recent layer in this multilayered tradition that goes back centuries and incorporates devotional, ritual, and tantric aspects.[6] BMH can be seen as an example of a *tantric reconfiguration*, as it uses what are in religious studies often called *tantric elements* (mantra, *yantra*), without being directly rooted in any existing historical tantric tradition.[7]

BMH as a New Way to Engage with Health from Within the Jain Tradition

It is important to stress that in many ways, BMH is essentially new. I argue that the difference between previous practices that ascribed the power to influence worldly affairs to the verses of the *Bhaktāmar Stotra* and BMH as a *tantric reconfiguration* lies in the latter's systematized, democratized, and—to an extent—commodified nature.[8] First, BMH brings together elements of different functional strata of the textual tradition, reconfigures them, and presents them in a new, systematized way. Arguably, the process toward systemization was started early on with the attribution of different mantras and *yantras* in the commentaries, but it has now come to fruition, with a clear exhaustive list of uses for each verse and succinct instructions for the use of its associated mantra, *ṛddhi* (shorter version of the mantra), and *yantra*. The publication of these instructions in the form of manuals and cards further establishes and to an extent fixates the system. The table below gives an example of the content related to one verse of the *Stotra*.

Table 2.1. Example of Systematized Bhaktāmar Healing (BMH) Practice for Śloka 23

Śloka 23*	Oh Lord, sages believe that you are the supreme being, You have the bright color of the sun, you are spotless, and you are beyond the realms of darkness. One conquers death by only following your path. O Lord of Ascetics, there is no better path leading to salvation.**
Commentary Guṇākara fourteenth century	Once, there was a great sage who meditated upon the mantra derived from this *śloka*. The goddess Cakreśvarī was pleased, and decided to grant him the power to defeat wicked gods. He ends up pacifying the goddess Durgā (summary based on Lefeber 1995).
BMH Manuals	Manju Jain (2016) and Priya Jain (2017)
Mantra	*om namo bhagwatī jayāwati mama samīhitārtham* । *mokṣa saukhyaṃ kuru kuru swāhā* । *om hrīm shrīm klīm sarwa siddhāya shrīm namaḥ* ।
Ṛddhi	*om hrīm arham namo āsi-visānam (jhraum jhraum namaḥ svāhā)*
Yantra	The associated *yantra* is provided in the BMH manuals.
Use	Safety of the body from evil spirits (and to win in court cases)
Procedure	After purification, at an auspicious occasion, being clothed in white, facing to the north and keeping the mantra there, an auspicious pitcher may be placed, and a candle kindled. The yantra is worshipped and then the *ṛddhi* and mantra syllables are adored 4,000 times with white rosary for evincing the mantra (qtd. from Manju Jain 2016).

* त्वामामननूतमिुनयः परमं पुमांस। मादत्यिवर्णममलं तमसः परस्तात् ॥
त्वामेव सम्यगुपलभ्य जयंतमिृत्युं। नान्यः शविः शविपदस्य मुनीन्द्र! पन्थाः ॥२३॥
[tvāmānananti munyaṃ paramaṃ pumāṃsa mādityavarṇamamalaṃ tamasaḥ parastāt, tvāmeva samyagupalabhya jayanti mṛtyuṃ nānyaḥ śivaḥ śivapadasya munīndra panthāḥ]
** The translation provided here is by Vinod Kapashi (Kapashi 2007, 97), which is based upon a selection of translations and commentaries (Kapashi 2007, 90–91).

Second, the BMH system is democratic, both in the sense that it is not an elitist movement but clearly wants to appeal and be accessible to common people and in the sense that its healers aspire to reach a broad, even global audience. BMH does away with any secret knowledge or any prerequisites of higher understanding or spiritual advancement on the part of the prospective patient/devotee. Whereas the *Bhaktāmar Stotra* as a devotional text is well-known and disseminated by Jain monks and nuns, who may also derive powers from its repeated recitation (*Bhaktāmara-siddhi*; see Kapashi 2007, 148), the spiritual healing system that emerged from the text is very much a lay affair. The small group of spiritual entrepreneurs at its core consists exclusively of lay Jains and is growing as more healers are trained. Although the necessity of guidance by an experienced mantra healer for any first attempt at putting BMH into practice is emphasized, the availability of free, downloadable manuals in multiple languages and of online and offline chanting courses clearly illustrates the accessible nature of this knowledge.

Third, the systematization and democratization discussed above are in a sense both prerequisite to and part of BMH's commodification and branding and related to the systematization and the aspirations to reach a broad audience just discussed. BMH, with its manuals, mantra cards, workshops, etc., has become commodified, integrated in, and available on the marketplace of spiritual wellness and healing. This marketplace is made up of different systems offering similar outcomes and, often, similar services (Jain 2014, 91–92). To function in this setting, BMH needs to be visible and enticing to potential consumers. Those who feel attracted to BMH, be it after an encounter with their online sources, a referral by a friend, or an introduction by a spiritual healer, can book services, attend virtual and onsite workshops, and download or buy books, mantra cards, copper *yantras*, etc. Although not all healers ask for remuneration for their services, the marketing of services and products to a wider audience is not only a question of compassion but also of good entrepreneurship (see Jain 2014, 92).

Explaining the Curative Efficacy of BMH

A first immediately visible layer of discourse in BMH manuals and websites denotes the power of the mantras as magic (using words like miraculous, miracle, magic, magical, and on some of Bhaktamarmantrahealing.com's Hindi pages, *jādū*). Drmanjujain25.com refers to the hymn as "48 magical mantras." The *Jaina Method of Curing* manual also speaks of the "miraculous benefits of chanting" the *Bhaktāmar Stotra* (Jain 2016). Bhaktamarmantrahealing.com presents the system as "48 Magical Solutions for all your problems." This is followed by a more specific listing of the potential benefits of the healing system:

> Experience the delight of Bhaktamar Mantra Healing and enjoy fantastic health, abundant wealth, harmonious relationships and professional success. Bhaktamar Mantra Healing is the magical gateway to cure so-called incurable diseases like cancers, kidney problems, heart and lung diseases, chronic skin problems, mental illness and addictions, and much more. Bhaktamar Mantra Healing solves your financial crisis and legal problems and makes your life peaceful and productive.[9]

Such claims seem to illustrate an approach to the *stotra* that has moved beyond the purely devotional and hints at the magical or tantric. However, this discursive layer is superficial. References to magic are mainly found in titles or in introductory paragraphs, indicating that magic may be used as a placeholder for more complex explanatory narratives. Indeed, reading further into the more detailed descriptions of the healing system, these magical powers are explained in myriad ways, and the placeholder terms such as "magic" make way for a mélange of religious, devotional, spiritual, and biomedical narratives.

Although research on Jain *tantra* indicates the presence of intra-doctrinal explanations for the power of mantras to effect this-worldly change,[10] these intra-doctrinal explanations are rare in BMH manuals and online sources. In fact, with the exception of some social media accounts, BMH sources tend to use a broader, nonsectarian discourse focused on spirituality, and thus eclipse specifically Jain soteriological and philosophical concepts. This tendency toward a less specific, more universal discourse does not mean Jainism is entirely absent from digital sources on BMH. First, the Jain tradition is recognized as the source of the healing system. The story of the composition of the *stotra* by

Mānatuṅga is often retold (e.g., on the Bhaktamar Stotra App), as are some of the miracle narratives that have been developed in the commentary literature. Within these retellings, religious figures of different soteriological categories (e.g., lay, mendicant, gods, goddesses, Jinas) are presented. Additionally, some healers pay explicit homage to Jain teachers who have inspired them, thus including Jain mendicants into the (margins of) BMH (e.g., Dr. Manju Jain opens her manual by paying homage to Digambara Ācārya Sri Vidyasagar Maharaj; see Jain 2016). Lastly, the Jain code of conduct is commonly—though not always explicitly—referred to as a lifestyle inspired by the Jain rules of conduct considered to be beneficial for general health and well-being, and a healer who limits themselves to a vegetarian diet with no alcohol is presumed to be able to effect more successful healing.[11]

By using general language, rather than specific Jain or Jain sectarian terms, and by emphasizing the importance of "faith" in an unspecified god or godlike entity as well as faith in the healing system itself rather than explicating any karmic transactions that may be at work in the background, the discourse moves from the religious to the spiritual, defined as the common experience behind different religious traditions (Manju Jain 2016, 296). "This hymn develops spiritual power. But it is absolutely necessary to have reverence or conviction for its practice . . . If we have no reverence for the mantra, if there is no attraction to it, no belief, there will be no result, even if it is correctly applied and properly pronounced."[12] Through this discursive universalization, BMH connects with other spiritual practices, either because they share some methods or because spiritual entrepreneurs tend to offer a range of healing services. Bhaktamarmantrahealing.com refers to other healing practices, such as astrology, *kuṇḍalinī*, cakras, colors, reiki, and prāṇic healing. The Global Bhaktamar Group WhatsApp group reiterates these connections by also presenting events and activities regarding, among others, numerology and face reading. The *Jaina Method of Curing* has six pages devoted to reiki practices (Manju Jain 2016, 302–307). This embedding in the field of spiritual wellness is reinforced by the participation of BMH's healers in national and international conferences on holistic, integrated, and spiritual healing, which is prolifically advertised on websites, in manuals, and on social media platforms.

In line with other global spiritual practices, scientific terminology and links with different branches of conventional science are plentiful on BMH's websites and in its manuals. These discourses connected to science range from references to and quotes from international scientists, crossovers into physics, and the appropriation of scientific and biomedical discourses. On bhaktamarmantrahealing.com, a page on the power of *Bhaktāmar* and faith starts with the following statement: "Scientists also accept that it is not possible to achieve success even in a secular work without any religious belief."[13] It proceeds to present the opinions of different American scientists about the power of prayer and belief. That most scientists quoted are American or European can be read as an attempt to engage with Western audiences. The excerpt cited above also indicates that science cannot solve everything, positing BMH not in opposition to science, but rather beyond it.[14]

When the specific therapeutic powers of mantras and *yantra*s are discussed, the discourse often moves between the spiritual/devotional and the scientific. Soundwaves and vibrations provide a link between effective mantra recitation and physics. "When we chant a mantra whole heartedly, it unifies us with our mind, body and soul. The vibrations of Mantra reach our nervous system and percolate to the various organs through motor nerves and the whole system give a feedback to the brain through sensory nerves that the body is rejuvenating. Each cell feels the vibration of mantra and thus mantra healing becomes effective."[15] When discussing the power of *yantra*, the chemical properties of copper similarly offer a link to biochemistry.[16]

The combination of biomedical and religio-spiritual terminology is typical for manuals and websites on BMH. However, some sources aspire to a closer connection to conventional biomedicine than others. Such aspiration is most obvious in the work of Manju Jain and comes to the fore mostly in her healing manual and website. The *Jaina Method of Curing* (Jain 2016) and the website drmanjujain25.com include material describing the author's experimental research in palliative care, with cancer patients and with schoolchildren. The healer's scientific credentials are further emphasized by mention of her work with different medical clinics and practitioners (from skin care to cancer),[17] her presence at psycho-oncology conferences, and her doctorate in alternative medicine from Zoroastrian College. The web pages and chapters that present this material use not only scientific terminology but also a degree of scientific methodology, which places BMH in a closer relation to conventional biomedicine. Within this framework, the putative effects of BMH are explained in a different, more subdued way, echoing academic medical literature on the potential salutogenic effects of spiritual healing, such as stress relief, and promoting a sense of agency (e.g., Levin 2009; Alling 2015).

To further an understanding of BMH as both an exponent of a long and established tradition within Jainism and a technology that seeks to move beyond any religious affiliation, Andrea Jain's discussion of modern yoga and consumer culture in *Selling Yoga* (2014) provides an interesting comparison—even more so because it includes a discussion of a Jain yoga system, *prekṣā dhyāna* (Jain 2014, 70). Jain describes how "postural yoga proponents market postural yoga as a universal and scientific system that anyone can adopt as part of his or her larger worldview and practice" (76). The aspiration to be universal implies a degree of *deterritorialization*, *detraditionalization* (Heelas 1996), or even *deculturalization* (Roy 2010) of practices. The emphasis on general devotional and spiritual elements, rather than specific Jain religious elements that emerges from the discourse analysis discussed, can be seen as indicative of this. The appropriation of biomedical and wellness discourses aligns with the aspiration to be both universal and scientific, and to support an interpretation of BMH as a therapeutic practice that is not exclusively linked to any religion or worldview but can appeal to and be practiced by people from very different places and backgrounds—including lay Jains, Jains in the diaspora, and non-Jains.

Concluding Thoughts: Toward a Productive Clash of Engagements?

As indicated in the description of the *Bhaktāmar Stotra* tradition, BMH has received very little scholarly attention. My 2022 article, which was actually written at the end of 2020, was an attempt to break new ground and add BMH as a new element to ongoing discussions on how Jainism is a living tradition wherein Jains continue to apply, interpret, and subtly adapt suitable elements to engage with the context they inhabit. The research on which the article was based was conducted between 2016 and 2020, and it consisted of participant observation at events; the analysis of manuals, websites, and social media accounts related to BMH; and in-depth interviews with practitioners (healers as well as patients). Often, these interviews were deeply emotional. One businessman in his forties who was sponsoring an elaborate *bhaktāmar pūjā* in his local *derāsar* related how he came to believe in the efficacy of this form of healing:

> We watched my wife's health deteriorate as the regular treatment for her cancer did not catch on. She was in hospital for weeks, and I had started preparing our sons for the worst. And in these situations, you know, you look for anything that might help. So I consulted this Bhaktamar doctor. It was her advice to conduct a Bhaktamar puja and chant mantras—we all chanted together in the hospital. And it worked. The chemo seemed to gain in effect, and she made a recovery which surprised even her doctors. Against all odds.

The research that forms the basis of my writing on *bhaktāmar* healing was thus collaborative in nature and made possible only by the openness, kindness, and generosity of my respondents. However, as I started analyzing the resultant data, operationalizing the critical analytical tools I have been trained in, and looking for relevant scholarly literature from which to draw useful comparisons and theories, the chapter became increasingly difficult to write, as I became painfully aware of the frictions that exist between my respondents' points of view and modes of practice and the exigencies of my own academic practice. Clearly, the scholarly endeavor to historicize and contextualize, to nuance and critically analyze, will not, cannot, and does not always correspond to the needs and sensitivities of a Jain practitioner or activist.

Throughout the chapter, I ended up using concepts such as *tantric reconfiguration* and *spiritual consumer culture* (following Jain 2014), as within a scholarly discussion they can be helpful in conceptualizing and understanding BMH as both an exponent of a centuries-old living tradition and an essentially new technology; both a devotional practice and an entrepreneurial one. The use of such terms enabled the article to enter into broader conversations with other disciplines and bodies of research and thus enhance its range and usefulness in the cumulative practice of scholarly knowledge production. However, this profuse application of academic "etic" terms rather than sticking to "emic" terms and narratives used by practitioners of BMH seems to show scant regard to those generous respondents who helped me make sense of this Jain curative practice in the first place. Indeed, I doubt whether my respondents would recognize themselves and their practice in these descriptions at all.

Furthermore, the striking juxtaposition and intermingling of religious, spiritual, medical, and scientific explanatory narratives posed a similar problem. As a scholar, I found this multivocality exceedingly telling. However confusing it may seem at times, this multiplicity of explanatory narratives serves a purpose: It underscores this relatively new practice's connections to other, more established institutions, practices, and fields on the one hand, and it offers different perspectives for a wide variety of potential practitioners to connect to on the other. However, in making explicit this multivocality I also became very aware that my analysis could easily be read as a critical dissection of this—for some Jains at least—very emotionally invested practice. The process of adding words like "putative" and "self-proclaimed" to any health-related claims that had not been proven according to biomedical science (which from a scholarly and ethical perspective is necessary) completed what I felt to be the process of alienation between me as a scholar on the one hand and my informants on the other.

My motivation to share this insight into what was a very personal process of seeking a balance between different perspectives should be read as an attempt to illustrate, to unpack, and to an extent help normalize the feeling of duplicity or "feeling torn" (see Miller's introduction to this volume), as well as to further the conversation regarding productive ways in which those involved in the emerging discipline of engaged Jain studies can deal with the frictions that give rise to these feelings. Writing about engaged practices, be they Jain or otherwise, from a scholarly perspective is hard. It is hard because hurting or breaking the confidence of respondents and informants who enabled the research in the first place is the very last thing an engaged scholar wants to do. However, when engaging in engaged Jain studies, scholars will encounter instances such as these, where despite the cordial contacts and collaborative research strategies, friction does arise. Some topics will be more prone to friction than others (e.g., see Miller's example of Aryika Jnanamati and her flat-earth advocacy in the introduction of this volume), but this should not lead us to shy away from research on any form of (engaged) Jain practice. Indeed, keeping in mind the history of scholarly myopia that was addressed by John Cort in his "Models of and for the Study of the Jains" (1990) and reiterated by Paul Dundas in *The Jains* (2002; originally published in 1992), as well as in the introduction to this volume, it is only just that we strive to have scholarship on Jainism reflect the rich diversity of the Jain traditions and the engaged practices that have emerged from them.

Rather than steer clear of friction, we, that is the activist, the scholar, and/or the devotee, must seek to foster a mutual understanding of the frameworks we work within. Along the lines of the Jain principle of *anekāntavāda*, we should be explicit about our own perspective and its exigencies, but recognize the existence and at least contextual validity of the other relevant frameworks that come with their own set of rules and customs. The inevitable friction should become a mutually recognized difference in practice between collaborators who share an engagement with Jainism, as well as with contemporary environmental and societal challenges. Where different frameworks meet, in scholarly work on activism for example, it is best practice to be explicit about how these different frameworks interact throughout the different phases of engagement—from motivation and research design to data-gathering to publication. Although this openness and the self-reflection it requires are by no means easy, this is a crucial practice required from all parties involved, both Jain and non-Jain, if we are committed to making engaged Jain studies work as a vibrant, inspiring, and intellectually honest (sub)discipline.

Notes

1. The research this work is based upon was funded by Research Foundation—Flanders (FWO), grant 12T7320N—and was conducted at the Department of Languages and Cultures of Ghent University, Belgium.

2. Although most mantras are connected with physical or mental health, some are said to be effective in other fields of life, such as success in business, legal proceedings, and exams.

3. Some of the material discussed in this chapter appeared as part of Tine Vekemans, "#MagicMantras: Bhaktamar Mantra Healing between Jainism and the Spiritual Marketplace," *International Journal of Hindu Studies* 26, no. 2 (2022): 189–214. It has been reprinted here with the kind permission of the original publisher.

4. For an overview of attempts to put a date to the compilation of the *stotra*, see Kapashi 2007, 79.

5. The 2012 edition, which includes an older Hindi translation by Nathuram Premi and an English translation by Manish Modi, is very useful (Modi 2012). Vinod Kapashi's book on the nine sacred recitations also includes a serviceable translation and some commentary (Kapashi 2007).

6. Both Ellen Gough (Emory University, Atlanta) and Aashi Jain (Florida International University) have worked on aspects of BMH, but at the time of writing, no works had been published.

7. Recent scholarship on *tantra* in different religious traditions tends to forego the sensationalist colonial representations in favor of an approach that foregrounds contextualized practices involving "tantric elements"—such as mantras (verbal spells), *yantra*s (diagrams), *mudra*s (hand movements), specific rituals, body practices, secret esoteric knowledge, etc.—that have a putative impact on either the advancement of the tantric practitioner on the path to liberation or the mundane circumstances in which the practitioner finds themselves (Brooks 1990; White 2000, 4–5; Urban 2001, 7–8). For recent work on mantras and other tantric elements in Jainism, see Ellen Gough's excellent book (Gough 2021) and encyclopedia contributions (Gough 2020a; 2020b).

8. These three aspects of BMH are reminiscent of Hugh Urban's three transformations of an esoteric tradition. Urban (2001) discusses how part of the Bengali Kartābhajā sect undergoes a progressive process of exotericization and institutionalization (204), resulting in a popularized, "deodorized," and commercialized version (9). As a tantric reconfiguration rather than an ongoing tantric tradition, BMH's democratization does not amount to exotericization as described by Urban, nor does its commodification reveal any attempts to "deodorize" any previous practices.

9. https://bhaktamarmantrahealing.com/.

10. For example, the mantra invokes a non-liberated deity who will then intervene on the devotee's behalf, or the mantra effects a change in an individual's karmic balance, which in turn impacts upon any negative karmic effects in the devotees' current and future lives (see Cort 2000b, 417; Qvarnström 2000, 597; Dundas 2002, 213).

11. https://bhaktamarmantrahealing.com / what-is-bhaktamar-stotra /.

12. "bhaktamar aur vishwas ki shakti" [translated from Hindi by the author]. https://bhaktamarmantrahealing.com / bhaktamar-faith /.

13. [Translated from Hindi by the author]. https://bhaktamarmantra healing.com / bhaktamar-faith /.

14. This complex stance, i.e., accepting science and scientific discourse while at the same time positing that "Western" science with its reductionism and matter-spirit dualism is of limited use in fully explaining spiritual healing, resonates with ideas developed by Meera Nanda (Nanda 2003, 98; 2016).

15. https://bhaktamarmantrahealing.com / faq /.

16. https://bhaktamarmantrahealing.com / healing-benefits-of-copper /.

17. The ethical issues relating to the integration of faith-healing practices in modern medical practice are a topic of debate. Those institutions and medical practitioners that allow integrated faith healing tend to foreground the autonomy and wishes of the patient, the potential benefits (in the form of personalized attention and possible placebo effect), or at least the absence of negative effects. However, those less inclined to allow faith healing within the framework of modern medicine point out possible negative health effects (e.g., of prolonged fasting) and warn that faith healings' admission in the medical setting may inadvertently have a legitimizing effect (Sarkar et al. 2014). Recently, an attempt to ban the Jain ritual of *sallekhanā* (fasting to death) reignited similar discussions about the place of religious health and bodily practices in modern medicine (Braun 2008).

References

Alling, Fred. 2015. "The Healing Effects of Belief in Medical Practices and Spirituality." *EXPLORE: The Journal of Science and Healing* 11 (4): 273–280.

Annant World. n.d. "Bhaktamar Mantra Healing." Accessed December 1, 2020. http://www.bhaktamarmantrahealing.com.

Balbir, Nalini. n.d. "Bhaktāmara-stotra." Accessed December 1, 2020. http:// www.jainpedia.org / themes / principles / sacred-writings / highlights-of-jainpedia / bhaktamara-stotra / index.html.

Braun W. 2008. "Sallekhana: The Ethicality and Legality of Religious Suicide by Starvation in the Jain Religious Community." *Medicine and Law* 27 (4): 913–924.

Brooks, Douglas Renfrew. 1990. *The Secret of the Three Cities: An Introduction to Hindu Śakta Tantrism*. University of Chicago Press.

Cort, John E. 1990. "Models of and for the Study of the Jains." *Method & Theory in the Study of Religion* 2 (1): 42–71.

———. 2000a. "Manatungacarya Aur Unke Stotra / Anusandhan." *Journal of the American Oriental Society* 120 (2): 293–249.

———. 2000b. "Worship of Bell-Ears the Great Hero, a Jain Tantric Deity." In White, *Tantra in Practice*, edited by David Gordon White, 417–33. Princeton: Princeton University Press.

———. 2001. *Jains in the World: Religious Values and Ideology in India*. Oxford University Press.

———. 2005. "Devotional Culture in Jainism: Mänatuṅga and His Bhaktämara Stotra." In *Incompatable Visions: South Asian Religions in History (Essays in Honor of David M. Knipe)*, edited by James Blumenthal. Center for South Asia, University of Wisconsin.

Dhanki, Madhusudan, and Jitendra Shah. 1999. *Mānatuṅgācārya Aur Unke Stotra*. 2nd ed. Shardaben Cimanbhai Ejyukeshanal Risarch Sentar.

Dundas, Paul. 2002. *The Jains*. 2nd ed. Routledge.

Gough, Ellen. 2020a. "Jain Mantras." In *Brill's Encyclopedia of Jainism Online*, edited by John E. Cort, Paul Dundas, Knut A. Jacobsen, and Kristi L. Wiley. Leiden: Brill.

———. 2020b. "Jain Maṇḍalas and Yantras." In Cort et al., *Brill's Encyclopedia of Jainism Online*.

———. 2021. *Making a Mantra: Tantric Ritual and Renunciation on the Jain Path to Liberation*. University of Chicago Press.

Granoff, Phyllis. 1998. "Cures and Karma: Healing and Being Healed in Jain Religious Literature." In *Self, Soul and Body in Religious Experience*, edited by A. Baumgarten et al. Brill.

Heelas, Paul. 1996. *The New Age Movement: The Celebration of the Self and the Sacralization of Modernity*. Blackwell.

Jacobi, Herman. 1876. "Zwei Jaina-stotra." *Indische Studien* 14. Deutsche Morgenländische Gesellschaft.

Jain, Andrea R. 2014. *Selling Yoga: From Counterculture to Pop Culture*. Oxford University Press.

Jain, Manju. 2016. *Jaina Method of Curing*. International School for Jain Studies / SBW Publishers.

———. n.d. "48 Magical Mantras." Accessed December 1, 2020. http://www.drmanjujain25.com.

Jain, Priya. 2017. *Faith Based Healing . . . Bhaktamar Stotra*. International School for Jain Studies.

Kapashi, Vinod. 2007. *Nava Smaraṇa: Nine Sacred Recitations of Jainism*. Hindi Granth Karyalay.

Lefeber, Rosalind. 1995. "Jain Stories of Miraculous Power." In *Religions of India in Practice*, edited by D. Lopez. Princeton University Press.

Levin, Jeff. 2009. "How Faith Heals: A Theoretical Model." *EXPLORE: The Journal of Science and Healing* 5 (2): 77–96.

Modi, Manish (trans.), and Mānatuṅga. 2012. *Bhaktāmarastotra*. Hindi poetic trans. and gloss. by Pandit Nathuram Premi, English trans. by Manish Modi. Hindi Granth Karyalay.

Nanda, Meera. 2003. *Prophets Facing Backward: Postmodern Critiques of Science and Hindu Nationalism*. Rutgers University Press.

Qvarnström, Olle. 2000. "Jain Tantra: Divinatory and Meditative Practices in the Twelfth-Century Yogaśāstra of Hemacandra." In White, *Tantra in Practice*.

Roy, Olivier. 2010. *Holy Ignorance: When Religion and Culture Part Ways*. Columbia University Press.

Sarkar Siddharth, Sreekanth Sakey, and Shivanand Kattimani. 2014. "Ethical Issues Relating to Faith Healing Practices in South Asia: A Medical Perspective." *Journal of Clinical Research & Bioethics* 5 (4).

Urban, Hugh B. 2001. *The Economics of Ecstasy: Tantra, Secrecy, and Power in Colonial Bengal*. Oxford University Press.

Vekemans, Tine. 2022. "#MagicMantras: Bhaktamar Mantra Healing Between Jainism and the Spiritual Marketplace." *International Journal of Hindu Studies* 26 (2): 189–214. Edited by Xenia Zeiler and Sravana Borkataky-Varma.

White, David Gordon. 2000. *Tantra in Practice*. Princeton University Press.

Part II
Social Engagement in the Diaspora

3

Engaged Curation

Challenges, Experiences, and Potentials from a Museum Exhibition About Jainism

JOHANNES BELTZ

Several major Jain art exhibitions have recently taken place globally (Fowler 2023; Flügel et al. 2023; SOAS 2023). A central feature of these exhibitions included varying degrees of direct engagement between public museum curators and local and global Jain communities in the envisioning and carrying out of each project. Within this context, this chapter explores the notion of engaged Jainism from a museum curator's perspective. It reflects on the author's experience of presenting Jainism to a largely non-Jain, Swiss audience in a non-Jain setting in collaboration with the Swiss and global Jain communities, within the context of the 2022–2023 public (and secular) art exhibition titled *Being Jain* (German: *Jain Sein*) at Museum Rietberg, in Zürich, Switzerland. This exhibition ran concurrently with, and yet completely independently of, other Jain exhibitions taking place around the globe in 2022 and 2023.

This chapter discusses how, at Zürich's Museum Rietberg, we worked with the Jain community using a form of "engaged curation" to collect and present Jain art to an audience largely unaware of the Jain tradition's existence. This chapter discusses the challenges we faced but also presents curatorial strategies and practices through which these challenges were addressed. In the end, this chapter reveals the innovative strategies we used to make Museum Rietberg's *Being Jain* exhibition relevant in order to generate an impact on our diverse public audiences, both Jain and non-Jain alike.[1]

Preparing an Exhibition on Jainism at Museum Rietberg

Museum Rietberg was founded in 1952 by the city of Zürich as a museum of non-European art. The city had received the collections of Eduard von der Heydt, who had bought numerous works of Asian, African, American, and Oceanic art on the Western art market during the 1920s and 1930s. Among his collections, Indian art covering a wide range of areas, times, and materials was of special importance.

Right from my early days at the Rietberg I was fascinated by the Jain art works in our collection. I still remember the moment when I encountered the majestic marble statue of the Jina Ṛṣabha and decided to dedicate an exhibition to this outstanding piece of art. Rietberg had indeed already hosted a Jain exhibition in 1974 that was organized by the newly appointed former director Eberhard Fischer (Fischer 1974). When I joined the Rietberg I was able to systematically acquire more donations and to make Jain art an important focus of the collection activities in the museum (Balbir and Beltz 2017).

About ten years ago, I took the first steps to put my idea into practice and started talking to our former director Albert Lutz and to colleagues about an exhibition on Jainism at our museum. However, other projects requiring immediate attention had already reached my desk. When in 2019 I restarted working with my co-curators on our new Jain show, we were aware that an exhibition on Jainism in 2022 would have to be significantly different from earlier shows. We asked ourselves how we could curate an exhibition on ancient artworks related to a minority religion, which is largely unknown in Switzerland, and also how we could make such an exhibition relevant to our audiences.

To address these challenges, we decided and acted upon five general strategic decisions. First, the exhibition should combine the past with the present. It would present significant art works showing the large range of material culture of this religion, from precious illustrated manuscripts to temple statues or ritual bronzes. The scenography and design would aim to render the exquisite exhibits accessible beyond their historic context, with artworks juxtaposed with contemporary photographs, interviews, and films illustrating how Jains in India use similar objects in their daily practice (see figure 3.1 and figure 3.2).

Second, the exhibition would be done in collaboration with Jains from all over the world, and from the Swiss Jain diaspora, thereby showcasing the diversity within the Jain community. To avoid sectarianism, our curatorial team would interview numerous and diverse Jains and give them the opportunity to express their individual opinions. Our selection would result in a wide range of perceptions and religious behaviors from monks and nuns, lay people, the old and the young, men and women, Jains from India, and diasporic Jains.

Figure 3.1. Main entry to *Being Jain* (*Jain Sein*) exhibition, with two Jina images flanking a documentary film screen. *Source:* Museum Rietberg. Used with permission.

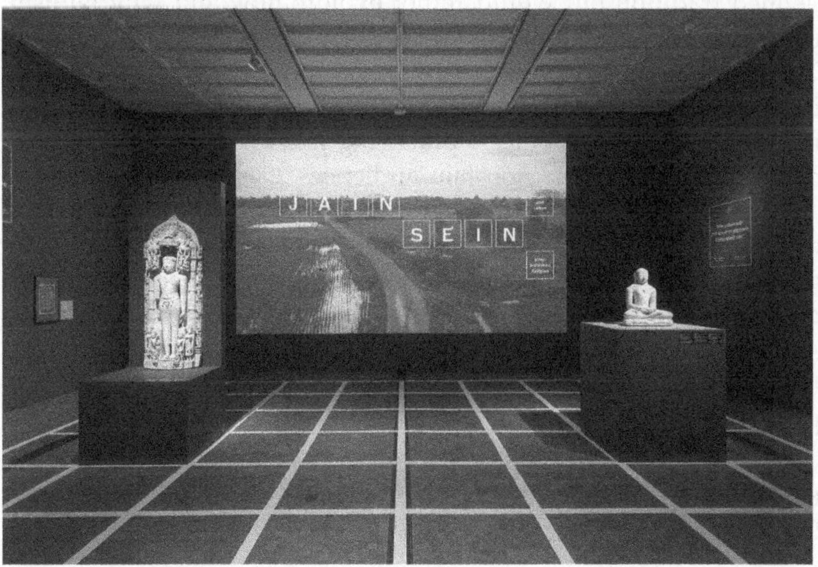

Figure 3.2. Image from one of the documentary films featured in the museum. *Source:* Museum Rietberg. Used with permission.

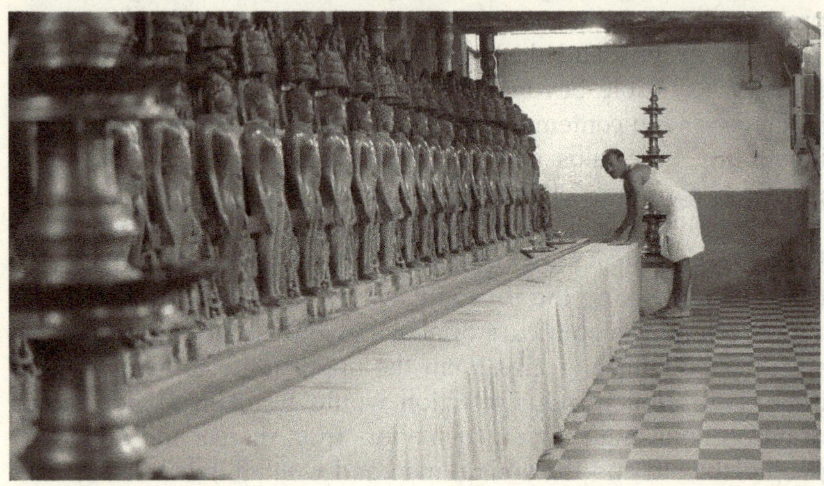

Third, the exhibition would not aim at providing an encyclopedic overview of all traditions and schools of Jainism from the beginnings of its 2,500-year (or perhaps much longer) history. Thus, the exhibition would not essentialize Jainism as a fixed and defined tradition but would rather explore how and why Jainism is perceived as meaningful today by Jains all over the world. The selection of objects would therefore not only be informed by its aesthetic quality or art historical significance, but also by the meaning each piece held for practicing Jains, whether in the past or present and for our non-Jain audiences.

Fourth, the exhibition would focus on the relevance of Jain ethics for contemporary society. In the context of climate change, global and regional conflicts, and increasing social inequalities, our curatorial team decided to focus on the themes of renunciation and nonviolence as most relevant for our local audiences, inviting them to think about global challenges in light of basic Jain ethical principles, though without indoctrinating them into the tradition.

And finally, fifth, the exhibition would be a participatory project. Throughout the exhibition, the curatorial team would try to reach out to diverse audiences and let them participate. In this process, "And You? The Game of Questions" was developed (more to follow). The publications for the exhibition would follow the same line: A beautifully designed and readable introduction to Jainism asked questions about our life and presented answers by Jain practitioners (Beltz et al. 2022). In addition, a short and concise paperback introduction summarized academic research in language accessible to a general audience (Krüger 2022).

Following these strategic decisions throughout the curatorial process, the curators, Jains, and the museum's public audiences would become "engaged" on at least four different levels. At the first level, we worked with the Indian government to borrow and present art works featuring the material culture of the Jains from a historical perspective. Twenty magnificent art works from several Indian museums traveled for the first time out of India (Beltz et al. 2023). On the second level, we screened films featuring our interviews of contemporary practicing Jains who would bring their lifeworlds into the museum setting for public viewing. To this feature of the exhibition, however, we added the third level of engagement by explicitly asking our audiences how they related to questions pertaining to Jain ethics such as renunciation or nonviolence in their own daily lives and in light of global challenges. And finally, fourth and of paramount importance, we the curatorial team and our public audiences became directly engaged with the diasporic Jain community as we conceptualized, assembled, and carried out the exhibition itself. In this final instance, Swiss Jains had the opportunity to share their tradition and values with our public comprised of primarily Swiss audiences. But so too did our public audiences gain an opportunity to reflect back to our Jain interlocutors many difficult questions of critical and social importance. In this way, not only did our audiences learn about Jain ethics, but our Jain participants had an opportunity to reflect on both the promises and challenges of applying their way of life to contemporary issues.

As Miller's introduction to this volume rightly points out, and for many reasons that will become apparent in this chapter, it is most often not appropriate, both historically and in the present, to conceive of an "engaged Jainism" that resembles anything like the socially and politically motivated forms of socially "engaged Buddhism" that have been well-documented over the past several decades in Buddhist scholarship. I therefore use the term "engaged curation" in a very specific sense here to capture the four primary activities outlined in the previous paragraph, and to highlight the many frictions that emerged as Jain ways of knowing and being in the world encountered critical public discourse at the museum in Switzerland.

Engaged Curation: Collaborating with Jain Institutions and Individuals

Among the four engagements outlined in the previous section, the work with the Jain diaspora was of crucial importance. The role played by diaspora communities is frequently alluded to in current debates on Orientalism, migration, inclusion, and decolonization. The argument is often put forward that immigrants from the countries in which the collection holdings originated should be more directly addressed and invited to become partners in joint projects, including in museums. In this regard, I was already collaborating with members of the Indian diaspora in Switzerland by 2003. As part of the exhibition *Ganesha: The God with an Elephant's Head,* the museum invited Hindus from all over Switzerland to celebrate the Ganesh Chaturthi festival on the museum grounds—with Indian music, food, and performed rituals. A spectacular highlight of this event was the immersion of a Ganesha idol in Lake Zürich during the "Long Night of the Zürich Museums."[2] In a procession, the museum audiences were invited to take an image of Ganesha down to the lake and to assist with its immersion (Eitle 2003).

This first engagement with the Hindu diaspora was further nurtured in the large-scale exhibition *Hindu Zurich,* which was shown at the city's town hall in 2004. The active involvement of Hindus living in Zürich was the guiding principle of this exhibition, and they contributed to a presentation of their religious community that included interviews, films, photographs, and a selection of objects. An exhibition "about" Hindus in Zürich thus became an exhibition developed in engagement "with" representatives of the Zürich diaspora (Beltz 2005a). These were not the only instances of this type of engagement. In 2018, Swiss Buddhists were invited to collaborate with Museum Rietberg on the exhibition *Next Stop Nirvana: Approaches to Buddhism* (Beltz 2021).

From my early experiences of working with diasporic communities, it was obvious that a show on Jainism would not manifest without substantial engagement with the Jain community in which I established numerous contacts as information regarding our intentions to create a Jain exhibition spread. One of the main differences from our prior experience, however, concerned the character and size of the Swiss Jain community. Compared to Buddhists and Hindus, Jains represent a small community in Switzerland, consisting of roughly thirty families and one hundred total people.[3] The members of this small community are often well-educated, some are highly paid and wealthy, and some belong to the global business elite. The community is spread across Switzerland, primarily in larger cities like Geneva or Zürich. Almost all Swiss Jains are of Indian origin, and have carved out a tenuous community identity in Switzerland.

In her 2012 PhD thesis, Mirjam Iseli had studied the Swiss Jain community, documenting the following primary phases diachronically. Though the first Jain migrants came to Switzerland in the 1970s, the first attempts to organize regular meetings and rituals began much more recently in 2008 (Iseli 2012, 155). As a result, some Jains started perceiving themselves as a discrete community within Switzerland, distinct from the Hindu fold. Indeed in 2008, some new community structures were built; Jains organized certain rituals together, invited religious specialists to Switzerland, and created a Google group. As a result, a sense of belonging to a specific religion was manifested and a specific Swiss Jain identity was formulated, though it remained ambiguous and fluid regarding its relationship to Hinduism.

Following the formation of this new Swiss Jain identity, Iseli (ibid., 226ff.) observed that the community progressively disintegrated from 2012 onward, culminating in the dissolution of any community structures. The reasons for this dissolution were manifold. Often times, the mobility of expats traveling with Swiss work visas (which are highly limited and difficult to obtain) led to their eventual departure. Acculturation of, affiliation to, and identification with a global Jain identity (rather than a local

Swiss Jainism) as well the diversity of the community and the limited numbers of practicing Jains further contributed. Iseli (ibid., 230–231) points out that the absence of communal structures and the inaccessibility of religious experts who were permanently accessible and present to support the community caused further disintegration. Only recently in 2022 has the community experienced a limited revival in Switzerland, with the installation and ritual praise of a Jain idol in the Divine Light Zentrum (a Hindu temple) in Winterthur that is managed through a WhatsApp group through the efforts of a prominent member of the Swiss Jain community.[4]

The lack of a cohesive Swiss Jain community was palpable throughout the exhibition. When organizing events, it was often difficult to reach out to the community to mobilize volunteers. Outside of our Tandem Tours and scheduled public talks, it was also a challenge to raise interest in our events and to mobilize Swiss Jains to join, as for example when we celebrated Mahavir Jayanti within the premises of the museum and had only a small number of Swiss Jains who participated. In fact, the largest support came from non-Swiss Jain individuals and institutions.

Two partnerships must be highlighted. First, the members and scholars of our advisory board have been a constant source of encouragement and practical advice.[5] Second, Arihanta Institute, an online Jain university based in California, was another indispensable source of support that enabled us to build our network and to get into contact with practicing Jains globally. In collaboration with Arihanta Institute, the curators conducted seven in-depth interviews with Jains from all over the world.[6] In the interviews, the interviewees talk about how they apply Jain teachings in their daily lives. Excerpts from the interviews were included in the exhibition's accompanying publication.[7] From these interviews and the many engagements between the Jain community, our public audiences, and the curatorial team, several primary Jain discourses emerged.

Global Discourses in the Local Swiss Jain Community

Though Swiss Jains' participation was limited during the exhibition, the museum did engage with members of the local Jain community on several specific occasions, including in advisory meetings, scheduled talks, and interactive tours that we called "Tandem Tours 'What Does It Mean to Me?'" in the exhibition. In these many interactions, the curators invited Jains to talk about themselves and to present their thoughts and ideas to public audiences. Talking with and listening to members of the Jain community, I came to understand that community discourse is centered around a few areas that are perceived of as having major importance pertaining to questions of ethics and daily practices. By outlining some results from an analysis of interviews, talks, and my diverse interactions with Jains at the exhibition, I attempt here to elucidate the ways Swiss Jains perceive themselves as being Jain (in accordance with the title of the exhibition).

First and most importantly, many Swiss Jains stressed the fact that Jainism is not a religion but rather a "scientific" way of life. This claim promotes Jainism as a scientific approach to reality, objective and true, and not as a religion (Prajna et al. 2016). This "scientization" (Auckland 2016; also see Miller's introduction to this volume) is a rhetorical trope, which is used widely by many modern religious movements. It transforms perceptions of the universe and metaphysics as well as ritual behavior such as meditation, fasting, or notions of purity and impurity into "scientific" practices. For example, in one of the events, a Jain justified the persistence of caste restrictions among Jains by highlighting the fact that social distancing was an effective, scientific way of protecting yourself from infections, such as for example COVID. The logic they proposed was that social distancing in accordance with caste restrictions limits physical contact and contamination and is therefore not only rational and scientific but in support of public health. These types of assertions made by Swiss Jains are grounded in the fact that Jains do indeed continue to practice caste restrictions in India (Rashkow 2013; Sanghavi 2013). Additionally, Jains are perceived as an exclusive community wherein intermarriage and conversion are not a common practice, nor are they encouraged (Jain 2019). In light of these social facts, commitments to casteism at times manifested during conversations with Swiss Jains, who were born in India, such as in the case I have presented here.

Among other popular notions quoted in discussions were the concepts of *ahiṃsā* (non-harming), *aparigraha* (non-possession), *syād-vāda* (a doctrine expressing the uncertainty of any statement), and *anekānta-vāda* (tolerance for other perspectives). However, apart from these well-known Jain principles, several Swiss Jains saw themselves as part of a modern, enlightened, and rationalized universal Jainism (Cort 2020; Iseli 2015). This Jainism is seen as a response to ecological and social challenges in contemporary society. Publications from non-Jain academics (often with a background in theological training) reinforcing these concepts by combining them with fundamental notions of ecology, nonviolence, and environment (Chapple 2001; 2002) and also with medical care, healing, and health (Donaldson 2019; Donaldson and Bajžel 2021) were featured in the museum gift shop.

One notable contrast that emerged in these discourses around non-possession and non-harming was the visible success and impact of the living Jain community on a global scale in the world of business. In many discussions in the exhibition and in most all guided tours, the public often asked how Jains justify their enormous accumulation of wealth in the hands of a small community, particularly with regard to India's rampant poverty and the well-known connections between one's wealth and one's environmental impact. It is indeed no secret that most Jains belong to India's top tiers of wealth. According to Prakash Jain, "[T]he Jains have themselves begun to take pride in their affluence and their contribution to the national exchequer. Thus, it is claimed that despite comprising 0.5% of India's population, the Jains' contribution to the country's GPD is about 25%. The Jains' share in direct income tax revenue is about 24%. About 46% of the share market is held by the Jains. They also own up to about 28% of the private property in India" (Jain 2011, 121–122). Financial institutions and large media houses also have Jains at their helm (Konikkara 2023, 47).

Audience members were surprised that these questions are not discussed within the community, or if they were, they were often rationalized according to Jain karma theory and other beliefs around caste as we have already seen. Wealth and success would for example be justified as markers of good karma. The rhetoric and controversial character of these claims became most visible during the allegations against Gautam Adani in January 2023 for cronyism and stock manipulation.[8]

Interestingly, or perhaps expectedly, in the globalized,

"universal" Jainism espoused at the museum, certain central Jain doctrines *lost* their relevance. For example, the complex Jain cosmography mapping heavens and hells, the related and equally complex doctrine of Jain karma and liberation, the ancient Jain belief that the world is flat, and even Jain ritual practice itself were contested or omitted in discourse.

Throughout my interactions with the community, it became clear that the community discourse was often disconnected from social and political realities (Vose 2022), often apologetic and at times fundamentalist. These observations were not a surprise but are general phenomena and characteristics of diasporic religious communities. Our invited Jain speakers encountered the rhetorical challenge of convincing public audiences of the relevance of their tradition without appearing to uncritically promote religious propaganda, a difficult task wherein the latter often nevertheless prevailed. To demonstrate this highly rhetorical dimension in Jain discourse at the museum and the important religious significance attributed to this discourse, I present now the Jain practice of vegetarianism as an example. Among all notions and references to the Jain tradition, vegetarianism was omnipresent and popped up in almost all conversations about Jain identity at the museum.

Vegetarianism: The Rhetoric of an Identity Marker

"Much of what you have been saying this evening is about food and vegetarianism, but is there some other way that Jainism is relevant for society today?," asked one member of the public audience to our invited Swiss Jain speakers during one of the museum's scheduled Tandem Tours.[9] The practice of not eating meat indeed dominates the image, discourse, and self-perception of the Jain community both globally and in Switzerland, and this central element of Jain practice became one of the predominant discourses at the museum as Jains engaged with the curatorial team and local public audiences. Almost all of the Jains that I interviewed reported to be vegetarian, insisting that this fact distinguished them most clearly from all other religions. Jains explained their vegetarianism as a practical consequence of their commitment to *ahiṃsā*, or non-harming (Miller and Dickstein 2021).[10] In our interviews, most Swiss Jains reported to abstain from meat, fish, shellfish, and eggs in their daily diet. Some even said they avoid certain root vegetables because one would, by destroying the root vegetable, simultaneously destroy the basis of life of the entire plant. Moreover, when harvesting root vegetables, one risks destroying microorganisms on the plant and in the soil. Consequently, potatoes, onions, and garlic are often absent from the menu of the Jains.

Jains involved in the museum project also conveyed how they practice the renunciation of violence in the secondary markets of the non-food sector. Many avoid products made of leather or cosmetics that are made from animal products. As we learned, standing up for animal rights is important to some Jains, as is supporting animal hospitals and protecting endangered species and wild animals in India.[11] An ecological vision of the world can be derived from this commitment to preserving and protecting animal life and the environment, and this vision was often shared by Swiss Jains in the exhibition activities.

Nevertheless, these and other oft-repeated food rules manifest quite differently in daily practice. Many Swiss Jains also admitted that they eat root vegetables including potatoes, a staple food for most anyone living in Switzerland, because abstaining from eating them would make their life difficult. I even met a few Swiss Jains who admitted discretely not only that they were flexitarians but also that they enjoyed eating meat regularly.

With these varying Jain commitments to the renunciation of meat, leather, and other animal products expressed during the exhibition in mind, it is important to consider the wider and very complex sociopolitical context in which they were being made. For example, the question of the consumption of dairy, a central part of most Jain diets, cannot be addressed without carefully considering dairy's relationship to cow slaughter. Yamini Narayanan (2023) recently pointed out the inherent contradictions of India being the world leader in milk production and in protecting cows. In this scenario, public attention is routinely diverted from the gruesome reality that involves the maltreatment of bovines and buffaloes, the humane-washing of gendered sexual and reproductive violence to animals, clandestine trafficking, and slaughtering. In addition to cow slaughter, dairy makes a large and measurable contribution toward producing greenhouse gases that are driving climate change. For

Swiss Jains living in a country with a large dairy industry itself, many of these same forms of harming remain linked to anyone's consumption of dairy in Switzerland (Kinzner et al. 2023).

When Jains such as those who participated in the exhibition claimed that vegetarianism is a truly nonviolent mode of nutrition while consuming milk, yogurt, etc. they seemed to ignore their participation in these very real forms of harm. Similarly, when making well-intentioned appeals for the banning of cow slaughter, they seemed to ignore the political and often violent complexities of many Muslim, Christian, and Dalit communities for whom this practice remains a vital economic and cultural activity (Ulrich 2007; Shepherd 2019). That being said, the members of the Swiss Jain community with whom the curatorial team worked to create the exhibition did not insist on "forcing" their lifestyle or vegetarianism onto others. Indeed, while planning for certain public events that would include food, several Swiss Jains requested the opposite: The public should be given the *option* to eat vegetarian food at public events, but they should not be forced to do so. This idea even carried itself into the museum's café menu (Richard 2023), where vegan and vegetarian options were provided for daily visitors with a sign indicating that these options were part of the overall exhibition plan.

In addition to issues such as caste and economic privilege already mentioned, the frequent mention of the Jain practice of a vegetarian diet as an expression of nonviolence is but one example of the seemingly contradictory discourses that the curatorial team and public audiences encountered at the museum as members of the Swiss Jain community brought their well-intentioned viewpoints into public discourse. As a public museum, however, the scholarly curatorial team had the dual obligation to respectfully engage the religious perspectives of this minority religion while also responsibly placing these perspectives within critical-analytical frameworks (see Miller's introduction to this volume). Thus, in the end, we had to conceptualize an exhibition that could be a space for the expression of the epistemological viewpoints of Jains living in Switzerland without objectifying these viewpoints while simultaneously maintaining a commitment to scientific epistemology, given the museum's status as a Swiss public institution. We were thereby tasked with creating a space for discussions around contemporary applications of Jain ethics like nonviolence, renunciation, and tolerance with our local audiences with whom we hoped to engage in conversation with the aim of creating a participatory exhibition that was critical and educational but also open to and respectful of the living Jain tradition. But how to achieve such a fine balance between emic, etic, and public perspectives in the exhibition plan?

Engaging with Museum Communities and Audiences

One of the other primary challenges we faced as we promoted the exhibition to the Swiss public was the simple fact that Jainism is a religion that is largely unknown in Switzerland. The Swiss Jain community was also too small and too exclusive to mobilize larger audiences in Switzerland to attend. How, then, could we make an exhibition about Jainism interesting and relevant to our local audiences, while balancing empathetic and critical approaches?

In the context of global challenges such as climate change, global and regional conflicts, pandemics, and the many other issues we face as a global society, we decided to focus on engaging our audiences with Jain ethics as the key narrative, a practice not typically encountered in an art museum. How might Jain concepts such as tolerance and nonviolence offer answers to our many global challenges? And how could we bring these Jain principles into conversation with these challenges without imposing normative, uncritical religious discourse on our public audiences?

The solution that we developed was an interactive game at the center of the exhibition that would encourage a diversity of opinions and freedom of choice following one's exposure to basic Jain ideas through the pieces of Jain artwork, history, and ethical principles situated throughout the exhibition (see figure 3.3).

We wanted to invite our audiences to talk about ethical behavior and everyone's responsibility in society considering Jain ideas, though without proselytizing. What made this game so interesting for our purposes was the fact that it had been historically used in India as a teaching tool by different religious communities including, but not limited to, Hindus, Buddhists, and Jains. In the Jain tradition, the Game of Knowledge (*jñan-chaupār*) provided a playful way to illustrate the Jain concept of liberation: The players

Figure 3.3. "And You? The Game of Questions" featured as an interactive game at the center of the exhibition. *Source:* Museum Rietberg. Used with permission.

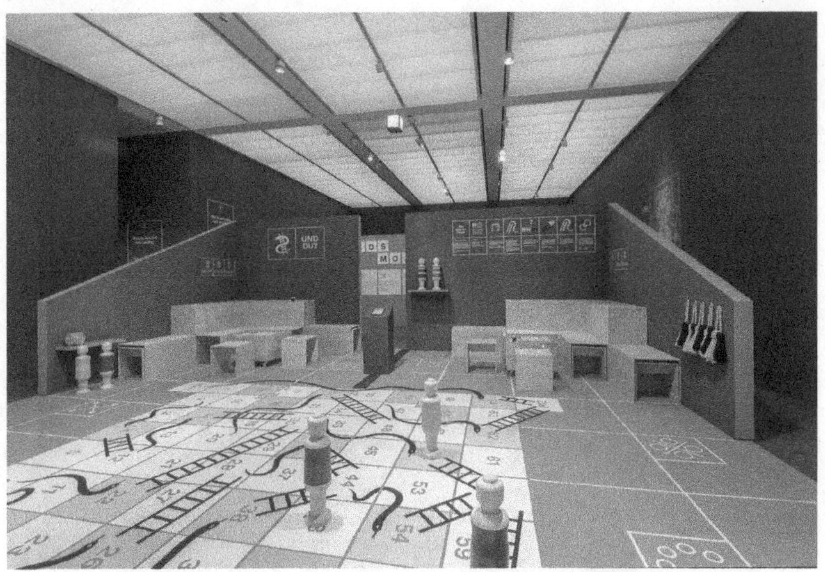

start with little knowledge and achieve more the further they move up on the game board, climbing ladders but also potentially sliding down snakes when engaged in karmically problematic behaviors. In more recent times, the game has also been developed in Europe and North America as Snakes and Ladders, and thus would, as we rightly suspected, be easily recognizable by our local audiences (see figure 3.4).

As a game of questions intended to provoke thought rather than to indoctrinate, exchange and interaction between all the co-players of the game became the central goal. When someone landed on a certain square provoking an ethical question to be asked, for example, they would have to answer the question: "Do you eat meat?" All players would then answer this question to themselves, while the player who had landed on the spot on the game board would have to guess how most of the other players answered the question. As soon as the player had given their assessment, the other players would reveal their answers. If the

Figure 3.4. Members of the public play "And You? The Game of Questions" at the center of the exhibition. *Source:* Museum Rietberg. Used with permission.

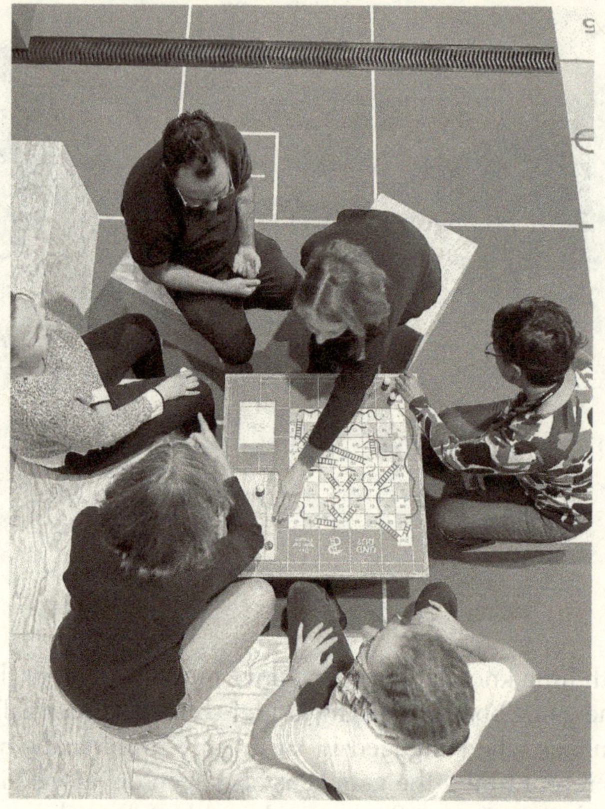

player guessed correctly, they would be able to climb the ladder, advancing higher on the board. If their guess was wrong, a snake would lead them down to a lower level. The first player to reach the last space first would win the game.

One of the key elements of this game was the engagement around daily ethical questions that it prompted, requiring self-reflection but also the need to guess how co-players think and act in daily life and whether or not players shared the same values. The game also included an online app, through which people could not only play from anywhere in the world with an internet connection but could also upload new questions of ethical relevance accessible to all.[12]

In addition to the game, we created a series of podium talks within the exhibition and the game area itself. In this intimate but playful environment we organized talks to discuss ethics concerning ecology, food, violence, or death, for example. For these talks, we always invited one practicing Jain to present the Jain perspective together with ordinary people, rather than elite experts. To facilitate interaction, we asked professional moderators to animate the discussion. Along with these facilitated discussions, many also noted in our guest book how deeply moved they were by the documentary films in the exhibition featuring, among other topics, the Jain ritual practice of fasting to death (*sallekhanā*).

In the end, our efforts were rewarded by the positive feedback from our audiences, which, amounting to 26,000 total visitors, included a much younger crowd than the museum would typically attract. The combination of art with reflections, discussions, and calls for engagement between the Jain and non-Jain communities were some of the key elements that helped us to achieve this success. In the end, this exhibition was another milestone in terms of innovative curating, receiving appreciation and reviews by the international press (Ali Khan 2023; Goswamy 2023). In light of this overall success, I will now offer some brief concluding remarks concerning our practice of "engaged curation" at the museum.

Conclusion

The present volume explores the notion of engaged Jainism in the field of Jain studies. Being familiar with the concept of engaged Buddhism from my earlier research on Dalits in India (Beltz 2005b), I was surprised to see this label used in the context of Jainism, and as previously mentioned, I therefore use the term "engaged curation" in a very specific and limited sense. The term "engaged Jainism" could be used to describe certain global Jain initiatives on veganism and nonviolence, and new tendencies within the Jain community could be compared to Buddhist modernism and reform movements. However, engaged Buddhist movements have generally been far more encompassing, radical, and above all socially and politically relevant than any of their Jain counterparts. As our process of engaged curation throughout the exhibition showed us, and as I have tried to briefly convey in this chapter, *Being Jain* simultaneously implies manifold promises and solutions but also challenges and potential pitfalls that may limit their effective impact.

Indeed, as Jains conveyed the promises of their tradition's ethical principles to public audiences through the exhibition considering our shared global challenges, public audiences simultaneously reflected back what they perceived as still mostly unanswered dilemmas surrounding the community's lived social realities and practices. As a secular institution whose job is to educate rather than indoctrinate, this down-to-earth, non-utopian outcome of our engaged curation at Museum Rietberg certainly did not solve the many global challenges our exhibition sought to grapple with. More modestly, however, it did open an honest dialogue between Jains and non-Jain publics wherein both parties hopefully left inspired, changed, and educated.

Notes

1. The exhibition *Being Jain: Art and Culture of an Indian Religion* was presented at the Museum Rietberg in Zürich from November 18, 2022, to April 30, 2023. The Parrotia Foundation, Max Kohler Stiftung, Arham Social Welfare Foundation, and Star Worldwide Group have been most generous in their financial support for the exhibition. A great thank you goes to Patrick Krüger, Harsha Vinay, Marion Frenger, and Michaela Blaser for working with me on that project. Without their contributions, neither exhibition nor catalogue would have been possible, and the project could not have been realized.

2. On that occasion, museums and cultural institutions remain open late into the night. Visitors can acquire a common entrance pass that grants them free access to all institutions as well as to public transport throughout the night. The first event of that kind took place in Berlin in 1997; the city of Zürich introduced it three years later.

3. According to several internet sites and statistics, roughly five to seven million Jains live today in India and in small communities across the world: https://www.pewresearch.org/religion/2021/09/21/population-growth-and-religious-composition/.

4. For more information about the Divine Light Zentrum's questionable history in Winterthur during Swami Omkarananda's lifetime

(1929–2000), see Strauss 2004, chap. 4.

5. We are grateful to the advisory board for their critical support of the project: Prof. Dr. Ana Bajželj, Prof. Dr. Nalini Balbir, Prof. John E. Cort, Prof. Dr. Christopher Chapple, Dr. Robert J. Del Bontà, Prof. Dr. Saryu Doshi, Dr. Eberhard Fischer, Prof. Dr. Peter Flügel, Prof. Dr. Julia A. B. Hegewald, Dr. Sulekh C. Jain, Dr. Shugan Jain, Dr. Andrea Luithle-Hardenberg, Prof. Dr. Christopher Jain Miller, Dr. Jasvant Modi, Dr. Narendra Parson, Sushil K. Premchand, and Prof. Dr. Steven Vose.

6. Our thanks go to Dhanesh Kothari, Sanjay Gubbi, Parveen Jain, Samani Chaitanya Pragya, Shalin Jain, Manoj and Anupama Jain, and Nisha Mehta.

7. The full interviews are available in English at https://www.arihantainstitute.org/jains-in-society.

8. Gautam Adani is a highly successful and wealthy Indian businessman and the founder and chairman of the Adani Group, one of India's largest conglomerates with diversified interests in various sectors. He figures prominently in many Jain platforms as a role model and authority. See, for example, https://www.jainsamaj.org/content.php?url=Shri_Gautam_Adani.

9. This question was made by a member of the public audience in our tandem tour on March 15, 2023.

10. Roughly nine-in-ten Indian Jains (92%) identify as vegetarian, and two-thirds of Jains (67%) go further by abstaining from root vegetables such as garlic and onion. These dietary practices extend outside the home; more than eight-in-ten Jain vegetarians also say they would not eat food in the home of a friend or neighbor who was nonvegetarian (84%) or in a restaurant that served nonvegetarian food (91%); https://www.pewresearch.org/short-reads/2021/08/17/6-facts-about-jains-in-india/4/7.

11. Interview with Sanjay Gubbi; https://www.arihantainstitute.org/jains-in-society/3-sanjay-gubbi-phd.

12. cf. https://unddu.rietberg.ch/en/game/.

References

Ali Khan, Murtaza. 2023. "An Exhibition that Highlights Jainism and its Ethics." *The Sunday Guardian*, June 25. https://sundayguardianlive.com/lifestyle/an-exhibition-that-highlights-jainism-and-its-ethics.

Auckland, Knut. 2016. "The Scientization and Academization of Jainism." *Journal of the American Academy of Religion* 84 (1): 192–233.

Balbir, Nalini, and Johannes Beltz. 2017. "Jain Art at the Museum Rietberg." *Jaina Studies, CoJS Newsletter* 12 (March): 50–53.

Beltz, Johannes. 2021. "Next Stop, Nirvana? Measuring the Success, Impact, and Sustainability of a Buddhist Art Exhibition" *Orientations* 52, no. 4 (July–August): 59–65.

———. 2005a. "´Hinduistisches Zürich: Eine Entdeckungsreise´: Bericht zur gleichnamigen Ausstellung im Stadthaus Zürich, 22.10.04–28.2.05." *Internationales Asienforum* 36 (3–4): 251–263.

———. 2005b. *Mahar, Buddhist and Dalit: Religious Conversion and Socio-Political Emancipation in Contemporary Maharashtra*. Manohar.

Beltz, Johannes, Michaela Blaser, Marion Frenger, Patrick Felix Krüger, and Harsha Vinay, eds. 2022. *Being Jain: Art and Culture of an Indian Religion*. Hatje Cantz.

———. 2023. *Being Jain: 20 Masterpieces from India, 10 Select Works of Art from the Rietberg Collection*. Museum Rietberg.

Chapple, Christopher Key. 2001. "The Living Cosmos of Jainism: A Traditional Science Grounded in Environmental Ethics." *Daedalus* 130 (4): 207–224.

———, ed. 2002. *Jainism and Ecology, Non-Violence in the Web of Life*. Harvard University Press.

Cort, John E. 2020. "Jain Society: 1947–2018." In *Brill's Encyclopedia of Jainism*, edited by John E. Cort, Paul Dundas, Knut A. Jacobsen, and Kristi L. Wiley. Brill.

Donaldson, Brianne. 2019. "Bioethics and Jainism: From ahimsa to an Applied Ethics of Carefulness." *Religions* 10 (243). https://doi.org/10.3390/rel10040234.

Donaldson, Brianne, and Ana Bajželj. 2021. *Insistent Life: Principles for Bioethics in the Jain Tradition*. University of California Press.

Eitle, Erik. 2003. "Zwischen Prozession und Party." *Tages-Anzeiger*, September 8: 13.

Fischer, Eberhard. 1974. *Kunst und Religion in Indien: 2500 Jahre Jainismus*. Museum Rietberg / Helmhaus.

Flügel, Peter, Heleen de Jonckheere, and Renate Söhnen-Thieme, eds. 2023. *Pure Soul: The Jaina Spiritual Traditions*. Centre for Jaina Studies.

Fowler 2023. "Visualizing Devotion: Jain Embroidered Shrine Hangings." Fowler Museum at UCLA. https://fowler.ucla.edu/exhibitions/visualizing-devotion.

Goswamy, B. N. 2023. "Of Salvation and Redemption Through Principles of Jainism." *The Tribune*. June 4. https://www.tribuneindia.com/news/features/of-salvation-and-redemption-through-principles-of-jainism-514000.

Iseli, Mirjam. 2012. *Entstehung und Auflösung der Schweizer Jaina-Gemeinschaft, Gemeinschaftsbildung in der Diaspora*. Tectum Verlag.

———. 2015. "Mein Jainismus, dein Jainismus? Unser Jainismus! Tendenzen Eines Universellen Jainismus in der Schweiz." *Zeitschrift für junge Religionswissenschaft* 10. https://doi.org/10.4000/zjr.328.

Jain, Prakash, C. 2011. *Jains in India and Abroad*. International School for Jain Studies.

Jain, Shugan Chand. 2019. *National Report. A Sociological Study of Jain Community. Executive Summary (Survey 2017–2019)*. International School for Jain Studies.

Kinzner, Elvira, Ji Min An, and Thomas Gruber. 2023. "The Milky Way: An Ecological Transition of the Dairy Industry." *Territorial Project, mas-utd.arch.ethz.ch*. https://www.mas-utd.arch.ethz.ch/Programme/Student-Work/Dairy-Pastures.

Konikkara, Aathira. 2023. "Divided Times: The Untangling of Samir and Vineet Jain's Empire." *The Caravan* 15 (12): 24–48.

Krüger, Patrick Felix. 2022. *Der Jainismus. Eine indische Religion der Gewaltlosigkeit*. Reclam Verlag.

Miller, Christopher Jain, and Jonathan Dickstein. 2021a. "Jain Veganism: Ancient Wisdom, New Opportunities." *Religions* 12 (7): 512. https://doi.org/10.3390/rel12070512.

Narayanan, Yamini. 2023. *Mother Cow, Mother India: A Multispecies Politics of Dairy in India*. Navayana Publishing.

Prajna, Samini Chaitanya, et al., eds. 2016. *Jain Philosophy: A Scientific Approach to Reality*. Bhagwan Mahavira International Research Center.

Rashkow, Ezra. 2013. "Jain Endangerment Discourse." *Department of History Faculty Scholarship and Creative Works*, 21. MSU Digital Commons. https://digitalcommons.montclair.edu/history-facpubs/21.

Richard, Katja. 2023. "Jain-Food im Museum Rietberg: So Köstlich Kochen die Strengsten aller Vegis." *Blick am Sonntag*, January 15. https://www.blick.ch/life/jain-food-im-museum-rietberg-so-koestlich-kochen-die-strengsten-aller-vegis-id18224507.html.

Sanghavi, Hemali. 2013. "Jains and Caste System: Conceptual and Comparative Perspective." *GRA: Global Research Analysis* 2, no. 2 (February): 119–120.

Shepherd, Kancha Ilaiah. 2019. "Freedom to Eat: The Fight for Beef as a Democratic Right." *The Caravan*, November 1. https://caravanmagazine.in/reportage/fight-beef-democratic-right.

SOAS. 2023. "Pure Soul: The Jaina Spiritual Traditions." SOAS University of London. https://www.soas.ac.uk/puresoul.

Strauss, Sarah. 2004. *Positioning Yoga: Balancing Acts Across Cultures*. Routledge.

Ulrich, Katherine. 2007. "Food Fights: Buddhist, Hindu, and Jain Dietary Polemics in South India." *History of Religions* 46, no. 3 (February):

228–261.
Vose, Steven M. 2022. "Normalizing Nationalism Through Social Media in Transnational Jain Communities." *The Immanent Frame*. November 30. https://tif.ssrc.org/2022/11/30/normalizing-nationalism-through-social-media-in-transnational-jain-communities/.

4

Engaged Jain Yoga

Narendra Kumar Jain's *The Seven Stages of Enlightenment* on the Berlin Wall

CHRISTOPHER JAIN MILLER

"The artistic language is an ineffable language, which many intellectuals do not even understand," asserted Narendra Kumar Jain in 2021.[1] Jain made this statement during an interview about his contribution of the mural, *The Seven Stages of Enlightenment* (1989/2009), to the Berlin Wall's popular East Side Gallery (see figure 4.1). As I desperately grasped to understand this ineffable language while gazing at Jain's mural for the first time, I was immediately captivated by the entangled layers of history, politics, and culture that his mural also clearly conveyed. Thus, while I will briefly attempt in the conclusion of this chapter to translate the artist's ineffable language, I will spend more time here attempting to disentangle other historical, cultural, and political layers in Jain's work to help us understand and appreciate his contribution to Berlin's East Side Gallery open-air mural project. These layers include the legacy of Indian modern art to which Jain is connected, India's historic relationship to West and East Germany, the Berlin Wall as a site for the production of artistic works and visual culture during and after the Cold War, and relevant history concerning the reception of yoga in India, Europe, and Germany.

Figure 4.1. The 2009 version of Narendra Kumar Jain's *The Seven Stages of Enlightenment* (*Die sieben Stufen der Erleuchtung*) at the Berlin Wall's East Side Gallery (2023). *Source:* Provided by the author with friend Christian Handler.

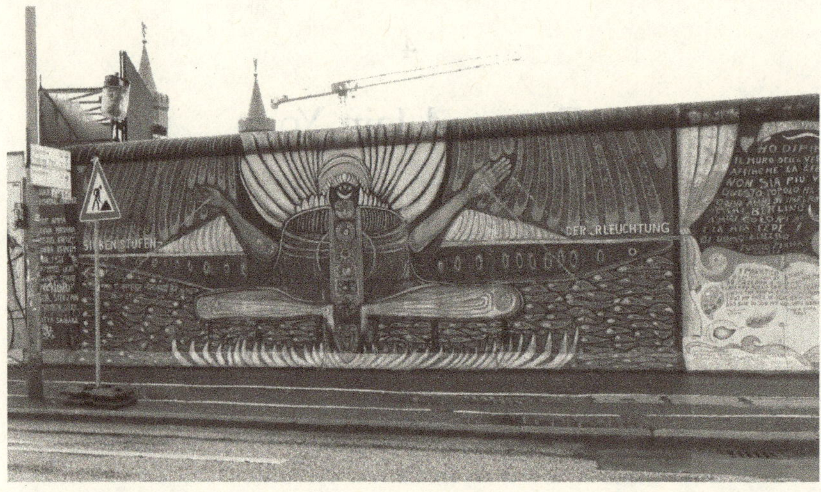

A limited number of recent studies have outlined the history of Indian modern art and artists, leaving us with a "still nascent understanding of a complex period in Indian art history" (Brown 2009, 21) to which this chapter will add one further contribution. Furthermore, existing historical studies of Indian modern art tend to focus on popular art and artists in India up until the year 1990. This chapter considers a piece of Indian modern art at the threshold of this historically significant time period during a year that initiated a decade of dramatic change for both Europe and India. In 1989, Narendra Kumar Jain, an artist and yoga teacher born into the Jain religious tradition, found himself directly engaged with Cold War politics and the international artistic culture that was operating on both sides of the Berlin Wall both before and after its fall. To consider Jain's artistic creation as merely derivative of this context, however, risks missing precisely how he harnessed it in order to visually communicate to his public audiences in Berlin his Indian culture's own situated truths grounded in yogic, tantric, Jain, Hindu, Buddhist, and other Indian philosophical understandings of what comprises freedom and enlightenment. Because Jain was born into the little-known Jain religious tradition, he found a place to bring other available Orientalist ideas into engagement with Berlin's broader visual culture, thereby proactively capitalizing upon the available structures and categories available to him as a member of the Indian diaspora.

As this chapter will show, Jain was indeed engaging his cultural truths, mediated as they were through his colonial and romantic Orientalist inheritances, with the concerns of Western understandings of freedom and enlightenment. I draw here from an online archive of existing German articles and video interviews wherein Narendra Kumar Jain explains the reasons for his visual choices as he navigated the particular representational freedoms he had access to as a member of Berlin's Indian diaspora. Through the choices he made, Jain painted an important and yet overlooked contribution to the Berlin Wall's East Side Gallery, *The Seven Stages of Enlightenment*, during the critical year of 1989, and then again in 2009 when he refurbished his mural.

Studying Indian Modern Art and Visual Culture at the Berlin Wall

Narendra Kumar Jain created his first version of *The Seven Stages of Enlightenment* (*SSE*) in 1989 at an important historical juncture, immediately before India began to change its political and economic relations globally as a result of the fall of the Berlin Wall. His refurbishment of the mural twenty years later in 2009 is also revealing, as his artistic choices at that time demonstrate the evolution of India's relationship to Europe and the so-called West as well as the new "representational freedoms" (Khullar 2015, 19) Jain had at his disposal two decades after the Berlin Wall's fall. With these considerations in mind, Jain's *SSE* presents an important case study in the history of Indian modern art.

By using the term "modern" in this chapter, I consider Jain's *SSE* to coincide with what art historians might refer to as "modern art," a movement that deliberately sought to undermine the post-Renaissance realist tradition in Western culture.[2] But I most specifically intend in this chapter to identify a particular ethos conveyed by "modern" art as it has been produced by pre- and post-independence Indians to express notions of Indian nationalism, ancient Indian wisdom, and authenticity that are nevertheless in tension with, following Brown, a concurrent impulse to convey "a particular approach to the world embodied in an epistemology of progress, a faith in universals, the primacy of the subject, and a turning away from religion toward reason" (Brown 2009, 4) as well as toward forms of cosmopolitanism and secularism that are broadly representative of Euro-American ideals (Brown 2009, 9–10; Khullar 2015, 220; Kumar 1999, 14).

As we consider Jain's *SSE*, it will benefit us to pay close attention to what Mitter identifies as the Indian "artist's agency . . . by analyzing art practices and reception as a cultural document that is historically situated" (Mitter 2008, 541). As one of these "cultural documents," Jain's *SSE* participated in the artistic "critical exchange between Western and non-Western cultures" (Khullar 2015, 18). Alongside the consideration of Jain's art within its national framework, we must simultaneously probe the manifold "worldly affiliations" (Khullar 2015) and entangled "trans-border histories" (Sunderason 2020, 250) pertaining to a particular piece of urban Indian diasporic art while maintaining a commitment to understanding its "deeply locational formations" revealed by its granular history, specific cultural inspirations, and local political influences (ibid., xi, 4, 34–36). Studying Indian urban art on the Berlin Wall in such a manner helps us see how Jain's artistic aspirations conveying an idealized, ancient Indian yogic culture have become imprinted in Berlin's post–Cold War urban environment. In these tensions between a seemingly universal yogic culture and the cosmopolitan European city as a symbol of modernity, progress, and development, we encounter, as Brown argues, the "in-between status of Indian modernism: between the local and the international, the Indian and the Euro-American, the ancient past and the 'not yet' " (Brown 2009, 132).

Drawing from Edward Said's work concerning "affiliations," Khullar encourages us to study these apparent tensions in Indian modern art through the analytical frame of "worldly affiliations" wherein "affiliation denotes a historical process by which a national art world came together and became conjoined with an international art world" (Khullar 2015, 14). Studying Indian modern art through the framework of "worldly affiliations" requires careful attention to "social relations and material conditions," and helps us overcome the tendency to view Indian art through the prism of the nation state alone (ibid.). Narendra Kumar Jain's transnational "affiliative network" (ibid., 24) influenced and indeed enabled him to paint his *SSE* on the Berlin Wall, while simultaneously opening an opportunity for him to share his own culture's historically situated truths.

The Seven Stages of Enlightenment

According to one of the East Side Gallery's primary organizers, David Monty, the *SSE* was completed in October 1989, before the fall of the Berlin Wall (Gründer 2019). The 1989 *SSE*[3] stands prominently in second position next to the first mural of the East Side Gallery, which was reserved for a message from the United States containing Hans Bierbrauer's image of the Statue of Liberty symbolizing and celebrating the democratic freedom shared between Europe and the United States (see figure 4.2). Jain's adjacent *SSE* visually mediates the yogic journey toward enlightenment and

Figure 4.2. Hans Bierbrauer's *Untitled* (1990) at the first position on the Berlin Wall at the East Side Gallery, with Jain's *Seven Stages of Enlightenment* immediately adjacent to the right (2009). *Source:* Image courtesy of photographer Mark Turner, CC BY-NC-SA 2.0.

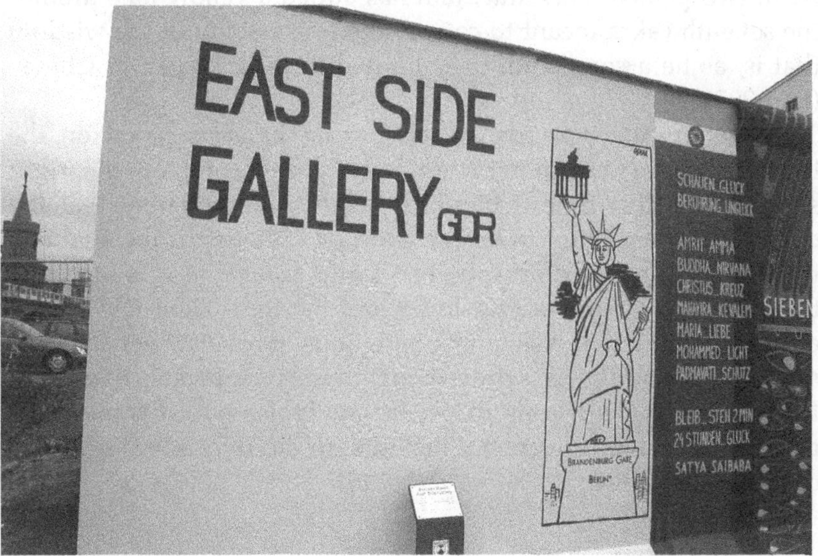

spiritual freedom via transnational yoga's popular seven-cakra model of the yogic subtle body.

The 1989 *SSE* conveys this message of freedom with a colorful meditating red Buddha seated above a lotus flower in a cross-legged lotus position with seven cakras containing flowers with varying numbers of petals running vertically from the center of the bottom of his body to the top of his head. The yogi's arms reach up into the air, with the right hand depicting *jñāna-mudrā* and the left hand an open palm. These primary features from the 1989 version of the *SSE* remain intact in the 2009 refurbishment of the mural, though Jain adds several important details in this final iteration. Indeed in 2009, when many of the original artists were invited to refurbish their 1990 murals, Jain added more stunning colors, sharper details, new images, and a variety of written expressions to the image (see figure 4.1), all of which were intended to connect "Indian Mythology and Wisdom with Western Religions and Philosophy" and to show how "according to Hindu belief, the practice of yoga makes it possible to progress through the stages of enlightenment which promise a better existence without suffering" (Jain 2021).

One notable change to the 2009 *SSE* is that the first five cakras starting from the bottom now contain associated Sanskrit seed syllables, while the sixth cakra located at the meditating red Buddha's third eye contains the well-known sacred syllable *oṃ* (with two petals). This time, Jain has added a yellow halo around the seventh cakra meant to convey the universality of the wisdom that is, as he asserts, "not only limited to India, Japan or China" (Jain 2021).

The Buddha's hands are also again in *jñāna-mudrā* on the left side of the mural with an open palm again on the right side, though this time it becomes much more apparent that the open hand was meant to be the hand of Christ with the stigmata representing the West and the hand in *jñāna-mudrā* was intended to be the hand representing India and the East. Here Jain makes clear something that was more ambiguous in his 1989 version: The meditating Buddha is synthesizing these two perspectives (i.e., East and West) as he sits in perfect equipoise with his eyes and face—both of which were not included in the 1989 mural—gazing down at the viewer.

The linguistic additions of the 2009 version of the *SSE* are also revealing, especially given Jain's express commitment to the "ineffable language" of art. These additions pithily convey interfaith, nationalistic, and Jain sentiments in a mix of German, Hindi, and Sanskrit on the left side of the image underneath a newly added Indian national flag. Names of Buddhist, Christian, Jain, Muslim, and Hindu religious figures included in the refurbished mural articulate Jain's express desire "to contribute to mutual understanding and cultural exchange," and it is notable that he now explicitly includes, as he mentions in a 2021 interview, "the Wisdom of the Jain teacher Mahavira" (Jain 2021).

Likewise, on both sides of the Buddha image a number of spiritual aphorisms highly suggestive of closely related ontological, metaphysical, and karma theory concepts found in Jain tradition are now written vertically. Following basic Jain philosophy, these aphorisms suggest that we all possess an independent, individual soul that is inherently omniscient and blissful, though tarnished by our individual karma and therefore unrecognizable to us in our ordinary experience. Only by correcting our conduct to align with Jain and yogic principles, both of which are grounded in an ethic of nonviolence (*ahiṃsā*), can we "become happy," as Jain puts it, and ultimately recognize the independence (*kevala/kaivalya*) and freedom of our soul. Finally, across the image we find the mural's title prominently written:

> "SIEBEN STUFEN DER ERLEUCHTUNG" ("Seven Stages of Enlightenment")

According to Jain, "Seven stages means seven chakras . . . the seventh is full enlightenment. And I tried to interpret them in my Indian manner . . . I wanted to combine my Indian philosophy with German Philosophy" (Jain 2021). When Jain was asked, during a video interview in 2019, "Which level of enlightenment have you reached?," he replied, "That I cannot say, it is a yogi's secret" (Jain 2019).

Along with these seven cakras, Jain's *SSE* combines several popular elements from Indian philosophy into one eclectic message of spiritual freedom. The classical non-dual cakra system and the Buddha from the 1989 version is overlaid in 2009 with Jain's ontological and metaphysical commitments taken from Jain philosophy. His inclusion of the Indian national flag and other world religions in 2009 also signals his commitment to his Indian national identity as well as his home country's pre-2014 religious pluralism and inclusivism including his own Jain tradition's popular commitment to remaining open to other philosophical perspectives (*anekāntavāda*). While each of these elements of Jain's piece can be situated in the history of transnational yoga, global Indian religiosity, and Western reception of Indian art (Davis 1997; Faure 1998; Singleton 2008; White 2014; Cort 2000; 2020), I focus our attention here on the core visual message of Jain's piece, the seven cakras, which in the mural materialize his seven stages of enlightenment.

Seven Cakras in Transnational Yoga

Jain's interpretation of the seven-cakra system reflects the classical six- and seven-cakra system often taught in transnational modern yoga culture, which itself has textual origins in the tenth-century tantric text titled *Kubjikāmatatantra*. This text disseminated, for the first time, a similar six-cakra system as part of its non-dual tantric system that became a template for many tantric yoga systems that would follow into the present.

Jain's understanding of the yogic subtle body including the cakra system also reflects common models that were reified in the crucible of the Indian *bhadralok*'s (Jacobsen 2018) encounters with colonial and romantic Orientalist influences, wherein elite Indians and Europeans co-constructed an idealized, textually mediated yogic body from preexisting South Asian practice lineages and Sanskrit yoga scriptures in the early twentieth century (Green 2008; Singleton 2010; Burchett 2019; Miller 2024). Those involved in these projects were selectively gleaning material from medieval tantric and *haṭha-yoga* texts that had already begun to internalize external sexual Kaula tantric practices within the yogic subtle body (Mallinson 2011, 779–780). They were also drawing from the extant "*bhakti* sensibility" influencing North Indian forms of yoga practice, which was highly compatible with British Victorian sensibilities (Burchett 2019, 169).

I have elsewhere captured the transnational dissemination of these transformative yoga systems as "engaged alchemies," a term also meant to encapsulate the processes through which yoga gurus and teachers have brought yogic subtle body logics into novel social environments transnationally (Miller 2024, 1), just as Narendra Kumar Jain has brought the cakras to the Berlin Wall.

Perhaps most prominently, in 1919 Arthur Avalon (Sir John Woodroffe) democratized the internalized seven-cakra system in Western and Indian culture through his still highly influential English publication of the sixteenth-century tantric text *Ṣaṭcakranirūpaṇa*, "Description of the Six Cakras" (the text actually describes seven cakras), a scripture from Kaula Śaivism's Southern Transmission through which the cakras lead a spiritual practitioner to an experience of nonduality. Shortly thereafter, Charles Leadbeater, a member of the Theosophical Society, popularized the cakras for an international audience in his 1927 book *The Chakras*. Compared to Avalon's work, Leadbeater's "was more heavily influenced by Western harmonial ideas of psychic forces and various astrological ideas" (Foxen and Kuberry 2021, 66). As Foxen and Kuberry note, the cakras would then "go through several stages of combinations and recombinations from the 1920s onwards, mostly by Western authors but a few by self-styled Indian yogis teaching in North America" (ibid.).

Similar speculations concerning the cakra system were also taking place in continental Europe as the popular system landed in German-speaking regions. During his own phase in the Theosophical Society, anthroposophist Rudolf Steiner mapped the Sanskrit names of the cakras onto the Western astral body (Astralkörper) in 1909 (Steiner 1909; Fuchs 1990, 49).

Steiner's work, as well as the later "anthroposophically-oriented" work of Werner Bohm in his book titled *Chakras* (1953), was explicitly mediated through sources from the Theosophical Society (Fuchs 1990, 49–50). Predating Leadbeater's 1927 book *The Chakras*, however, Steiner had also already described "special abilities" like clairvoyance that occurred from the activation of the cakras using various practices apparently independent from the Theosophical Society's influence (ibid., 50).

While some of Steiner and Bohm's contemporaries including psychoanalyst Richard Rösel saw "no real basis" for the cakras in modern scientific applications of yoga (ibid. 72), the system later found popularity and authority in other yoga organizations including the German Yoga Society (Deutsche Yoga Gesellschaft, est. 1970), which by 1982 included "Mystical Physiology (cakras, etc.)" in their curriculum (ibid., 156–158). Yoga Vidya (est. 1992), a major yoga organization in Germany founded upon the teachings of the famous Swami Sivananda Saraswati (1887–1963), also still uses, as Sivananda himself had, Avalon's translation of the *Ṣaṭcakranirūpaṇa* to teach the cakra system in Germany today.[4] All of this is to say that Jain's *SSE* clearly inherits, but also capitalizes upon, the popularity of what has now become a well-known transnational yoga system, which commonly conveys a spiritual journey through seven cakras on the path toward spiritual liberation and enlightenment.

Narendra Kumar Jain, the Berlin Wall's Yogi Artist

Born in Delhi in 1937, Narendra Kumar Jain is, following the 2009 linguistic additions he made to the *SSE*, a self-described "Indian fortune teller, yogi, painter, and art historian."[5] Following a lectureship position at the University of Agra that began in 1963, Jain first came to West Berlin in 1967 at the invitation of the German Academic Exchange Service (Deutscher Akademischer Austauschdienst) for a one-year study visit at the College of Arts (Hochschüle der Künste) and then served a one-year guest professorship at Heidelberg College (Jain 2019).[6] Also employed as an artist, he eventually created the popular Berlin mural known as *Weltbaum* (*World Tree*) with Polish-German artist Ben Wagin in 1974 before completing the *SSE* in 1989 (Jain 2021).

According to Jain, his background in yoga began with training at the age of two with his mother in India. There, his father Shri Chandu Lal Jain Aktar worked as a lawyer, was a poet, but also served as a nonviolent freedom fighter alongside Gandhi against the colonial British. At a convention Jain attended with his father when he was only five years old, he claims to have learned the lotus position from Gandhi himself, recalling in a 2009 interview, "I was very restless, jumping around. Gandhi spoke to me soothingly and showed me the lotus position. I was so excited that I stayed seated for two hours" (Meixner 2009).[7] Jain continued his yogic pursuits, apparently even spending "weeks wandering alone in the Himalayas" in an area known to have tigers, where, one day while "sitting in a cave and meditating," he recounts his experience of remaining in meditation even when he felt a tiger breathing on his neck (ibid.).

Following his early yogic pursuits, Jain arrived in Germany amidst an influx of thousands of students and laborers from India in the 1960s and 1970s who came to both East and West Berlin to work and study in the fields of engineering, medicine, and business (Goddar 2000).[8] Among all those who immigrated, Jain was a rather unique exception as he was both a yoga teacher and an artist (ibid.). A news article from 2000 reports that Jain had already taught thirty thousand people yoga in Berlin by 1972, most of whom were Germans. By 2009, the same year Jain refurbished the *SSE*, we find that his yoga studio is considered "probably the best" in Berlin and that some might even consider him as "Berlin's best yoga teacher" (Meixner 2009). By this time he had evidently "introduced around 70,000 people worldwide to the magic of yoga" (ibid.). Jain's apparent success did not emerge in a vacuum, however, as the stage for his yoga teachings had already been set in the centuries preceding his arrival.

The Reception of Yoga in Germany

By the time that Jain arrived to Berlin in 1967 and painted his subsequent mural on the Berlin Wall in 1989, yoga—in manifold forms—had already long been a part of German culture on both sides of the wall (Fuchs 1990; n.d.). Early on in the eighteenth and nineteenth centuries, German Indologists had studied Sanskrit texts, while those who were influenced by Romanticism among them and groups including the Anthroposophical Society created various points of reception for yogic systems to enter mainstream German culture. As Alter has shown, the popular system of German Nature Cure became a critical "transnational conjuncture" for yogic and German ideas surrounding health and wellness to meet in the early twentieth century (Alter 2000, 82). Around the same time, and in the wake of German Theosophical speculations around yoga, Europe was "inundated with a flood of 'esoteric' literature" while "numerous groups, lodges and circles competed for the favor of the public and praised their promising 'secret techniques'" (Fuchs n.d.).[9] Within this context, as Fuchs observes, "The techniques of Indian yoga served as a welcome addition to the esoteric 'menu'" (ibid.), which included the cakras. In the 1950s, the German Gymnastics and Sports Association (Deutschen Turn- und Sportbundes) of the German Democratic Republic (GDR) nevertheless declared a "yoga ban," although the changing political climate between East and West Germany in the early 1970s included reforms that made "many GDR officials more friendly towards yoga" (ibid.). Consequently, a shift begins in the late 1970s that opens the door for yoga in East Germany. As Fuchs highlights, "By the mid-1980s at the latest, yoga courses had become established in almost every larger city in the GDR" in both public and private settings and were taught within secular and therapeutic frameworks (ibid.).

Both West and East Germany had thus already been well prepared for Jain to paint his yogic mural on the Berlin Wall in 1989. When he finally began to paint the *SSE* in the spring of 1989, he brought with him the historically mediated understandings of yoga, the cakras, and Indian spirituality outlined in this chapter. He nevertheless also encountered there a fitting social and historical moment that was well prepared to receive him and his work.

The Berlin Wall: A Site of Creative Speculation and Place of Engagement for Artists

The Berlin Wall was built in the long aftermath of the Potsdam Conference in 1945, where post–World War II Germany was divided between the Allied powers of the United States, Great Britain, France, and the Soviet Union (USSR). Beginning in the early 1960s, East Germany began to construct a wall to thwart its residents from escaping to West Berlin, creating a dangerous border environment where many people lost their lives as they attempted to escape from the GDR's communist regime to West Berlin's symbolic island of freedom.

Due to all of the important political and cultural encounters that have transpired there, scholars considering the Berlin Wall have broadly described its location as "a site of creative speculation" (Gerstenberger and Braziel 2011, 13) and a "a place of *engagement*" for "*engaged* forms of cultural diplomacy" that eventually gave rise to "countercultural communities and expressive spaces beyond governmental oversight" (Farber 2020, 3, 7, 15–16, emphases added). In this context, artists were working *together* on both sides of the wall (Farber 2020, 5, 7; Mesch 2008, 20; Hockenos 2017).

Following the wall's fall on November 9, 1989, "the subcultures of East and West collided in the ruins of eastern Berlin" where, as Hockenos observes, the "boundless untended spaces invited improvisation" (Hockenos 2017, 7). The Berlin Wall's East Side Gallery would become one of these spaces inviting improvisation from artistic legacies from all over the world, including the legacy of Indian modern art in Narendra Kumar Jain's *SSE*.

In the years preceding Jain's invitation to join the East Side Gallery project, the Berlin Wall had already begun to undergo artistic modification from the encouragement of West German authorities (Gray 1985, 40), and, according to Gray, the "ubiquitous graffiti and sloppy images that previously abounded" were "giving way to more serious, complex and powerfully painted communications" as "professional artists as well as students" were "in the process of making the wall into one of the most extraordinary political statements in the world" (ibid., 39).

As a part of these coordinated efforts, David Monty, Heike Stephan, and Christine Maclean coordinated the East Side Gallery open-air mural project by inviting 118 artists from twenty-one countries to paint 105 murals in the period leading up to the Berlin Wall's eventual fall. These artists intended to "open up different perspectives on life in the divided city, the fall of the wall and German unity" (Stiftung 2023a), and a large section of the wall has remained standing as a place to preserve these perspectives into the present.

What makes Jain's contribution to the East Side Gallery particularly important is that he began to paint his mural in East Germany, the border of which was the Spree River, in March of 1989, before the fall of the Berlin Wall on November 9, 1989. Crossing the Oberbaum Bridge (Oberbaumbrücke) each time to paint the mural on the wall just on the other side of the river, Jain was entering potentially dangerous territory in East Berlin. He nevertheless commenced his mural in the spring of 1989 with the encouragement of his German colleague David Monty, who had connections to the East German border guards, as well as on the grounds that he had an Indian visa and passport, which in principle allowed him to legally enter East Berlin (Jain 2019). Since India belonged to the Non-Alignment Movement and did not side with the United States or the Soviet Union during the Cold War, Indians could more freely travel between East and West Germany in ways that members of other nations could not. These enabling factors are significant, as they demonstrate the complex international political landscape in which Jain was working and how Jain's work was particularly enabled through his "affiliative network" (Khullar 2015, 24) that had depended on him as an Indian artist to help accomplish the East Side Gallery's goals to paint the Berlin Wall.

Despite the potential dangers awaiting artists of all kinds (Ladd 1997, 26), Jain accepted Monty's invitation. Shortly thereafter, he took his Indian passport and "could freely go over the Oberbaum Bridge" with his "car and begin the first painting" (Jain 2019). While painting in early 1989, Jain recalls, "it was forbidden in the GDR to even speak about yoga, or to paint yoga, and for this reason I was frequently insulted" (Jain 2021). By the time he decided to paint the *SSE* on the East Side Gallery Wall, Jain seemed to be well aware, as we will later see, of his non-aligned Indian culture's apparent role in mediating the Cold War's divisions through a particular form of enlightenment that he had inherited not just from yoga's transnational history but also from multiple legacies of Indian modern art.

Indian Modern Art, Neo-Tantrism, and Muralism in Pre- and Post-Independence India

Early colonial encounters between Europe and India found Europeans either marking the often divine subjects found in Indian religious art as "Much Maligned Monsters" or, at other times, showering praise on "the Indian tradition," which they "exalted for its spirituality" (Mitter 1992, xix, 3).[10] As Mitter observes, "These somewhat contradictory threads continued to exist together and were often interwoven in the descriptions of a particular traveler" and "persisted even into the modern period" (ibid., xviii, 2). Alongside these "contradictory threads," starting around the mid-nineteenth century, the British constructed a binary between

Indian art and Western art, framing the former as decorative and the latter as naturalistic. Some nineteenth-century "enlightened Indians" such as India's "first modern Indian artist" and oil painter Raja Ravi Varma (1848–1906) consciously aligned themselves with this hegemonic Orientalist discourse and began to paint following the style of Western academic realism while nevertheless retaining a proud commitment to including Indian subject matter in their work (Kumar 1999, 14–15). In doing so, Varma and others laid the foundations for what became an anti-colonial, nationalist Indian culture that was Hindu and Sanskritic in nature, even as it had internalized Orientalist portrayals of Indian spirituality (Mitter 1994, 201). As Brown has observed following Mitter's work, "This genealogy of Hindu iconic painting (including the problematic subtext that Hinduism stands in for all religion in India) undergirds the works of the postindependence period" (Brown 2009, 47). Both Brown and Mitter's observations here help us more definitively understand Narendra Kumar Jain's explicit choice to portray yoga primarily within the available structures of "Hindu belief" (Jain 2021) rather than that of his own Jain tradition.

As Kumar writes, the colonial encounter between India and the British amounted to "a collaboration as much as a confrontation" (Kumar 1999, 15). Even those in opposition to "enlightened Indians," such as anti-colonial artists and intellectuals belonging to the Bengal School including Abanindranath Tagore (1871–1951) and Nandalal Bose (1882–1966), themselves internalized colonial and romantic Orientalist discourse as they "sought to establish the decorative impulses of Indian art as emblematic of a spiritual superiority over the materialistic culture of the West" (Khullar 2015, 42–43; Sunderason 2020, 12).

Nevertheless, not all artists in India agreed with the nationalist approaches heretofore described. Though at first a nationalist himself, Rabindranath Tagore soon became an internationalist who sought to assimilate Western culture and the arts into his own Indian culture (van der Linden 2013, 128). Tagore encouraged eclecticism and an even playing field between various cultures wherein both would be changed in their artistic encounters, while neither culture would lose its unique identity (Kumar 1999, 17). Western-trained Hungarian-Indian painter Amrita Sher-Gil (1913–1941) and some who would follow her also sought to "cultivate an art that was organic and vital, connected to the past and to the West" and "to generate a national culture synthesizing East and West in the wake of colonialism" (Khullar 2015, 12, 43, 47). Sher-Gil "believed," as Khullar stresses, that "the task of great art was to establish a connection between national and international community" (ibid., 43, 56). Others including Jamini Roy (1887–1972) followed a similar impulse, constructing "a pan-Asian unity on the basis of a largely imagined common past," which enabled them to "bypass traditional Indian art without forgoing their Indian identity or embracing internationalism unequivocally" (Kumar 1999, 16–17). The Bombay Progressive Artists Group (est. 1947) and K. C. S. Paniker (1911–1977), who headed the Progressive Artists Association in Chennai (est. 1944), continued from the 1940s to take seriously the charge that Indian art should *integrate* itself with international forms of modern art (ibid., 18).

Following India's independence in 1947, the preexisting twin obligations to develop a national identity and yet maintain a commitment to modern, artistic internationalism continued to influence the development of Indian artists. Thought provoking for our purposes here is the emergence of neo-tantric art, which, through the work of artists such as the Bombay Progressive Artists Group's S. H. Raza (1922–2016), emerged during a period when images of icons, gods, and goddesses were in vogue.

Neo-Tantric Art

Neo-tantric art inspired "a geometric symbolism that connects the broader universe to the microlevel of the body and the local," with the work of Raza and others making its way to major cities and artistic communities in Europe and North America (Brown 2009, 13, 45, 83). By 1962, neo-tantric artist Jagdish Swaminathan (1928–1994), who painted the popular *Color Geometry of Space* series (1967), established Group 1890 in New Delhi as India's capital city began to emerge as a popular meeting point for both national and international artists (ibid., 15). Common elements found in this neo-tantric genre included sexual symbols as well as "mystical abstraction marked by the use of Indic symbols such as the *bindu* (dot), *surya* (sun), *naga* (serpent), and *yantra* (cosmic diagram)" (Khullar 2015, 175).

Within this neo-tantric movement, K. C. S. Paniker's famous *Words and Symbols* (1966) combines Indian words and symbols in a rather partially complete way. As Brown writes, Paniker's "work demonstrates the fundamental impossibility of summing up 'India' and instead focuses on the fragmented nature of the country's postcolonial condition" while also making "obvious the problems with excerpting one moment of India's past to stand in for Indianness as a whole" (Brown 2009, 85–86). Paniker's neo-tantric piece thereby "engages directly with the question of knowledge making, mounting a critique of science and knowing that centers both colonial efforts to control India and the development of modernity itself" (ibid., 158).

Another important artist inspiring neo-tantric art was G. R. Santosh (1929–1997), whose later 1973 work *Untitled* "represents the wider movement of neotantric art" (ibid., 49) and is diametrically opposed to the fragmented spirit of Paniker's work. Characterizing Santosh's paintings is a "philosophical interpretation committed to the purity of metaphysical categories" wherein "the objects, symbols, and practices" apparently "transcend time" and "present a unified South Asian cultural heritage" (ibid., 51). His appeal to tantra combined with Western abstraction, as Brown shows, provided Santosh with "a universal yet Indian conceptual and visual well from which to drink" and through which he "and the other neotantric artists find an idiom that allows them to tap into the constructed authenticity of Indian spirituality so popular in Western culture in the late 1960s and early 1970s" (ibid., 51, 53).

Inspired also by new academic research considering tantra, the genre of neo-tantric art expanded among Indian artists in the 1960s and 1970s where it continued to combine Western abstraction with Indian symbolism (Kumar 1999, 19). While Indian artists were contending with the simultaneous sentiments to develop respectable art within the "secular, reason-driven space of enlightenment," neo-tantric artists were maintaining a commitment to "the spiritual, iconic, and religious" and in doing so were, at least in some ways, working against the "central stream" by combining these sentiments in their work (Brown 2009, 48).

Within the context described in this section, Narendra Kumar Jain's 1989 *SSE* reflects the essentializing, neo-tantric impulse and style of artists such as G. R. Santosh while clearly not reflecting, we should note, the intentionally fragmented nature of Paniker's work. And in addition to his neo-tantrism, Jain's work can also be further contextualized within the concurrent tradition of Indian muralism.

Indian Muralism

During the same period during which Indian artists were developing neo-tantric art, others were also experimenting with muralism. Decades before the activist community mural projects taking place in the countercultural United States in 1967 (Barnett 1984), however, Indian muralists had already been greatly inspired by the political mural movement with origins in early twentieth-century Mexico. Mexican muralism, a form of art that was intended to educate the illiterate concerning the history of Mexico following the Mexican Revolution, indeed had a significant transnational influence on Indian muralists including, for example, Satish Gujral who had studied muralism in Mexico with the famous artists Diego Rivera (1886–1957) and David Siqueros (1896–1974) in the 1950s (Khullar 2015, 22). Gujral subsequently expanded on the influence of his Mexican teachers and "expressed his desire for murals to connect with the built environment and architecture of the city" in India (ibid., 152).

Like Gujral, Indian artists including K. G. Subramanyan (1924–2016) and Benodebehari Mukherjee (1904–1980) at Kala Bhavan also began to use murals as a way to engage and communicate with a larger public in India (ibid.; Kumar 1999, 17–20). Subramanyan's mural project *The Wheel* (1969) at Gandhi Darshan, for example, demonstrated how "modernist grids and homespun weaves could coexist in postcolonial India" and that artists needed to "negotiate a balance between the ideologies of the handmade and the mechanical," that is, between the concerns of the traditional and of the modern, in their muralism. Subramanyan undertook such projects in the 1960s and 1970s in order to "engage a public for art" in the face of India's accelerated urban and economic development, aiming toward "synthesis" and the conjoining of "opposed forces" of tradition and modernity (Khullar 2015, 152, 163).

Influenced by the Mexican mural movement of the 1920s, artists in India from the 1950s onward expanded the meanings, styles, and uses of murals in public spaces both in India and eventually, globally. By the 1980s, a new eclecticism had emerged in Indian art, and a crucial transition begins wherein it is no longer "conceived as the unfolding of a sensibility" and "self-expression" but was rather undertaken to create art as a conscious intervention *into* history (Kumar, 21, emphasis added).

Trained in art and art history in India and Germany, Narendra Kumar Jain emerges from this context. Like his neo-tantric artistic predecessors, his *SSE* draws from popular neo-tantric and yogic philosophies popularized in the crucible of colonialism and materializes these philosophies during a particular historical moment with his mural at the Berlin Wall. Rather than challenging notions of Indian authenticity as some of his neo-tantric predecessors may have (Khullar 2015, 175), however, Jain's work capitalizes on an opportunity to reinforce well-known stereotypes of Indian culture for his European diasporic audience (Brown 2009, 49–51). And rather than using sexual imagery from what might be considered left-handed tantric traditions as some of his neo-tantric contemporaries had, Jain's work presents instead an internalized tantric approach to enlightenment that was democratized globally in the colonial encounters between India and Europe in the early twentieth century (and which, we might add, reflects the ethos of Jain tantra more broadly). As I argue in the concluding section to this chapter, Jain's *SSE,* though clearly absorbing these manifold historical influences, was nevertheless a conscious, synthesizing intervention into his own particularly critical historical moment.

Conclusion

Khullar's engagement with Said's notion of "affiliations" focusing on artists' social relations and material conditions shows us how Indian modern art "is *constituted by* the world," though Khullar also draws our attention to Spivak's notion of "reworlding," which, just the opposite, "shows how the world is produced by and through the imagination" and thus how Indian modern art simultaneously "*constitutes* the world" (Khullar 2015, 22, emphases added). Combining both Said's (materialist) and Spivak's (idealist) approaches, Indian art history, according to Khullar, "would elucidate the process of translation by which the world is made visible in the image and the image becomes a world, invoking a world of other images" (ibid.). Following Khullar here, the question that remains then is how, if at all, the *SSE* "*constitutes* the world" and might in fact be "reworlding" (ibid., emphasis added).

Consider then how Jain's *SSE* is flanked by two prominent murals depicting seemingly universal Western messages of freedom, liberation, and enlightenment. To the right of Jain's mural in third position at the gallery, we find Italian artist Fulvio Pinna's (1948–) *Hymn to Joy* (1990), which "celebrates liberation from dictatorship" and "the freedom of the East Germans" (see figure 4.3) (Pinna 2021).[11] Pinna's express intention here is "to remind everyone that all people are *born free*, but many have to live in bondage" (ibid., emphasis added).

To the left of the *SSE* is a mural that was reserved for a message from the United States. Here we find Hans Bierbrauer's (1922–2006) caricature of the Statue of Liberty in New York, where

Figure 4.3. Fulvio Pinna's *Hymn to Joy* (1990) to the right of Jain's *Seven Stages of Enlightenment*. *Source:* Robert Harrison, Alamy. Used with permission.

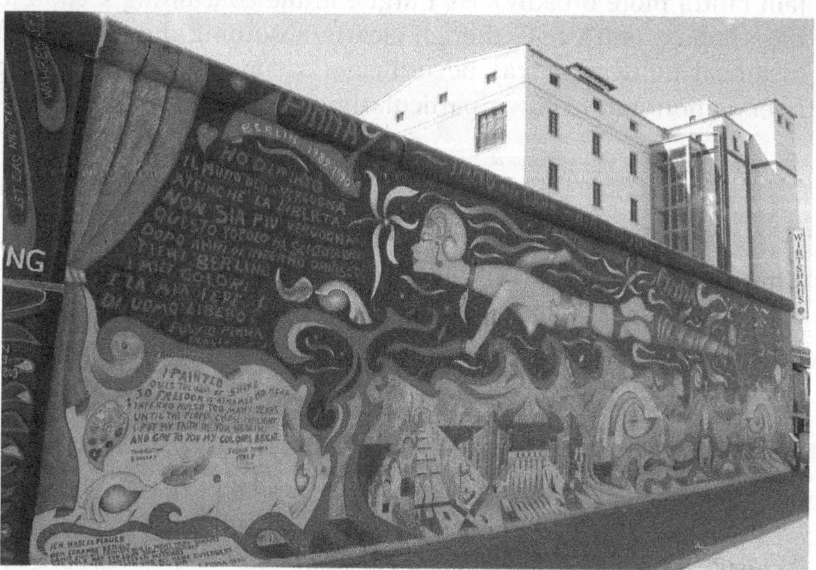

we observe Libertas, the Roman goddess of liberty, holding the Brandenburg Gate (Brandenburg Tor), a symbol of German freedom, instead of her customary torch. Bierbrauer's image, which replaces the torch with Berlin's cultural symbol of post–Cold War freedom, conveys a message not unlike the flame Libertas proudly holds in New York in the same hand (see figure 4.2). According to the United States National Park Service, the flame "is a symbol of enlightenment," which "lights the way to freedom showing us the path to Liberty . . . 'Liberty Enlightening the World' " (National Park Service 2022).

These murals flanking Jain's *SSE* at the East Side Gallery celebrate forms of freedom and liberation born from the European and American Enlightenments, which had also produced the seemingly universal but now fractured pursuits of modernity: a commitment to reason, progress, universal truth, knowledge, secularism, happiness, justice, and democracy. Jain's *SSE*, situated as it is between other works conveying various iterations of these pursuits, but also among messages from other cultures from around the world, suggests another type of progress and universal truth grounded in the layers of Indian history, culture, and philosophy I have disentangled in this chapter.

Rather than beginning from Pinna's starting point where "people are *born free*" (Pinna 2021, emphasis added), Jain's mural expresses the Pan-Indic cultural notion that assumes that people are instead perpetually *reborn into bondage and suffering*. And rather than conveying Libertas's "symbol of enlightenment" (National Park Service 2022) born of the European and American Enlightenments, in Jain's model freedom from suffering comes only after a progressive journey through seven cakras that finally amounts to a particular type of *yogic enlightenment*.

Apparently capitalizing on an old Orientalist binary, the yogi's outspread hands in Jain's *SSE* convey a form of transcendent yogic enlightenment as they unite the colonially constructed binary between East and West. That being said, and given Jain's special Indian status and citizenship in a country belonging to the Non-Alignment Movement coupled with his consequent privileged access to the east side of the Berlin Wall before its fall, East and West also take one further, and perhaps more obvious meaning in Jain's work. As the two seemingly opposed worlds of East and

West Germany remained divided by a slab of concrete surrounded by danger, Jain capitalized on India's non-aligned political status in the lead-up to the wall's fall, which gave him the opportunity to bring yoga's popular unifying message to the second position on the East Side Gallery in 1989 before other artists were even able to begin their work. Inseparable from his social and material conditions in pre– and post–Cold War Berlin, Jain harnessed this opportunity for cross-cultural communication of his own country's seemingly universal yogic path to enlightenment and unification within the structures, categories, and representational freedoms available to him. The self-proclaimed fortune-teller yogi's *Seven Stages of Enlightenment* was thus simultaneously mediated *but* perhaps also prophetic, was clearly *constituted by* Berlin and India's past while also *constituting,* in advance of the wall's fall, a free world that might experience enduring enlightenment, unification, and freedom from suffering through the cakras' seven stages of enlightenment.[12]

Notes

1. Quotations from the video interview (Jain 2021) are translated to English by the author from German.

2. See, for example, Mesch's definition of modern art (Mesch 2008, 1).

3. An image of the 1989 *SSE* (labeled with "1990" along with all the other murals) is available here: https://www.eastsidegalleryexhibition.com/artworks/jain-die-sieben-stufen-der-erleuchtung/.

4. See, for example, Yoga Vidya's interpretations of the text here: https://wiki.yoga-vidya.de/Shat_Chakra_Nirupana.

5. English translations from the original German are the author's own.

6. English translations from the original German are the author's own.

7. English translations from the original German are the author's own.

8. English translations from the original German are the author's own.

9. For an excellent summary of Fuch's work, visit http://www.yoga-akademie.de/YoInDeutsch.htm#_ftnref1. English quotes from Fuchs are the author's translated from German at this link.

10. Note that Mitter's work focuses primarily on European reception of Hindu art.

11. Quotations are translated to English by the author from the original German.

12. Special thanks to Justin Malachowski from the faculty of cultural studies at the University of Leuphana for reading an initial draft of this chapter and providing feedback.

References

Alter, Joseph S. 2000. *Gandhi's Body: Sex, Diet, and the Politics of Nationalism.* University of Pennsylvania Press.

Barnett, Alan. 1984. *Community Murals: The People's Art.* Art Alliance Press.

Brown, Rebecca M. 2009. *Art for a Modern India, 1947–1980.* Duke University Press.

Burchett, Patton E. 2019. *A Genealogy of Devotion: Bhakti, Tantra, Yoga, and Sufism in North India.* Columbia University Press.

Cort, J. E. 2000. "'Intellectual Ahiṃsā' Revisited: Jain Tolerance and Intolerance of Others." *Philosophy East and West* 50 (3): 324–347.

———. 2020. "Jain Society: 1947–2018." In *Brill's Encyclopedia of Jainism Online*," edited by John E. Cort, Paul Dundas, Knut A. Jacobsen, and Kristi L. Wiley. Brill.

Davis, Richard H. 1997. *Lives of Indian Images.* Princeton University Press.

Farber, Paul M. 2020. *A Wall of Our Own: An American History of the Berlin Wall.* University of North Carolina Press.

Faure, Bernard. 1998. "The Buddhist Icon and the Modern Gaze." *Critical Inquiry* 24 (3): 768–813.

Foxen, Anya, and Christa Kuberry. 2021. *Is This Yoga? Concepts, Histories, and the Complexities of Modern Practice.* Routledge.

Fuchs, Christian. n.d. "Anmerkungen zur Geschichte und Gegenwart des Yoga in Deutschland." Accessed August 4, 2023. http://www.yoga-akademie.de/YoInDeutsch.htm#_ftnref23.

———. 1990. *Yoga in Deutschland: Rezeption, Organisation, Typologie.* W. Kohlhammer.

Gerstenberger, Katharina, and Jana Evans Braziel, eds. 2011. *After the Berlin Wall: Germany and Beyond.* Palgrave Macmillan.

Goddar, Jeannette. 2000. "Unsere Götter warden wir nie aufgeben." Taz de. https://www.taz.de/!1226445/.

Gray, Cleve. 1985. "Report from Berlin: Wall Painters." *Art in America* 73:39–41.

Green, Nile. 2008. "Breathing in India, c. 1890." *Modern Asian Studies* 42 (2/3): 283–315.

Gründer, Ralf. 2019. "Interview mit David Monty." East Side Gallery. http://eastsidegallery.net/dave-monty-alias-sigfried-schoenfelder/.

Hockenos, Paul. 2017. *Berlin Calling*. New Press.

Jacobsen, Knut. 2018. *Yoga in Modern Hinduism: Hariharānanda Āraṇya and Sāṃkhyayoga*. Routledge.

Jain, Narendra Kumar. 2019. "Narendra Jain: 'Sieben Stufen der Erleuchtung.'" Berliner-mauer.de. Video interview. https://www.berliner-mauer.de/dr-narendra-jain-interview-23-12-2019.

———. 2021. "Die sieben Stufen der Erleuchtung." East Side Gallery Ausstellung. Video interview. https://www.eastsidegalleryausstellung.de/kunstwerke/jain-die-sieben-stufen-der-erleuchtung/.

Khullar, Sonal. 2015. *Worldly Affiliations: Artistic Practice, National Identity, and Modernism in India, 1930–1990*. University of California Press.

Kumar, R. Siva. 1999. "Modern Indian Art: A Brief Overview." *Art Journal* 58 (3): 14–21.

Ladd, Brian. 1997. *The Ghosts of Berlin*. University of Chicago Press.

Mallinson, James. 2011. "Haṭha Yoga." In *Brill's Encyclopedia of Hinduism*, edited by Knut A. Jacobsen. Vol. 3. Brill.

Meixner, Silvia. 2009. "Yoga bis uns schwindling wird." Morgenpost. https://www.morgenpost.de/printarchiv/biz/article104481689/Yoga-bis-uns-schwindling-wird.html.

Mesch, Claudia. 2008. *Modern Art at the Berlin Wall: Demarcating Culture in the Cold War Germanys*. Tauris Academic Studies.

Miller, Christopher Jain. 2024. *Embodying Transnational Yoga: Eating, Breathing, and Singing in Transformation*. Routledge

Mitter, Partha. 1992. *Much Maligned Monsters: A History of European Reactions to Indian Art*. University of Chicago Press.

———. 1994. *Art and Nationalism in Colonial India, 1850–1922*. Cambridge University Press.

———. 2008. "Decentering Modernism: Art History and Avant-Garde Art from the Periphery." *The Art Bulletin* 90 (4): 521–548.

National Park Service. 2022. "Statue of Liberty National Monument New York: Get the Facts." https://www.nps.gov/stli/planyourvisit/get-the-facts.htm#:~:text=What%20does%20the%20torch%20represent,%22Liberty%20Enlightening%20the%20World%22.

Pinna, Fulvio. 2021. "Hymne an die Freude." East Side Gallery Ausstellung. https://www.eastsidegalleryausstellung.de/kunstwerke/pinna-hymne-an-die-freude/.

Singleton, Mark. 2008. "The Classical Reveries of Modern Yoga: Patañjali and Constructive Orientalism." In *Yoga in the Modern World:*

Contemporary Perspectives, edited by Mark Singleton and Jean Byrne. Routledge.

———. 2010. *Yoga Body: The Origins of Modern Posture Practice*. Oxford University Press.

Steiner, Rudolf. 1909. *Wie erlangt man Erkenntnisse der höheren Welten?* Philosophisch-Anthroposophischer Verlag.

Stiftung, Berliner Mauer. 2023a. "East Side Gallery: Ausstellung." https://www.eastsidegalleryausstellung.de/.

Sunderason, Sanjukta. 2020. *Partisan Aesthetics: Modern Art and India's Long Decolonization*. Stanford University Press.

van der Linden, Bob. 2013. *Music and Empire in Britain and India: Identity, Internationalism, and Cross-Cultural Communication*. Palgrave Macmillan.

White, David Gordon. 2014. *The Yoga Sutra of Patanjali: A Biography*. Princeton University Press.

5

Engaging Spaces

Jain Position and Identity in the Urban Space of Bangkok, Thailand

YIFAN ZHANG

The Jains, as urban dwellers in Southeast Asian social and cultural contexts, were for centuries actively engaged in trade networks crossing the Indian Ocean and Bay of Bengal, as well as in regional trading endeavors. The Jains residing in Bangkok who have made these oceanic journeys into Southeast Asia navigate their social and cultural environments amid the dual concepts of being identified and practicing self-identification, as well as amid internationalization and localization. Alongside the presence of capitalism, urbanism, and nationalism, these individuals maintain their Jain lifestyles through both overt and covert means, while also demonstrating innovative mindsets and practices as they engage their new social context in Southeast Asia.

This chapter will present ethnographic research that investigates "engaged Jainism" by analyzing the performance of "Jain-ness" as Jains navigate their urban and modern diasporic setting in Thailand. Notably, two Jain temples serve as central hubs for this diasporic community. Through interviews and participant observation both within and outside of these temple settings, this chapter describes what it means to be Jain in Thailand in the present, bearing in mind Thai Jains' historical engagements across the Indian Ocean. The perseverance of Southeast Asian Jain identity has much to teach us about how minority cultures and traditions might effectively employ strategies to ensure the survival of their culture as they engage with other cultures, such as, in this case, Thai culture. The case study presented here also illustrates the broader issue of the survival of minority traditions in diaspora, resistance to cultural hegemony, and how certain diasporic communities have managed to thrive in today's global era.

The Industry, the City, and the Community

The diamond and colored stone industry in Bangkok is a sector characterized by its dynamic nature (Scott 1994, 249–263). The industry in Bangkok has experienced significant growth since the 1980s, fueled by Thailand's economic development and favorable factors such as skilled artisans, cost-effective labor, natural resources, and government support. The Gem and Jewelry Institute of Thailand predicted a potential 10% growth in gems and jewelry exports for 2022, reaching a total export value of US $8.84 billion (Arunmas 2023). This thriving industry has attracted Jain entrepreneurs to establish and expand their businesses in Bangkok, connecting with commercial networks in the region.

The diamond and colored stone district in Bangkok spans across multiple streets and buildings within the Silom and Bang Rak districts in central Bangkok, offering a wide range of options. This location provides easy access to logistical, financial, and public amenities. In the bustling cityscape of Silom, Mahesak, and Charoen Krung, there are numerous well-known jewelry stores to explore. These stores, owned by individuals from various cultural backgrounds, play a vital role in the diverse commercial scene in the area. Every business community has its own unique specialization. For example, Gujarati Jains are known for their expertise in the diamond trade, Marwari Jains and various Muslim groups excel in dealing with colored gemstones, and the Sino-Thai community members focus on gold-related activities. From my field visits over several months in 2023, it is clear that the boundaries between different jewelry zoning areas are blurry in this context.

It is interesting to see how shops that focus on traditional jewelry like diamonds, gemstones, gold, and silver are located near stores that sell shark's teeth and ammonites. The wide variety of jewelry available in this area guarantees a steady stream of potential customers, no matter what type of jewelry is being sold.

This vast array of goods is at least in major part a consequence of the movement of individuals across borders and the establishment of diasporic cities, a phenomenon prevalent in contemporary society. The diverse ways in which individuals experience transnationality is a significant characteristic of globalization's multifaceted nature. In the case of the Jains residing in Bangkok, their individual and collective experiences of transnationality are shaped by their origins in India and their affiliation with specific religious sects. During a conversation with Sanjay Jain (interview, Oct. 23, 2023), a Marvari Jain entrepreneur specializing in colored stones, who has successfully established himself from Bikaner to Bangkok, he expressed his intention to return to Rajasthan to dedicate more time to caring for his elderly parents. Similarly, Manish Jain (interview Oct. 24, 2023), a Jain individual from Gujarat, shared with me his sentiment of having an equal preference for both Thailand and India.

During the early years of the new millennium, Backman observed that Bangkok, with its small Jain community primarily involved in the diamond trade, has expanded its presence globally to dominate diamond processing and handling. This development has positioned Bangkok as a prominent diamond center alongside traditional diamond capitals such as Antwerp, London, New York, and Tel Aviv (Backman 2005, 160–166). The intricate relationship between the city and its community in each of these places is dynamic, consisting of mutual influence and social transformation. The city, being a vibrant cultural and commercial hub, serves as a nexus where diverse nonlocal multicultural communities converge and coexist. In turn, these communities become integral components of the city's fabric, contributing to its ever-evolving nature. The Jains residing in Bangkok, regardless of their diverse origins in India, are contributing to the city's commercial sector with a distinct Jain flavor.

Thai society is often characterized as homogeneous. However, it is important to note that the emphasis on homogeneity has been consistently highlighted in official and other forms of discourse, which has resulted in the suppression of differences. It is therefore worth mentioning that multiculturalism has not been a prominent focus on Thailand's official agenda (Hayami 2006, 283–294).[1] Nevertheless, the presence of multicultural practices has been an undeniable aspect of Thailand's development, and it is therefore important to critically examine Thailand's cultural and religious diversity. In this regard, the Jain community in Bangkok, which is predominantly composed of individuals of Indian descent, offers a fascinating case study that sheds light on the continuous redefinition of the concept of the "other" in Thai society.

Jain-ness, Indian-ness, and Infusions of Thainess

The term "Jain-ness" has been previously discussed by Jain scholars as a means to describe the cognitive process of thinking in alignment with Jain principles (Rankin and Mardia 2013). Additionally, it has been used to elucidate the practical aspects of embodying Jain beliefs and living a Jain lifestyle (Rankin 2018). Previous academic discourse on the concept of Jain-ness primarily centered on its manifestation within the cultural context of India. However, Andrea Jain's research diverged from this trend by examining the construction of Jain-ness as a product of the social environment and familial background specific to Jain individuals. Additionally, her work explored the role of yoga and meditation practices in shaping the development of Jain-ness within the broader context of the contemporary religious landscape of Jainism (Jain 2014).

The topic of diasporic Jain-ness remains relatively unexplored. In my analysis, I contend that the manifestation of Jain-ness within the Thai social and political framework possesses distinct Thai characteristics. This includes the performative aspect of practicing Jainism, as well as the unique experience of being a Jain in Thailand while engaged with particular Thai cultural logics. The term "the theater state" is employed by the renowned anthropologist Clifford Geertz (1980) to elucidate the performative nature of the island of Bali, an island that exhibits distinct theatrical characteristics. In a similar vein, Peter Jackson (2004) explicitly designates Thailand as "a performative state," highlighting its inherent performance qualities. The Jain community in Bangkok demonstrates a favorable acceptance of the performative aspects of Thai national and cultural identity, strategically incorporating elements of both Jain-ness and Thainess to effectively navigate their diasporic business operations while maintaining a strong Jain identity.

For example, during my visit to the Jewelry Trade Center Thailand and my meeting with Bony, a Jain diamond entrepreneur, I observed the presence of a modest altar in his office. Positioned near the window, the altar featured a printed picture of the Jain sacred place known as Shatrunjaya Hill. Additionally, I noticed a portrait of the King of Thailand displayed on the opposite side of the office. It is worth noting that this practice of displaying such religious and national symbols is not unique to Bony, but rather a customary tradition among the Jain community in Bangkok within their business environments (Bony, interview, Sept. 13, 2023).

The manifestation of Jain-ness in a Thai environment encompasses both performative expressions and a grounded approach. The Jains residing in Bangkok endeavored to establish robust connections with the local civil society and educational institutions in Thailand's capital city. They achieved this by facilitating collaboration and support between several Thai scholars and the esteemed Jain studies organization known as the International School for Jain Studies (ISJS).

Over a span of approximately four years, from 2006 to 2010, the Jain communities in Bangkok, according to my informant Nomnian, assisted six Thai religious studies scholars (Nomnian, interview, Sept. 28, 2023). This collaborative effort resulted in an enhanced awareness and comparative understanding of Jainism among the concerned individuals (HereNow4U 2015). According to the former president of Jain Samaj Bangkok, who currently resides in Phuket, Thailand, it has been reported that following the conclusion of the ISJS summer program, a group of Thai academics successfully organized annual visits for their students to the Digambara and Śvetāmbara mandirs in Bangkok for multiple years (Jain, interview via online method, Sept. 19, 2023). The process of fostering mutual understanding between the predominantly Buddhist society in Thailand and the Jain community in Bangkok has begun, primarily driven by the efforts of the Jain community. This has resulted in the recognition of the significance of Jain beliefs and practices, particularly among Jain householders (*śrāvakas*) who are actively engaged in promoting and sharing their faith.

While the focus of this chapter is on the concept of Jain-ness within the context of Thailand, I will also examine negotiations between Jain identity and regional Gujarati identity as well as national Indian identity. This negotiation is carried out fluidly, skillfully demonstrating the coexistence of Jain-ness and Indian-ness, while simultaneously demonstrating Jains' respect for the nation's Thainess (and occasionally demonstrating their personal Thainess) as a technique to help the Jains in their business management as well as their personal lives.

Indian-ness

In the Thai context, the concept of "Indian-ness" is understood from the perspectives of both the Thai nation and the diasporic population with Indian origins. The inclusion of royal Hindu ceremonies and the assimilation of Hindu customs into daily Thai life enhance the localized interpretation of Indian-ness as experienced by the Indian diaspora, despite the fact that these two groups are typically classified differently by bureaucrats and Thais.

One can observe this situation directly at the grassroots level, through the perspectives of Thai believers and their Indian counterparts. During a conversation on the sky bridge near the renowned Erawan Brahma shrine, Geeta, an Indian woman who has lived in Bangkok for fifteen years, pointed out a noticeable similarity between Thais and Indians—the worship of Lord Ganesh, who receives an overwhelming amount of devotion from both groups (Geeta, interview, Oct. 6, 2023). However, despite the presence of certain quantifiable cultural and religious resemblances as perceived by both groups, the boundaries between Thai identity and Indian identity remain rather pronounced and distinct. During an interview conducted with a Thai brahmin at the Ganesh shrine situated on the river island of Phra Pradaeng, located at the Chao Phraya River across from Bangkok, my informant expressed their perspective on the Indian visitation practices at Thai Hindu shrines. He claims that Indians are seldom seen in Thai Hindu shrines. Interestingly, Thai devotees seem unconcerned about whether the holy location they visit is of Thai or Indian origin. In contrast, Indians prefer to keep deep connections with local Hindu temples (Anonymous Thai Hindu, interview, Sept. 3, 2023).

The Jain community in Bangkok, despite being recognized as one of the minor religious groups of Indian origin, has a dearth of official statistical information concerning its population size, as neither the Thai government nor the Jain community has provided any comprehensive data in this respect. Nevertheless, the current estimation is that there is a population of several hundred Jains residing in the vibrant city. The Jains can exhibit greater adaptability due to their community's comparatively smaller size. Their adaptability enables them to ensure that there is always some space available for the Jains, as the allocation of space is determined through cultural negotiation. This aligns with the Thai constitution, which explicitly prohibits discrimination based on religious beliefs and upholds the principle of religious freedom, as McCargo shows (2004, 155–170). Due to shared doctrinal and cultural affinities with mainstream Thai Buddhists and Indian Hindus, the Jain community in Bangkok establishes a common ground with both groups in terms of spatial negotiations. Their relatively obscure status and discreet nature have contributed to their predominantly community-based religious practices, distancing them from public religious discourses. Although Jainism is not officially recognized as one of the country's five religions, the Jain community in Bangkok has managed to find spaces within this bustling city to practice their faith nonetheless.

According to Nomnian, a former lecturer in religious studies at Mahidol University in Thailand who had engaged with the Jain community in the country, Jainism is likely to maintain a relatively limited presence in Thailand. This observation was attributed to the phenomenon of spiritual practices being simplified and commodified in the modern world, which renders the intricacies of Jain practices challenging to adhere to and comprehend (Nomnian, interview, Sept. 28, 2023). Although Jains have been involved in business activities in Bangkok for nearly thirty years, their focus in the city remains primarily on the Indian community, rather than on spreading Jain teachings and practices to a wider audience.

It is interesting to note that most Thai Buddhists have a limited understanding of Jainism, despite the shared historical background and doctrinal similarities. The difference in understanding between the two religious traditions highlights a clear distinction in how collective or individual identities are expressed. Indeed, in the city of Bangkok, a unique space has been created for Jains to establish their presence and celebrate their identity. I had the chance to observe the actions of a young Jain named Nandan Shah, which shed light on this negotiation. One day, Nandan decided to show his dedication to his faith by changing his WhatsApp status to reflect the Āyambil Oḷī, a Jain external austerity focused on practicing self-control over one's taste (Shah, interview, Oct. 5, 2023). This status update also emphasized the unique attire of the Jains, particularly the dhoti worn by males during their rituals. Nandan's actions were intended to inspire other Jains to wholeheartedly embrace their religion, culture, and beliefs. In addition, his focus on his Indian heritage highlights the unique nature of Jainism within the broader religious landscape of Bangkok.

Infusions of Thainess

The nuanced and impactful manner in which Thai culture has been disseminated, as well as its capacity to incorporate individuals with diverse physical characteristics, has garnered significant interest in past scholarship. Traitongyoo argues that the idea of Thainess has been purposefully managed to enhance the ethnic homogeneity of Thailand as a modern nation-state (Traitongyoo 2008). This assertion aligns with Winichakul's contention that the primary outcome of Thainess is the formation of a sense of "otherness" toward those considered not Thai within Thai society. When analyzing social identity in Thailand, it is therefore imperative to consider the concept of Thainess. The dichotomous mindset of "us versus them" operates through two distinct mechanisms: negative identification and identification. Negative identification pertains to the clear manifestation of Thainess when distinguishing otherness or un-Thainess. On the other hand, identification involves the deliberate selection of certain elements or norms to define Thainess, as Winichakul further elaborates (2013, 575–91).

The concept of Thainess was closely linked to the integration of the Chinese community into Thai society during the rise of Thai nationalism in the 1940s. Thai nationalists viewed Thainess as a desirable attribute that Thais should protect and foster, considering it as a positive form of nationalism (ibid.). Over time, the concept of Thainess has progressively expanded its scope to include not just the Chinese community but also other ethnic groups, including the Indian—and Jain—population under consideration.

According to Connors (2005), there has indeed been a shift in the concept of Thainess since the 1980s as it has been used to identify local cultures, diverse ethnic identities, and national identity to construct a concept of Thainess that is applicable in the global era. In the present-day environment, particularly following a significant surge in Thai nationalism during the initial decades of the twentieth century, the nationalistic sentiments associated with the concept of Thainess have gradually diminished, rendering its racial significance rather insignificant (Basham 2001, 107–136). The notion of Thainness is primarily seen as a social construct within the social and cultural settings of Thailand. The condition originates from the need to represent Thai identity in the face of global demands that are not Thai in nature, as shown by the modern concept of Thainess in Thailand. The prevailing Thai dominance in daily cultural activities defines the limits of Thainess mainly via the concepts of "royal nationalism" and "Buddhist nationalism" (Keyes and Shigeharu 2013). The essence of Thainess is manifested via the expression of Thainess within the context of the nation's principles of "Nation, Religion, King." Whether individuals or groups are Thai citizens or not, it has been customary for them to display their own interpretation of Thainess.

Soi Phuttha Osot's "Khaek" Feature and the Presence of Jain Mandirs

> Think of a city and what comes to mind? Its streets.
>
> —Jacobs 1961, 39

The needs of various modes of transportation, such as walking, riding, and standing, have historically been met by the design of streets. The general public favors streets that are conducive to these kinds of uses. In multicultural urbanity, streets are also places where people of various cultural origins can meet and interact with one another. People's intimate and formative experiences on the streets every day have the potential to help them overcome the social barriers that keep them apart (Knapp 2009). Whether viewed through the lens of modernism, which sees streets as something "from which to get from A to B, rather than a place to live in," or through the lens of postmodernism, which sees streets as places meant to foster and complement new urban lifestyles, streets are the terrain of social encounters, sites of domination and resistance, places of pleasure and anxiety (Fyfe 2006).

The alley called Soi Phuttha Osot (see figure 5.1) is one such place situated in the bustling Bang Rak district of Bangkok, providing easy access to the city's Silom Business area and the diamond and jewelry district. The alley ("soi" means alley in Thai), I observed, is incredibly diverse, always adapting to the

Figure 5.1. The location of Soi Phuttha Osot in Bangkok. *Source:* Imagery © 2024 Airbus, CNES / Airbus, Maxar Technologies, Map data © 2024; Google Maps 2024.

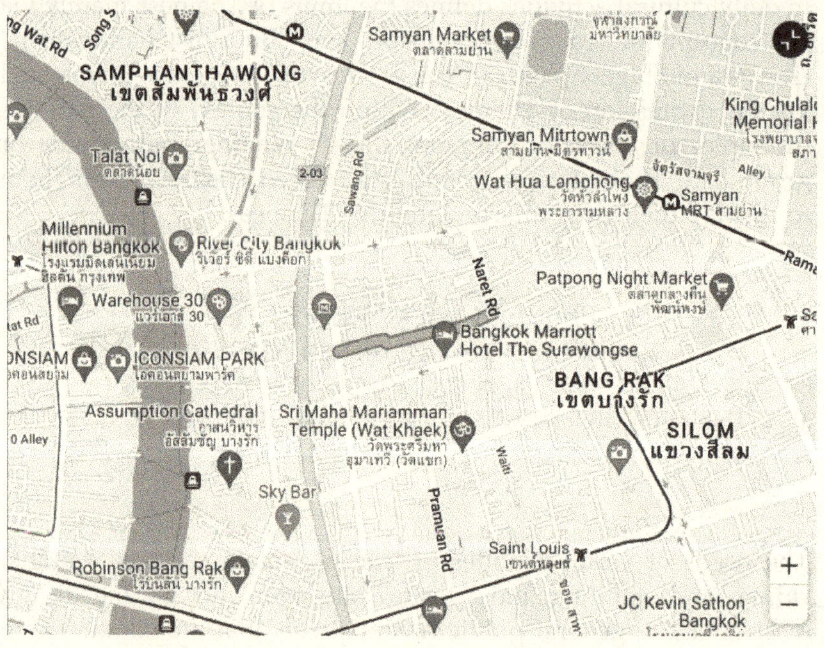

ever-changing mix of cultural elements. After spending more than a month in this lane, I have gained a deep understanding of the diverse multicultural environment here, especially with the two Jain temples.

It is important to note that Jains were the pioneers from South Asia who first selected this alley as the foundation for their homes and businesses. In an interview with Hitesh Jain (Jan. 13, 2024), a longstanding member of the Jain community in Singapore, he mentioned that during his visit to Bangkok in 1990, he observed that the Jain community had already integrated seamlessly into the alley and the surrounding lanes. The neighborhood in Soi Phuttha Osot, today predominantly inhabited by the Sino-Thai population in Bangkok, has gradually acquired a multicultural character over time.

Indeed, religious and ethnic groups abound on Soi Puttha Osot. Bangkok's Bangkok Mosque, Assumption Cathedral, Holy Rosary Church, Haroon Mosque, and Sri Maha Mariamman Temple are in the alley along Mahesak Road. The lane is home to Jains, Thais, Sino-Thais, Hindus, and Muslims. Jains and Myanmar Nepalese Hindus feed local Hindus and Jains. Asians rent from Sino-Thais, while Muslims dwell near the mosque. People of various religions worship and perform daily rituals in the lane, wearing their traditional garb.

Soi Phuttha Osot is widely recognized in metropolitan Bangkok as a prominent location with a significant South Asian demographic and cultural influence. This perception is shared not only by the Thai population but also by other South Asian individuals who have selected Bangkok as a destination for their professional and personal growth.

The coexistence of two Jain temples in the Soi Phuttha Osot region of Bangkok might be attributed to deliberate spatial negotiation rather than being a random occurrence. The presence of South Asian characteristics in Soi Phuttha Osot serves as a means to comprehend the cultural and religious manifestations of Jainism within the area. Jains, among other foreigners engaging the Thai cultural landscape in the area, comprise "Khaek" in the Thai language, which is defined in a mainstream Thai language dictionary as denoting both a "guest" and a "foreigner." The term possesses an ethnic connotation about individuals of Indian descent, occasionally misidentified by ethnic Thais as Nepalis, Bangladeshis, Pakistanis, Sri Lankans, and other South Asian populations (McDaniel 2013, 191–209).[2]

To provide a deeper understanding, it is worth noting that the Hindu shrines found throughout Bangkok, and potentially across Thailand, prominently display images of Brahmā and Indra, etc. These shrines, with Thai characteristics, are generally perceived as representative of the Thai identity rather than the Khaek identity. Conversely, Hindu shrines located in areas inhabited by individuals of South Asian descent are typically categorized as Khaek shrines. The alley currently serves as a residence for many South Asian communities, which is evident in its South Asian characteristics. This remains true despite the demographic shifts in ethnic and religious groups, particularly as perceived by the Thai population.

Jain and Jay discuss the collective construction of Indianness within Indian diasporic households, wherein parents play a significant role, but children have the potential to organically assimilate some aspects of Indian culture to a certain degree (Jain and Jay 1997, 873). The term "Indian culture" refers to a broad and inclusive concept that encompasses both the Jain and the Hindu religious cultures. The Jain community, as a collective, identifies strongly with their Indian heritage, which is an integral part of their Jain identity. Due to the fact that the majority of Jains are Indians, their cultural self-identification is primarily associated with being Indian. The Jains often participate in various Indian cultural activities, which serves as a way for them to establish their presence within Indian communities. This allows the Jains to showcase their affinity with the Hindus, though it is uncommon to see Hindus embracing Jain beliefs and principles.

Nevertheless, Jains have also deliberately chosen to reside in close proximity to one another, often on the same street and lanes or in the same buildings, in order to visibly or discreetly manifest their distinct Jain-ness. Thus, even as they showcase their affinity with Hindus and the Indian community in general, Jains have also established their own religious institutions, engaged in religious activities, and developed their uniquely Jain identity.

The establishment and evolution of an alley's culture and milieu have been shaped by previous and current residents. South Asian culinary influences began to appear in Soi Phuttha Osot gradually as Jain, Hindu, and Muslim residents worked to build a cultural ambiance in the alley. Due of its popularity with South Asians, the alley has taken on South Asian tastes. The South Asian community utilized the alley to preserve and exhibit their cuisine and culture. For instance, the Myanmar Nepalese Hindus play a significant role in the provision of vegetarian meals to the alley community. Additionally, they cater to the dietary needs of Jains by offering Jain-friendly menus. The two remaining vegetarian restaurants in the alley are also highly favored by Jain entrepreneurs and professionals, who regularly patronize these establishments during weekdays.

It is noteworthy that despite a significant number of Jains relocating from Soi Phuttha Osot to Sathu Pradit Soi 19 (Sathu Pradit Road Alley No. 19) to reside in close proximity to fellow Jains and improve their overall quality of life over the past decade, these restaurants have managed to maintain their popularity. The same holds for grocery stores in South Asia that are under the ownership of Hindu diasporas from the Indian and the Myanmar Nepalese population. The tapestry of South Asian cultural characteristics is intricately interwoven into the fabric of this lane, reflecting the diverse cultural details and connections that enrich the lives of its inhabitants.

Virang, a Jain entrepreneur residing in the Sathorn neighborhood of Bangkok, frequently commutes to a vegetarian restaurant called Shree Ganesh using his recently acquired motorcycle, accompanied by his Hindu colleagues from the workplace. During the period when I resided near the eatery, I would often visit during the midday hours to observe the restaurant's patrons. It became clear to me that this establishment is favored by young Jain entrepreneurs, such as Virang, who seek an environment conducive to partaking in vegetarian meals during lunchtime (Virang, interview, Sept. 20, 2023).

Through my observations, I was able to witness not only the existence of Jain camaraderie but also the profound interconnectedness between the Jains and Hindus, particularly those who share a common Gujarati heritage. As a multicultural setting, the process of negotiating and engaging space and place within the alley of Soi Phuttha Osot involves the Jains, among other residents and users of the alley, mutually influencing and shaping one another while nevertheless sharing common cultural attributes such as language. In Chan's work, he posits that intercultural understanding is best achieved through venues that encourage the critical examination and deconstruction of preconceived notions within a secure and impartial environment (Chan 2013, 149). While it is true that many Jains no longer see Soi Phuttha Osot as their primary place of residence, the alley continues to serve as such a site of cross-cultural engagement.

This phenomenon reveals an intriguing story of a vibrant process of change happening within this cultural environment, wherein the alley itself is currently undergoing a continuous process of transformation. In the wider area surrounding the alley, there is a noticeable shift toward embracing Islamic influences due to the fact that the alley and its extended areas have experienced a notable increase in the number of South Asians, especially those from the Muslim community. A significant number of people with Pakistani, Bangladeshi, and Indian backgrounds have opted to make this area their home. During the ceremonial inauguration of the Thai-Pakistan Friendship Mosque on October 29, 2023, near Soi Phuttha Osot, I observed that the event attracted a considerable amount of attention from different Muslim communities, including the Thai Muslim community, African Muslim community, and South Asian Muslim community. The varied participation added to the increasing Islamic influence in the alley as the ceremony unfolded.

In the face of coexisting with different societal norms, followers of Jainism in Bangkok display an impressive ability to uphold their devout lifestyles by employing a variety of strategies to navigate the dominant cultural environment they find themselves in, including creating new arenas of Jain influence. By preserving the old site of the Jain community centered around the two temples in the alley, we witness a demonstration of cultural change within the alley. Nevertheless, with the growing impact of Islamic culture and lifestyles in the area, many Jains made the decision to move south and form a new community with other Jains who share their beliefs. As old Jain places remain, new Jain sites are also coming into existence.

Reconstructing Jain-ness: Sathu Pradit Soi 19 as a New Jain Arena

When our focus shifts toward Sathu Pradit Soi 19 (Sathu Pradit Road Alley No. 19), alternatively referred to as Naradhiwas Soi

24 (Naradhiwas Road Alley No. 24), situated in proximity to the southern periphery of the urban landscape, we encounter a thoroughfare characterized by towering contemporary apartment complexes, globally oriented educational institutions, and dining establishments offering diverse culinary experiences.

Although the Śvetāmbara and Digambara temples in Soi Phuttha Osot continue to exist, the focal point of Jain activities is gradually relocating to Sathu Pradit Soi 19. This shift is driven by the desire to cater to the convenience requirements of the majority of Jain community members who reside in this area, as opposed to other locations within the city. Here we also need to pay attention to the Śvetāmbara Jains as the majority group of Jains in Bangkok, who have the majority voice in Bangkok's Jain community. Together, the Śvetāmbara and Digambara Jain communities established the Thai Jain Association (TJA) as a collaborative effort, though due to the significant numerical disparity between the two groups, the association is primarily led and represented by the Śvetāmbara Jains, making their presence more prominent in the association's name and activities.

The annual Paryuṣaṇa / Daśalakṣaṇa ceremony is commemorated in Bangkok by both the Śvetāmbara and Digambara Jain groups to foster communal cohesion. Although they share similar concepts of seeking forgiveness, they have different commencement dates. The celebration of the Śvetāmbara Jains took place on the premises of the Sino-Thai Pow Leng Association of Thailand (Lǔ xiān pǔníng tóngxiāng huì), which is situated near Sathu Pradit Soi 19 (see figure 5.2). The event's location is strategically positioned in close proximity, facilitating convenient pedestrian access for attendees.

The TJA took charge of the elaborate celebrations that spanned over a duration of eight days in early September 2023, as well as in previous years. In the year 2023, the Śvetāmbara Jain Paryuṣaṇa witnessed a noteworthy gathering at the main hall of the Phow Leng Association, with an impressive participation of over four hundred individuals. The venue experienced a state of full occupancy with more than 250 people, indicating a significant gathering of individuals belonging to the Śvetāmbara Jain community. Both male and female members, along with their children, were observed to be actively participating in the event. In a contrasting scenario, the corresponding Digambara event took place within the premises of the Digambara Jain mandir only, with

Figure 5.2. The location of Sathu Pradit 19 in Bangkok. *Source:* Imagery © 2024 Airbus, CNES / Airbus, Maxar Technologies, Map data © 2024; Google Maps 2024.

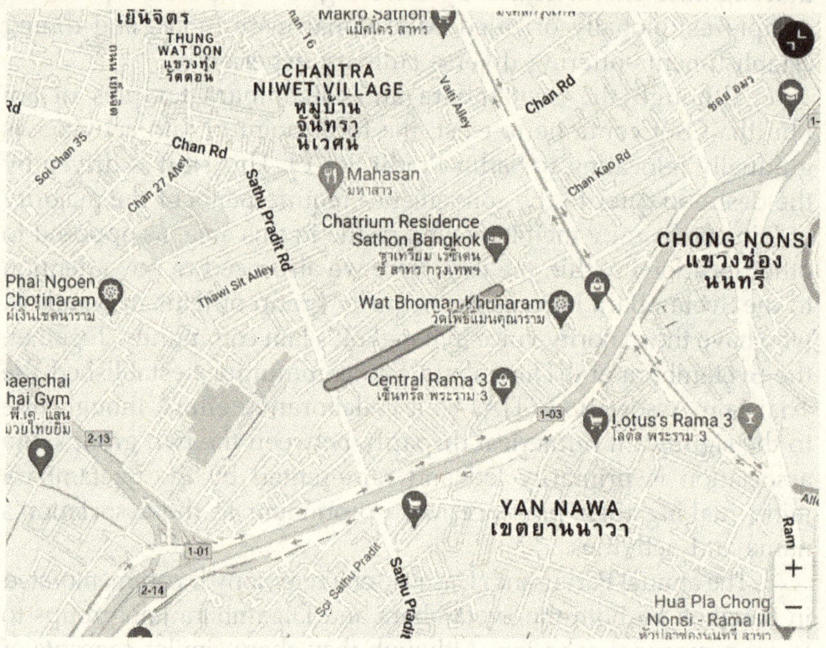

a significantly smaller number of community members. Notably, this occurred immediately after the conclusion of the Śvetāmbara Paryuṣaṇa, without the involvement of the Thai Jain Association as the organizing entity for the event.

The emergence of Sathu Pradit Soi 19 as a prominent location for the Jains in Bangkok signifies the potential for the alley to become the primary hub of Jain culture in this bustling metropolis. This alley indeed holds great significance as a space for the current expression of "Jain-ness" within the city. The story of the Jains and their relationship with this alley also serves as a noteworthy illustration of their dedication to fostering connections within their community, as well as a sign of their commitment to maintaining active engagement in broader cultural spheres in Bangkok. Moreover, it highlights their commitment to simultaneously preserving and upholding their unique Jain identity.

Conclusion

This examination of Jainism has provided a particular portrait of the development of contemporary Jainism in urban Bangkok, where Jains engage with multicultural communities even as they maintain a strong commitment to their own religious tradition. The Jains residing in Bangkok demonstrate a remarkable ability to navigate the intricate social and cultural dynamics of their environment, adeptly negotiating the interplay between the formation of personal identity and self-expression, while also skillfully managing the simultaneous phenomena of globalization and localization. This chapter has primarily focused on the grassroots level, reporting fieldwork observations to provide readers with a view into the intricate aspects of everyday Jain practice as the community continues to engage contemporary urban Bangkok.

Notes

1. Hayami's assertion regarding the growing recognition of diversity within the nation, particularly in the context of bettering the state's relationship with minority groups in the North, supports the argument that diasporic communities may exhibit greater flexibility and adaptability in their cultural and religious practices in the country's only mega city of Bangkok (see Hayami 2006).

2. "Khaek," as highlighted by McDaniel 2013, pertains to ethnicity rather than religion.

References

Anonymous Thai Hindu priest. Interview by Samut Prakan, author, at the island of Phra Pradaeng, September 3, 2023.

Arunmas. "Exports of Jewelry, Gems Set to Grow by 10%." *Bangkok Post*, August 9, 2023. https://www.bangkokpost.com/business/general/2625933.

Backman, Michael. 2005. "Diamonds, Jains, and Jews." *Inside Knowledge: Streetwise in Asia*. Palgrave Macmillan.

Basham, Richard. 2001. "Ethnicity and World View in Bangkok." In *Alternate Identities*. Brill. https://doi.org/10.1163/9789004488526_009.

Bony, interviewed by Samut Prakan, author, Bangkok, September 13, 2023.

Chan, Felicity Hwee-Hwa. 2013. "Spaces of Negotiation and Engagement in Multi-ethnic Ethnoscapes: The 'Cambodia Town Neighborhood' in Central Long Beach, California." In *Transcultural Cities: Border-Crossing and Placemaking*, edited by Jeffrey Hou, 319–334. Routledge.

Connors, Michael. 2005. "Ministering Culture: Hegemony and the Politics of Culture and Identity in Thailand." *Critical Asian Studies* 37 (4).

Fyfe, Nicholas. 2006. *Images of the Street: Planning, Identity, and Control in Public Space*. Routledge.

Geertz, Clifford. 1980. *Negara*. Princeton University Press.

Geeta. Interview by Samut Prakan, author, Bangkok, October 6, 2023.

Hayami, Yoko. 2006. "Introduction: Notes Towards Debating Multiculturalism in Thailand and Beyond." *Japanese Journal of Southeast Asian Studies* 44 (3): 283–294.

HereNow4U. 2015. Jain Summer School in India @ HERENOW4U. https://www.herenow4u.net/index.php?id=72686.

Jackson, Peter A. 2004. "The Performative State: Semi-Coloniality and the Tyranny of Images in Modern Thailand." *SOJOURN: Journal of Social Issues in Southeast Asia* 19 (2): 219–253.

Jacobs, Jane. 2020. "'The Uses of Sidewalks: Safety': From The Death and Life of Great American Cities (1961)." In *The City Reader*. Routledge.

Jain, Andrea. 2014. *Selling Yoga: From Counterculture to Pop Culture*. Oxford University Press.

Jain, Anju, and Jay Belsky. 1997. "Fathering and Acculturation: Immigrant Indian Families with Young Children." *Journal of Marriage and the Family* 59 (4): 873. https://doi.org/10.2307/353789.

Jain, Hitesh. Interview by Samut Prakan, author, Singapore, January 13, 2024.

Jain, Pramod. Interview by Samut Prakan, author, Bangkok (via online method), September 19, 2023.

Jain, Manish. Interview by Samut Prakan, author, Bangkok, October 24, 2023.

Jain, Sanjay. Interview by Samut Prakan, author, Bangkok, October 23, 2023.

Keyes, Charles F., and Shigeharu Tanabe. 2013. *Cultural Crisis and Social Memory: Modernity and Identity in Thailand and Laos*. Routledge.

Knapp, C. 2009. "Making Multicultural Places." *Project For Public Spaces* (PPS). http://www. pps. org/multicultural_places.

McCargo, Duncan. 2004. "Buddhism, Democracy and Identity in Thailand." *Democratization* 11 (4): 155–170.

McDaniel, Justin. 2013. "This Hindu Holy Man Is a Thai Buddhist." *South East Asia Research* 21, no. 2 (June): 191–209. https://doi.org/10.5367/sear.2013.0151.

Nomnian, Archphurich. Interview by author, Bangkok, September 28, 2023.

Rankin, Aidan. 2018. *Jainism and Environmental Philosophy: Karma and the Web of Life*. Routledge.

Rankin, Aidan D., and Kanti V. Mardia. 2013. *Living Jainism: An Ethical Science*. John Hunt Publishing.

Scott, Allen J. 1994. "Variations on the Theme of Agglomeration and Growth: The Gem and Jewelry Industry in Los Angeles and Bangkok." *Geoforum: Journal of Physical, Human, and Regional Geosciences* 25, no. 3 (August): 249–263. https://doi.org/10.1016/0016-7185(94)90030-2.

Shah, Nandan. Interview by author, Bangkok, October 5, 2023.

Traitongyoo, Krongkwan. 2008. *The Management of Irregular Migration in Thailand: Thainess, Identity and Citizenship*. PhD diss., University of Leeds.

Virang, Mehta. Interview by author, Bangkok, September 20, 2023.

Winichakul, Thongchai. 2008. "Nationalism and the Radical Intelligentsia in Thailand." *Third World Quarterly* 29, no. 3 (April): 575–591. https://doi.org/10.1080/01436590801931520.

Part III

Engaging with Business and Economy

6

Engaging Jain Ideas

Interdisciplinary Business Ethics Education

BENJAMIN ZENK

Business is the most popular postsecondary degree field in the United States by an increasingly large margin. In the 2020–2021 academic year, nearly one in five bachelor's degrees conferred in the United States were business degrees (US Department of Education n.d.). During the same period, nearly one in four of all master's degrees conferred in the US were business degrees (ibid.). Furthermore, according to the US Census Bureau, around one in three adults twenty-five and older in the United States had attained a bachelor's degree or master's degree by 2021 (US Census Bureau, n.d.). Each of these rates is growing. Business curricula are thus reaching a wider and wider audience in the United States, and likely around the world. As enrollment grows, one can expect that business curricula will have increasing influence locally, nationally, and globally.

Due to this influence, deficiencies of any kind in business school curricula are *very* likely to negatively affect the world at large. This puts the disseminators of these ever more popular curricula—universities, educators, publishers, accrediting bodies, etc.—in positions of consequence with respect to the urgent needs of humanity and the planet. As a faculty member in a college of business myself who teaches business ethics, I feel a particular urgency here. As a scholar of philosophy working with texts and concepts from the Jain tradition as well, I am interested in how engaging ideas from the Jain tradition with business education may constructively contribute to business curricula globally.

This chapter is motivated by these complementary impulses that culminate in a concern that holistic philosophical reflection is too often and too readily dispensed with in pedagogical practice in a business curriculum, particularly in business ethics curricula where the prominence of such reflection might be expected. Its aim is not to prescribe an alternative approach to business ethics education. Rather, it is to inquire into the conditions of an appropriately holistic and philosophical approach to such education and along the way to show that the Jain tradition offers philosophical resources that are uniquely poised to meet many of these conditions. The first section explores possible causes for a dearth of philosophical content in business ethics curricula and research and argues for a renewed focus on philosophical inquiry in this area. To this end, it revisits Donaldson and Preston's categorization of approaches to business ethics research as descriptive, instrumental, and normative, and offers an expanded and modified account of that categorization to emphasize the centrality of a philosophical approach. The second section explores how these revised categories might relate to educational practice, arguing that a philosophico-religious curriculum is particularly suited to supplementing the shortcomings of instrumental, descriptive, and prescriptive approaches to business ethics education. The third section explores resources from the Jain tradition insofar as they support a holistic, philosophical approach to business ethics education. The final section offers reflection on the goals of business education and the urgency of our need to critique them systematically.

Approaches to Business Ethics Research

Business ethics research is often subjected to extremely practical expectations. This in itself is not a bad thing. However, if the "practical" is pursued without reflexive questioning—without genuine meta-ethical dialogue about the origin and nature of value, without an authentic normative inquiry into appropriate criteria for good work, etc.—then the supposedly "practical" is woefully inadequate to guide a curriculum, especially one as massively influential as that of the various business disciplines.[1]

Unfortunately, popular writing in business ethics can be shortsighted in just these ways. Authors often instrumentalize the ideas and arguments they explicate. One can see this in many titles of popular work in business ethics. Articles from *Forbes* magazine include "Harnessing the Power of Diversity for Profitability" (Adams 2017) and "Doing the Right Thing Is Just Profitable" (Georgescu 2017). Each of these takes for granted what it means to do the right thing and that the primary justification for doing it is not found in normative premises, but in instrumental ones: It is profitable to be ethical. The wonderfully organized but likewise normatively deficient *Business Ethics* textbook from the well-known OER publisher OpenStax has an opening chapter titled "Why Ethics Matters." The only reasons given in this chapter for why ethics matters are that it "permits us to sleep well at night," that it will "engender trust among those with whom we interact," and that "customers, clients, employees, and society at large will much more willingly patronize a business and work hard on its behalf if that business is perceived as caring about the community it serves" (Byars et al. 2018). That is, we should be ethical because it will lead to higher self-esteem, improved reputation, and increased profitability. The rest of the chapter seems to confuse claims about what is presumably ethical with claims about why ethics matters. The arguments offered are nearly completely devoid of philosophical reflection and embody a problematic level of instrumentalism and prescription. Given how influential business curricula are, to the extent that such short-sightedness characterizes popular literature on business ethics, the same short-sightedness will likely be reflected in student learning.

In an article titled "History and Philosophy of Management at the University of Johannesburg: A New Direction for the Department of Business Management," strategic management scholar Professor Geoff Goldman suggests that his colleagues already recognize such pedagogical problems in the teaching strategies common to their disciplines. He observes that faculty lament a lack of appreciation for alternative methodologies, a forgetfulness of the philosophical underpinnings of disciplinary ideas, and a lack of incentive to engage in philosophical inquiry (Goldman 2009, 38).[2] Goldman concludes, "At the end of the day we want graduates who think innovatively, holistically, can see the outcomes of their decisions, who constantly question and challenge convention. We firmly believe that the ability to reason philosophically is a crucial ingredient in shaping the graduates that we want to produce" (ibid., 41). These shortcomings, according to Goldman, suggest that the curriculum is missing philosophical depth, and that our goal should be to remedy this by reinserting philosophy into the business management curriculum.

Indeed, what seems to be missing in academic work in business disciplines is an attention to philosophical foundations. It is missing meta-ethical inquiry—a direct and authoritative consideration of the nature, foundations, and scope of issues in these fields. It is also missing normative inquiry—an open-ended inquiry into the possible criteria for correct moral action in these fields. This may have something to do as well with a shift in hiring practices in business schools. As Jeffrey Moriarty has put it in his article "Business Ethics" in the *Stanford Encyclopedia of Philosophy*, "Business schools have hired psychologists to understand why people engage in unethical behavior and strategists to explore whether ethics pays." Moriarty adds that while considerations of the psychological motivations and strategic dimensions of ethics are interesting, they are "no substitute for normative reflection on what *is* ethical or unethical in business" (Moriarty 2021). I would add that they are no substitute either for normative reflection on what *is* ethical or unethical, full stop. No amount of information regarding the how or why of professionals' behavior will ever reveal whether that behavior is right. To explore that question, philosophical reflection is indispensable.

In their classic, seminal analysis of stakeholder theory, "The Stakeholder Theory of the Corporation: Concepts, Evidence, and Implications," Thomas Donaldson and Lee Preston (1995) argue that approaches to business ethics and stakeholder management in academic literature had split into at least three prominent approaches by the mid-1990s. They labeled these approaches "descriptive," "instrumental," and "normative." This widely cited categorization is extremely useful, since it allows the authors to bring into parsimonious focus exactly why certain approaches are insufficient.

They first explain that some research employs stakeholder theory "to describe, and sometimes to explain, specific corporate characteristics and behaviors" (ibid., 70). That is, some research simply describes what businesses do. This is the descriptive approach.

They then observe that other research employs the theory "to identify the connections, or lack of connections, between stakeholder management and the achievement of traditional corporate objectives (e.g., profitability, growth)" (ibid., 71). That is, some research considers whether and how the employment of stakeholder theory is instrumental to profit. This is what they have called the instrumental approach.

Finally, they point out that still other research employs stakeholder theory "to interpret the function of the corporation, including the identification of moral or philosophical guidelines for the operation and management of corporations" (ibid.). That is, some research attempts to justify stakeholder theory ethically. This is what they have termed the normative approach.

Their categorization helpfully frames the observation that normative justification is foundational to descriptive and instrumentalist accounts of stakeholder management and sound ethical reasoning more generally. However, there are two problems with this. The first is that the term "normative" in this categorization is a somewhat imprecise catch-all, given that meta-ethical, normative, and prescriptive or applied considerations seem to be included in it. The terms "ethical" or "moral" would perhaps be more suitably general. The second and closely related issue is that the normative category itself conflates at least two distinct separate aspects of business ethical scholarship: the prescriptive and the philosophical. Thus, I suggest that for the sake of exhaustiveness and conceptual consistency, we expand Donaldson and Preston's "normative" to two categories, the "prescriptive" and the "philosophical." This leads to a fourfold division:

1. Descriptive
2. Instrumental
3. Prescriptive
4. Philosophical

As hinted at in the newly proposed categories, some research justifies and *prescribes* a certain interpretation of stakeholder theory. This can be called the "prescriptive" approach and captures much but not all of what Donaldson and Preston seem to have signified with "normative." There is a distinct approach to business ethical scholarship that is not identical to the prescriptive but is also suggested by their explanation of the "normative." Some research is focused on open-ended *philosophical* ethical inquiry. It is inquisitive rather than prescriptive, but is nonetheless ethical in its orientation, finding and posing ethical questions rather than justifying and prescribing specific solutions. This can be called the "philosophical" approach. It is common in both research and teaching, and yet is not perfectly captured by Donaldson and Preston's threefold idea.

This modified categorization can be extended in yet another way, as has just been foreshadowed. While Donaldson and Preston's analysis is interested in how normative aspects of business ethics research underpin the descriptive and instrumental aspects, one can just as easily understand the prescriptive and philosophical as forming the basis for a plurality of approaches to teaching ethics. That is, in addition to business ethics scholarship, business ethics teaching can easily be considered to employ some combination of descriptive, instrumental, prescriptive, or philosophical approaches. Let's take a moment to substantiate what it would mean to teach business ethics in each of these four ways.

Approaches to Business Ethics Education

Business ethics education is approached descriptively to the extent that it describes or explains corporate or professional behavior. Whether in the form of case studies illustrating presumably good or bad behavior, or in the presentation and explanation of industry standards for business activity such as the Principles of Responsible Investment (PRI) in finance, Generally Accepted Accounting Principles (GAAP) in accounting, or International Organization for Standardization (ISO) standards more broadly, descriptive approaches explain what is presumably best for professionals and institutions to do without openly exploring whether and why they should do it. To designate an approach as descriptive is to point out that it fails to explore *why* certain values or behaviors should or should not be adopted beyond presumed self-evident considerations. It does not directly address questions of the nature or scope of ethical behavior or the criteria that may properly govern such behavior.

To educate students ethically along descriptive lines, and only those lines, is to commit oneself, and to commit one's students, to a version of the naturalistic fallacy in ethics. The naturalistic fallacy, similar in nature to Hume's Law, but distinctly put in the work of G. E. Moore, is the failure to recognize that "purely factual premises about the naturalistic features of things do not entail or even support evaluative conclusions" (Ridge 2019). Educators and students alike should recognize that the mere fact that someone or some firm *does* behave a certain way does not itself entail that they *should* behave in that way. To make that case, normative and meta-ethical inquiry and argument is necessary.

Business ethics education might also take an instrumental approach. An approach is instrumental to the extent that it utilizes descriptive data to make observations regarding the profitability of certain activities or frameworks in corporate management. Management research firm McKinsey and Company's diversity reports are prominent examples of tools that enable and express an instrumental approach. In their 2020 report on diversity, for example, it is observed that the "business case [for diversity in corporations] continues to strengthen. The most diverse companies are now more likely than ever to outperform less diverse peers on profitability" (McKinsey and Co. 2020). The business case is nothing other than the instrumental case. This is the prominent justification offered in the textbook mentioned above (Byars et al. 2018). Such an approach draws connections between presumably ethical activity and profitability, among other things.

Interestingly, McKinsey and Co. is the subject of a troubling and scathing critique on the satirical and comedic HBO series *Last Week Tonight with John Oliver* (Oliver 2023). In a 2023 episode, writers on the show highlighted the logical consequence of treating the "business case" as sufficient justification for a company's activity. One example offered is that McKinsey and Co. devised management strategies for Purdue Pharma to effectively get FDA approval of a new version of OxyContin, also recommending that the company turbocharge its sales of this drug. In a bizarre twist, McKinsey and Co. has also worked with the FDA (Hamby and Forsythe 2022). This suggests that they may have been in effect promoting the safe use of opioids and promoting their rampant over-distribution at the same time.

The theoretical problem with the business case is that it fails to directly justify *good* practice. Instead, it justifies any mode of practice that *works* to the end of profitability. In other words, the problem with an instrumentalist approach is that if the case for being ethical is that it is profitable, then when it is not profitable to be ethical, being ethical is no longer justified.

Furthermore, specific frameworks and methods for ethical decision-making tend to obscure their own traditional nature, their nature as having developed out of or having been inherited by way of an academic tradition. Neglecting this, one will be inclined to treat these methods as inherently objective and therefore superior to cross-cultural and indigenous ways of being, doing, and thinking, which are by contrast seen as traditional and subjective. A convincing and lasting approach requires a more sophisticated, normative, and meta-ethical analysis as well as access to insights beyond the inherited walls of one's discipline and culture.

A prescriptive approach to business ethics education goes a step further than the descriptive and instrumental approaches in terms of justification. It argues that for philosophically and normatively considered reasons, a certain business ethic is ideal. As an approach, this avoids the theoretical pitfalls of descriptive and instrumental approaches—committing the naturalistic fallacy in the case of the descriptive approach and a failure to establish any particular ethical theory in the case of the instrumental approach—but it retains its own pedagogical problem: Even a normatively defended prescription for business students and professionals to act in a particular way is problematic, since it offers merely one ethical dogma in the context of a slew of mutually incompatible but justifiable alternatives. One might consider this a version of the informal fallacy called "stacking the deck." In other words, in attempting to justify its own prescription, it will tend to eschew alternative accounts, even though those accounts may be just as plausible. To be sure, there may be some definite benefits to students learning a particular set of justified moral values—a consistent message, a teacher who exemplifies the values they preach, etc.—but the major drawback to this is that such prescriptions are pedagogically limited. They stack the deck against other justifiable approaches.

A thoroughly philosophical approach to teaching ethics in business is necessary to remedy the shortcomings of the other three approaches, and it is the necessary basis for those approaches. A philosophical approach widens the scope of ethical consideration by asking about the nature, limits, possible frameworks, and application of ethical ideas without the trappings of any particular jargon or preconceived goal. It embraces myriad controversies at the foundations of ethics, unlike the other approaches. A philosophical approach also foregrounds reflexive critique. It is thus open to challenging other approaches directly, pointing out fallacies at work in prescriptive, instrumental, and descriptive approaches. It asks whether ethics can be meaningfully explored at all. It promises to be less alienating than the other approaches to students of distinct and perhaps disagreeing traditions, in the end more compelling to students harboring skepticism about business ethics as usual. A philosophical approach will furthermore contextualize business ethical reflection in a context that is interdisciplinary in nature.

And yet, there are limitations to a philosophical approach in business ethics education. For example, there is rarely enough time in a semester or other course term to teach *systems* of ethics, unless dogmatically. Normative ethics is also predominantly anthropocentric (Brennan and Lo 2022). One must drift far from the mainstream in normative ethics to encounter ecocentric, biocentric, or land-centric ethics that challenge the status quo. Also, a focus on theory in philosophical ethics can seem overly abstract. An emphasis on abstract universals in ethical theorizing can result in a general disregard of human limitations and this can confound the practically-minded. As Mary Midgley (1996, 119) puts it in the case of business ethics, "Discussions of moral theory seem to look upwards, right away from the facts, at remote ideals, calling for a clarity and inflexibility which may well seem unattainable." Finally, philosophical, ethics-oriented education does not exhaust the interdisciplinary basis for ethical and cognitive reflection, which requires ontological, epistemological, hermeneutical, and other foundational inquiry, not to say anything of disciplines apart from philosophical subfields and even cross-cultural insights.

To this last point, business ethics education is naturally interdisciplinary. Outcomes of any inquiry into ethical and reliable thinking can apply across multiple fields—e.g., psychology, law, medicine, cosmology, axiology, anthropology, sociology, rhetoric, and mathematics. The foundations of business ethics education thus should be sufficiently broad to address this scope of application. Ultimately, business ethics education should address the question of what we are thinking *for*. Is the goal of ethical and cognitive inquiry *understanding* for its own sake? Are we thinking merely to develop tools for us to reach profitability goals, which are themselves not subject to scrutiny? There are limits in place for the descriptively, instrumentally, and prescriptively oriented business curriculum. We should eschew such limitations. In doing so, we will need to engage in philosophical ethical inquiry, asking foundational questions regarding who and how we ought to be. An earnest holistic consideration of such questions will lead us to hermeneutical questions regarding the nature and limits of understanding as well as to ontological questions regarding the nature of ourselves and our existence. In what remains of this chapter, I argue that the Jain philosophical tradition contains resources that can be employed and explored to facilitate just such a holistic consideration.

Jain Philosophy and Professional Ethics

The Jain philosophico-religious tradition outlines a way of life centered around nonviolence and vegetarianism, and in its philosophical system one finds an elaborate and plausible metaphysic that justifies and motivates these basic lived ideals. It offers an example of a holistically developed system of inquiry and understanding that addresses and explores issues of ethical, hermeneutical, and ontological import. Ethically, it advocates maximal nonviolence as an ethical ideal. Hermeneutically, it urges humility in interpretation based on an acknowledgment of the infinite aspects of any given thing and an individual's limited access to knowledge. Ontologically and metaphysically, it offers a pluralist conception of substances that are themselves bifurcated into living and nonliving. Bringing these ideas together, it suggests that the breadth of our understanding is causally related to the kind of action or non-action that we accrue throughout the course of our lives. In this way, it provides ample resources for educators to address the shortcomings of descriptive, instrumentalist, and prescriptive approaches to teaching business ethics.

In this section, a particular curriculum in professional ethics and Jain philosophy is outlined and explained. There are obviously many idiosyncratic ways in which one might go about developing a curriculum in Jain philosophy and professional ethics. I have chosen to do so on the basis of the arguments given above. In light of those arguments, a curriculum in professional ethics ought to expand philosophical inquiry in our classrooms in meaningful and challenging ways, in this case through Jain ideas and arguments.

It is not enough, however, to simply offer exposure to Jain ideas. One must avoid approaches that are merely descriptive, instrumental, or prescriptive. Availing oneself of these opportunities requires reading Jain philosophy not by way of a description of a historical curiosity, but as a living challenge to our assumptions; not as an explanation that someone *has* thought in a certain ways, but an exploration of *whether and why* such thoughts might be justified; not as a tool for effectively achieving one's business goals, but as an intrinsically valuable inquiry into truth, reliability, and coherence; not as a prescription for how one should be, but as an invitation to consider how one might be. Rather than merely giving examples of how individuals and firms have utilized Jain values (a descriptive approach), gathering evidence that connects Jain values with profitability (an instrumental approach), or proposing a Jain-inspired system of professional ethics for students to consider adopting (a prescriptive approach), this curriculum should provide opportunities for students to reflect upon and adjust the foundations of their own professional ethical outlook in conversation with plausible Jain ideas and arguments about how we ought to think, speak, and act (a philosophical approach). What follows is an outline of such a curriculum.

First, I propose that such a curriculum should begin by attempting to justify itself philosophically, as I have just done, assessing the limits of business ethics education. To summarize, conventional business ethics education is largely restricted to instrumentalist, descriptive, and prescriptive accounts, while responsible exploration of the topic requires normative philosophical exploration. A philosophical approach should explore ethical, hermeneutical, and ontological issues. It should explore ethical issues in the sense that it should contain a non-question-begging account of *why* one should act in a certain manner, professionally. That is, it should not simply presume that the answer to this *why* is self-evident. Ethically, it must critique descriptive, instrumental, and prescriptive accounts, appealing instead to broadly meta-ethical and normative inquiry. Hermeneutically, it should assess the limits of philosophical inquiry, and defer to other disciplines or inquiries when its own interpretive tools are insufficient. Ontologically, it should address foundational questions concerning the nature of our existence and our sense of the purpose of human life.

Second, I propose that such a curriculum explore texts and concepts in Jain philosophy and Jain ethics insofar as they serve to facilitate philosophical reflection on the limits of ethical inquiry, fostering dialogue on foundational issues. This will require systematic exploration. So, from a textual perspective, it is imperative that students explore a primary text or a reconstruction that attempts to arrange the entire range of Jain philosophy systematically. The *Tattvārthādhigama Sūtra* recommends itself here. In particular, the curriculum could focus on introducing through this text Jain notions of right worldview, knowledge, and practice (*samyag-darśana-jñāna-cāritrāni*); metaphysical pluralism (*anekānta-vāda*); epistemological non-absolutism (*naya-vāda*); and the practice of virtue cultivation (*vrata*).

Third, once a systematic introduction to this tradition is offered, ethical, hermeneutical, and ontological issues can be explored in turn and in mutual connection. For example, we can consider the necessity of harm or violence, the need for a balance between personal and professional morality, the moral tenability of the pursuit of affluence, the validity of anthropocentrism, the relationship between self-perception and ethical outlook, or the question of when it is appropriate to gracefully exit the realm of business activity.[3] Anyone familiar with the Jain tradition will recognize the salience of Jain philosophy in these areas. Imagine a student who takes for granted that violence to nonhuman animals is a necessary part of human nutrition, and that the goal of business activity should be the promotion of a higher standard of living for all. A holistic understanding of the Jain philosophical system will give this student ready access to plausible and integrated ontological and hermeneutical frameworks that suggest that we should strongly oppose such violence and understand the pursuit of affluence as misguided. It provides students with an internal interlocutor and a reference point for continued conversation within themselves.

In summary, the course would be divided into several modules, corresponding to the reasoning offered above:

- The Limits of Professional Ethics and Viable Alternatives
- The Jain Philosophical System
- Ontological Issues in Jain Philosophy
- Hermeneutical Issues in Jain Philosophy
- Ethical Issues in Jain Philosophy

More concretely, we can explore Jain ontology, especially notions of self and soul, in dialogue with anthropocentric understandings in professional and philosophical ethics. The biophilic and pluralistic ontological foundation of Jain philosophy in the notion of infinite souls finds expression in a non-one-sided hermeneutical strategy, which could be explored in detail next. Finally, the Jain normative ethic of nonviolence and non-possession should be explored as deriving from this holistic philosophical basis.

For example, the course could explore the scope of violence and how, in Jain texts, it is understood to extend to thought and word in addition to deed. It could explore the necessity of violence in the course of householder life and the relationship between violence and anthropocentrism. In terms of non-possessiveness, Jain texts can be read in a way that offers compelling critiques of affluence and the relationship between quality of life and standard of living, and as our colleague Atul Shah has put it, Jainism indeed offers a deep understanding of the nature and limits of money.[4] One can explore more applied normative connections, too. For example, Jain ethical vows pose unique questions regarding the conflict between moral life and professional life in the distinction between great and small vows, the relevance of and need for strategies for virtue cultivation, and the separation of life and work.

The argument offered here suggests that a suitable course in Jain professional ethics should pick up where prescriptive, instrumental, and descriptive approaches leave off, taking philosophical inquiry to be central to considerations. Once a clear and thorough reconstruction of the Jain philosophical system is provided, students can then explore the implications, limits, and viability of such a system with respect to controversies and questions at the core of professional ethics.

Conclusion

As global markets deal with inflation, recessions loom, and unemployment increases, we may anticipate higher university enrollment. Trends suggest that this will lead to still higher enrollment in business programs, too. To the extent that this trend is global, shall we celebrate or lament the fact that business and other vocationally oriented classrooms are increasingly among the most influential with respect to the philosophical worldviews of our youth? I think we can do our fair share of both, but there are some obvious reasons to lament this until a radical transformation of the curriculum is implemented. Wendell Berry has put the issue succinctly, observing that "we have before us the spectacle of unprecedented 'prosperity' and 'economic growth' in a land of degraded farms, forests, ecosystems, and watersheds, polluted air, failing families, and perishing communities" (2017, 69–70).

Business and other educational programs themselves, for the purposes of funding allocation and accreditation, will likely celebrate their enrollment increases as evidence that whatever each program may do differently, they are mostly doing it well. Nonetheless, it should be clear to anyone that the simple fact that an increasing number of people enrolling in a program does not mean that that program's curriculum is well-executed. Even if we suppose (perhaps rightly) that business curricula are by and large well-executed, it is still pertinent to note that doing *well* is not the same as doing *good*. Upward mobility for a larger percentage of students increases in postgraduate employment rates, better standardized test scores, more alums in managerial roles: All of these things are clearly *good* with respect to the livelihoods of our students and especially with respect to their embeddedness in capitalist economies. But all of these things—mobility, employment, qualified individuals—are also compatible with an environment in increasing peril, a shrinking middle class, an increased reliance on unhealthy systems of food production, and other morally questionable outcomes. I wish for my students to be antithetical to such problems, to be a danger to such problems, to be antidotes to the greed, overconsumption, and homogenization that such problems involve.

Ecological thinker and author David Orr worries similarly that modern education—because of its increasing emphasis on specialization over multifaceted knowledge, career over calling and purpose, and separation of the practical from the theoretical—runs the risk of unwittingly "unleash[ing] upon the world minds ignorant of their own ignorance" (Orr 2024, 17). Orr's argument is that modern education is too steeped in disciplinary silos, too instrumentally focused, and in general too myopic to facilitate the holistic vision required to address global problems. To this point, Orr insists that "the planet does not need more successful people . . . It needs people who live well in their places. It needs people of moral courage willing to join the fight to make the world habitable and humane. And these qualities have little to do with success as our culture has defined it" (ibid., 17). In other words, modern education is fixated on an unhealthy conception of success. It is possible to succeed at the expense of our neighbors, at the expense of our ancestors, at the expense of future generations, and even at our own expense. A better world requires the courage to live well in our places more than it requires this kind of success. Education provides the most reliable foundation for the widespread development of such courage, and since business curricula are the most prominent postsecondary curricula in the United States by a growing margin, addressing these issues in business education is extremely important.

But how to encourage this in each other? How to encourage it in our classrooms? I can only share my own pedagogical strategies insofar as I have attempted to justify them philosophically and insofar as they have worked for my students. I have argued here that business coursework ought to become broader, more reflexive and self-critical, and more embedded in the history of ideas. I believe that the study of philosophy as a way of life, the study of ways of life as philosophy, the study of philosophy religiously, and the study of religious texts philosophically are important ways in which, educationally, we can offer ourselves and our students opportunities to expand our worldviews. Jainism is just one of many traditions that offer opportunities for this, but in my view it is one that is uniquely suited to address some of the most important barriers to ethical and existential reflection in students of our business curricula.

Notes

1. While one may argue that such practical appeals are utilitarian in nature and thus are normative in their justification, the point here is that claiming that these appeals *could* be defended by way of utilitarian or consequentialist frameworks is different from claiming that they *are* defended or justified in this way. Utilitarian conclusions are instead often taken for granted as uncontroversial in business ethics literature, and very few sophisticated reasons are offered in their favor. These conclusions, and the reasons prominently appealed to in support of them, are not uncontroversial.

2. I must thank Aleksandra Jasinska for sharing this article with me during a conversation about her doctoral research at the University of Fribourg.

3. I thank Malay Patel for this last suggestion shared in his presentation at the Defining Applied Jain Studies Conference at Arihanta Institute (2023).

4. I thank Atul Shah for this insight shared during his presentation at the Defining Applied Jain Studies Conference at Arihanta Institute (2023).

References

Adams, Desmund. 2017. "Harnessing the Power of Diversity for Profitability." *Forbes*, July 26. https://www.forbes.com/sites/forbesbusinesscouncil/2022/03/03/harnessing-the-power-of-diversity-for-profitability/.

Arihanta Institute. 2023. "Defining Applied Jain Studies." https://conf.arihantainstitute.org/agenda.

Berry, Wendell. 2017. "The Total Economy." In *The World-Ending Fire: The Essential Wendell Berry*, edited by Wendell Berry. Counterpoint.

Brennan, Andrew, and Norva Y. S. Lo. 2022. "Environmental Ethics." *The Stanford Encyclopedia of Philosophy*, Summer 2022 ed., edited by Edward N. Zalta. https://plato.stanford.edu/archives/sum2022/entries/ethics-environmental/.

Byars, Stephen, and Kurt Stanberry et al. 2018. *Business Ethics*. OpenStax. https://openstax.org/details/books/business-ethics.

Donaldson, Thomas, and Lee E. Preston. 1995. "The Stakeholder Theory of the Corporation: Concepts, Evidence, and Implications." *The Academy of Management Review* 20 (1): 65–91. *JSTOR*.

Georgescu, Peter. 2017. "Doing the Right Thing Is Just Profitable." *Forbes*, July 26. https://www.forbes.com/sites/petergeorgescu/2017/07/26/doing-the-right-thing-is-just-profitable/#360853967488.

Goldman, Geoff. 2009. "History and Philosophy of Management at the University of Johannesburg: A New Direction for the Department of Business Management." *Philosophy of Management* 8 (1): 37–41.

Hamby, Chris, and Michael Forsythe. 2022. "Behind the Scenes, McKinsey Guided Companies at the Center of the Opioid Crisis." *New York Times*, June 29.

McKinsey and Co. 2020. "Diversity Wins: How Inclusion Matters." Accessed October 15, 2023.

Midgley, Mary. 1996. "Sustainability and Moral Pluralism." In *Utopias, Dolphins and Computers: Problems in Philosophical Plumbing*. Routledge.

Moriarty, Jeffrey. 2021. "Business Ethics." *The Stanford Encyclopedia of Philosophy*, Fall 2021 ed., edited by Edward N. Zalta. https://plato.stanford.edu/archives/fall2021/entries/ethics-business/.

Oliver, John. 2023. McKinsey & Company. *Last Week Tonight with John Oliver*. Created by John Oliver. HBO, season 10, episode 14.

Orr, David. 2004. *Earth in Mind: On Education, Environment, and the Human Prospect*. Island Press.

Ridge, Michael. 2019. "Moral Non-Naturalism." *The Stanford Encyclopedia of Philosophy*, Fall 2019 ed., edited by Edward N. Zalta. https://plato.stanford.edu/archives/fall2019/entries/moral-non-naturalism/.

"U.S. Department of Education, National Center for Education Statistics, Integrated Postsecondary Education Data System (IPEDS)." n.d. Fall 2011 through Fall 2021, Completions component. See *Digest of Education Statistics* 2022, table 322.10; and *Digest of Education Statistics* 2021, table 322.10.

"U.S. Census Bureau. n.d. Accessed June 4, 2023. US Educational Attainment in the United States: 2021. Table 2. Educational Attainment of the Population 25 Years and Over." *Selected Characteristics* 2021. https://www.census.gov/data/tables/2021/demo/educational-attainment/cps-detailed-tables.html.

7

Engaged Jain Business and Professional Culture

ATUL K. SHAH

One of the smallest religious communities of India today has one of the largest national and global footprints (per capita) when it comes to commerce and the professions. This record of success is not just contemporary but comes from a long tradition of business and public service, which is directly rooted in the teachings and permissible vocations for Jains.[1] In this chapter, we look at this history and tradition, and explore the rationale for the continued success in these fields. This chapter will also demonstrate to the wider business world, which is largely unaware of the Jains, that this is a community and tradition we have much to learn from, especially at a time of a profound crisis in sustainable development. By sustainable development, I mean development and business models that can literally be sustained in the broadest sense and are therefore not only limited to (though they may include), for example, environmental sustainability.

In this chapter, I write as an insider of the Jain tradition, adopting what Miller has identified as the constructive-reproductive model of engaged Jain studies, using what Cort would describe as an "internal model *for* the Jains" (Cort 1990, 55; see Miller's introduction in this volume). I draw from my experience of growing up among the Jains in East Africa who had migrated from India, as well as from my professional career as a qualified chartered accountant, an academic with a PhD from London School of Economics, and a long-standing research and education career in finance based in the United Kingdom.[2] During this time, I have actively spoken about the Jains. Throughout my education career, there was no mention of the Jains by any of my lecturers as an exemplar business and finance community, a lacunae I will address in this chapter by engaging the Jain tradition with the concerns of business and professional culture and ethics.

Secular Dichotomy and Its Perils

There is often a frown when religion is discussed in the business academy, where it is dismissed as unscientific and parochial, when in reality Jain wisdom and philosophy contain many fresh perspectives from which the business academy can benefit. I use this chapter to showcase the depth and breadth of Jain business science, which cannot be separated from religion and enhances our understanding of sustainable commerce and industry, at a time when we need solutions that have stood the test of time.

Contemporary business science is cultural, transactional, functional, and formulaic, with ethics and belief seen as marginal to the discipline and usually siloed as separate modules.[3] It has also become highly technical and specialized, especially in fields like accounting and finance, with the recent era of financialization enabling finance and its metrics to overwhelm and dominate other disciplines to a large extent, even when its own science is deeply flawed and problematic (cf. Zwan 2014; Shaxson 2018; Brooks et al. 2019). The divorce of culture and ethics is a root cause of many of the problems of the modern world—it enables irresponsible business leaders to enter into very powerful and influential positions (Kets de Vries 2012; Hare 1996). The huge concentration and abuse of power by multinational corporations, run by other people's money, where ownership and management are completely divorced (cf. Kay 2015; Korten 1995; Whyte and Wiegratz 2016), is deeply problematic.

In such a context, Jain business ethics become even more relevant, as culture and ethics are central to Jain commerce and not peripheral to it. The philosophy of inclusivity, which extends to all living beings, not just humans, makes such a perspective highly applicable, particularly given our contemporary challenges surrounding biodiversity loss, climate change, and environmental pollution. In this regard, some Western authors have called for a shift in business and economic science toward a holistic and inclusive perspective, where society and nature are not othered but instead seen as critical resources that need to be preserved and protected (cf. Daly and Cobb 1994; Ekins et al. 1992; and Elkington 1999). The Jain tradition of business and professional ethics has much to offer to this important task.

The chapter is organized as follows. First, we will examine the commercial history of Jains and the networks and institutions that helped support their progress and continue to do so. We will then go into the principles and ethics of Jains, which lend themselves to such sustained success and intergenerational networks and reputation, including an ability to keep wealth, not just make it. We explore the conduct and character of Jains, and the social capital that enables not just commercial training but also trust and relationships critical to lasting success. This combination of knowledge and networks has also shown itself to be applicable and robust in very diverse contexts that arise from globalization and migration. There is an intercultural intelligence and skill of assimilation and adaptation that again is worthy of much deeper research and analysis. Jain leadership is then elaborated as a grounded and humble practice, where power and greed are not allowed to overwhelm social responsibility and accountability. Finally, I draw out the central messages from this chapter for an engaged Jain studies where the living community and diaspora is a wide canvas for analysis and reflection on sustainable development.

There is a dearth of research and writing on Jain business history and ethics that one can draw upon,[4] and, furthermore, the research method in this chapter is subject to the particular history and experience of the author.[5] I have been an active community leader throughout my adult life, directly participating in engaging young Jains and professionals in the fields of business and ethics, and also a migrant with experience of three continents and a year spent in Washington, DC, as a visiting professor. My own life has been a story of social and entrepreneurial capital in movement and adaptation, and the active engagement with younger generations caught up in the crossfire between East and West. In some cases, I ask the reader to forgo the need for empirical evidence and to allow my personal, auto-ethnographic experience as a Jain with such life experience to shape a broader understanding of one of the oldest living business cultures of the world. Much of Jain culture and heritage stem from an oral tradition and an intimacy of community networks and knowledge that is difficult for a Western-trained scholar to comprehend.[6] We start by examining the business history of the Jains.

Jain Business and Community History

The surname Mehta is common among Jains and it means "treasurer," "accountant," and "administrator." These seem to be common professions in the early history of the Jains, when we often rose to ranks of the chief treasurer of kings or the top civil servants helping to run and manage their kingdoms. Given the (at least) three-thousand-year history of Jains, and the fact that India was a key global trading country until the eighteenth century, when a third of global trade was centered around it, commerce has played a growing role in Indian economic history. Even today, India has very quickly risen from the ashes of exploitation and empire to once again take a leading role in global trade and commerce. The skills of commerce have been part of India for centuries, with particular communities like the Gujaratis and Marvaris excelling in it.

Growing up in a migrant Jain community in East Africa, I experienced firsthand the role of commerce and industry in the shaping of the diaspora, with religion and community never far off and always deeply entwined. In the port town of Mombasa, which I sometimes refer to as the "New York of Africa," we built a four-acre Jain temple complex in the heart of the town, merely seventy years after migrating there. Next to it is Jain Street, where a lot of the import/export and trading businesses were located. The ritual of Chopda Pujan at Diwali, when traders come together to open new books of account and collectively pray for greater empowerment to serve and advance the economy and society, is etched into my memory. The language of trade and commerce was also commonly heard in community gatherings, such that when it came time to choose my career, accountancy seemed the only option so far as family and tradition were concerned.

Having migrated from Gujarat, the fact that we established ourselves in trade in a foreign country so quickly, and even learned the local language without any formal classes and training, shows an adaptability and assimilation skill that must have been honed over generations.[7] Even the local African workers who were employed in our businesses seemed very happy and contented, such was the way they were treated and respected. In East Africa, employees were seen as assets and colleagues, and the educated professionals promoted to managers.

Building Trust Through Adaptation, Open-Mindedness, and Assimilation

The temple in the heart of Mombasa was a vibrant hub of community, and we had an equally large social, sports, and welfare center not far away, where community luncheons and weddings were held.[8] During festival times, we had expert speakers and artists from India who were invited to entertain and inspire us toward more self-discipline, self-renewal, and living a responsible and reflective life. The open-air *medaan* in the grounds of the temple was often brimming with people from the whole town invited to listen to the lectures. It was an interfaith gathering without the label—such was the open-mindedness and generosity of the time. Audiences of two thousand were not uncommon, and the pin-drop silence was deafening to my child's ear, but memorable too. Here was interdependence in practice, with a respect for wisdom and knowledge, and an understanding that community lies at the heart of life and purpose.

Reflecting on this history, profit, wealth, and charity were rarely publicly discussed or elevated, and the "Sheths," the super-successful businessmen, were respected for their status but not given overwhelming importance in an inclusive community. Success in business was seen as arising from *puṇya* or karmic merit, and not attributed to self or ego or any special skills or acumen. In fact, for the prosperous, charity was seen as a duty, not a choice. In Mombasa, many top entrepreneurs also worked in various committees to serve the community, bringing their business skills to implement the vision.

Mutuality and Mentoring

Going back deep into Indian history, in times when transportation was arduous, local communities would have flourished through self-governance with the temple becoming a source of lifelong learning and training in wisdom.[9] It was a hub of social capital, trust, and networking without any need for special categories or classifications to the practice—trade simply happened naturally, and the loss of honor and reputation was a key self-regulator of conduct.[10] The fact that communities lived close to each other, and there was little media or technology to control communication, led to more direct oral and primary engagement that can only have helped reinforce trust and mutuality.[11] Institutions of education and training, where absent, were built and sponsored by Jain businesses all over India, and the same happened in Kenya, where I was taught in Jain schools at the nursery and primary levels and went to a secondary school endowed by a famous Indian philanthropist, Allidina Visram.

In the early days in Mombasa (1920s and 1930s), community leaders would go around each business in the evening, asking them what help they needed—such was the spirit of service and shared success. In his famous essay on the theory of the gift in Jain tradition,[12] Laidlaw analyzes Jain almsgiving as a pure, selfless act wherein expectation of return was ritually nullified. I experienced this spirit growing up in an immigrant landscape, and felt it to be alive and unspoken, with no need for a quid pro quo.

Someone who has grown up in an environment of materialism, individualism, and low social and community capital may find it difficult to understand such depth of trust and relationships, and may even feel suspicious or suffocated by the thought of it. This is where knowledge and analysis become limiting. Field experience through engaged participation and observation is critical to understanding the nature and layers of humility and mutuality that have been woven into the Jain culture for generations. Pure reading and critical study will not be sufficient. In fact, it can lead to misunderstanding and misrepresentation due to the individualist perspectives in which people would have been raised. "Cultural intelligence" requires a mindfulness of difference and active attempts to understand cultures in their own living contexts.[13] We now reflect on ethics and professionalism—principles that enable Jains to protect public interest and understand the limits of private wealth.

Jain Commercial Ethics and Public Interest Professionalism

The tenets of *ahiṃsā* (nonviolence), *aparigraha* (non-materialism), and *anekānta* (pluralism) embrace biodiversity and a respect for all life as being central to the Jain philosophy. Embraced within it is a profound understanding of the nature and limits of money—it is a means to an end but never an end in itself.[14] The Jain principle of *aparigraha*—non-possessiveness—explains that external objects or possessions are only temporary and transient, and we should not be obsessive and instead be generous in giving and sharing if we are to succeed materially. There is a responsible and accountable sense of ownership and enterprise, where purpose and meaning are central to trade, and wealth and metrics of profit are not allowed to overwhelm trust, relationships, and quality service to customers.

The role of knowledge and understanding is central throughout the life of a Jain, and learning is highly privileged and respected.[15] Jain ethics call for an ongoing reflexivity and mindfulness of one's actions and character, helping to check greed, waste, and extravagance in enterprise. Business leaders would regularly attend community events, provide needed financial support for charitable institutions, and engage with Jain monks and nuns to get more inspiration for their spiritual journey. The saints become role models and often themselves come from very successful business families, but after renunciation they live a simple nomadic life where they are not allowed to carry any money or have any possessions.

In terms of charity, it is often repeated that even though Jains are less than half a percent of India's population and even less in the diaspora, Jains provide a disproportionate amount of charity, showing that we understand the need for money to flow toward good causes. For example, JAINA's Academic Liaison Committee has engaged generous Jain donors to endow over thirty academic positions and opportunities in North America and Europe, providing the opportunity for scholars to build their academic careers and to be able to offer students education in the Jain tradition.

Two key ingredients of successful professionalism are knowledge and public interest protection. Jain ethics respect both, and the upbringing within a strong set of family values and an extended community helps significantly. Jain acculturation provides unique coaching in the importance of preserving public assets and institutions, and serving society to its own benefit, not the private benefit of the professional. This explains why Jains have become highly successful doctors, accountants, bankers, and business advisors all over the world. The culture, behaviors, and ethics have given them a significant career boost, as these aspects can rarely be taught in an institutionalized education setting.

The contemporary focus on greed and materialism as keys to business success is completely antithetical to the Jain understanding of commerce. Profit maximization has become enshrined into the science of economics and is celebrated as an ideal. The same attitude prevails when it comes to borrowing and leveraging—the higher the borrowing, the better the return to the shareholders of the business. The whole science of finance is based on the separation of the owners from the managers, and the huge rot and disengagement that results from businesses fueled by other people's money.[16] Furthermore, the climate crisis is leading to massive disruption in the science of commerce. Jain wisdom is not even known let alone respected by the new revolutionaries taking on these challenges, whose secular approaches could be greatly enhanced by considering Jain professional ethics.

In contrast, most Jain businesses are owner-managed so there is no separation of the shareholder and the management. Similarly, due to the understanding of interdependence woven into the central philosophy of Jains (*parasparopagraho jīvānām, Tattvārtha Sūtra* 5.21, generally understood to mean that "all living beings are worthy of compassion and respect and interconnected in the web of life"), Jain businesses have a high level of respect for different stakeholders like suppliers, customers, and finance providers.[17] The leadership that emanates from such principles is responsible and accountable, not because of any laws or rules, but because culturally and religiously, it is the right way to conduct business. Religion and community act as resources of conscience and self-regulation, and even trust is controlled by the need to preserve honor and reputation (*abru*). In my hometown of Mombasa, Kenya, the street adjacent to the temple was called Jain Street and trade was conducted as an extension of faith and community.

One of the most popular business professions for Jains is accounting and finance, either as chartered accountants or CPAs, or as bankers, financiers, and investment advisors. Their education and respect for knowledge makes them experts in their fields, and being raised in a caring and inclusive culture helps them to be mindful of others and to protect the public interest. Often the training and mentoring in these areas starts from the home and the community, with role models and mentors easily approachable and accessible. The self-discipline that comes from the ethical codes is a key reason for client satisfaction, referrals, and brand and reputation building. Hence Jains working in the professions are rarely unemployed.

A Jain accountant friend of mine in the UK, Bharat Dhanani, was once asked by a client for his business card. When he gave the client a card, the client said he wanted a whole box of them so he can give them out in his community and tell them that Bharat is the best accountant in the world! Such was the professionalism and trustworthiness exalted by Bharat, that the client felt moved to become his ambassador. A lot of Jain enterprises have grown in this organic way, without the need for lawyers or expensive marketing and sales campaigns. The size and scale of the business depends on the growth ambitions of the founders, and in many cases, they are contented to control the growth so that it remains manageable and controllable, even when other opportunities are presented.

One industry where the Jains have a global reach and influence is the diamond polishing industry, which they have come to dominate through perseverance and a strong focus on honesty and self-policing of contractual disputes or bankruptcies (cf. Lum 2014). They are not involved in the mining of diamonds, which does have a poor reputation due to child labor and exploitation in developing countries. However, this does not exonerate them from the significant violence, and there is little evidence of the Jain community actively addressing this issue and ensuring ethics and human rights in the entire supply chain. It contradicts their culture and character and suggests that in lucrative industries, ethics can be suppressed. Jains have developed sophisticated internal dispute resolution mechanisms, however, and these are effective and save vast amounts of legal costs.[18] Prior to the Jains, the Jews were the dominant community in the precious gems trade, and the Jains gained prominence due to their access to cheaper labor in India for the polishing of diamonds.

Overall, Jain wisdom, ethics, and lived experience become a lodestar of hope and a significant opportunity for the reform of business science—though Jains are not perfect, there is an idealism that directs their character and conduct, and a conscience that regulates their business leadership and practice in general. At a very basic level, the fact that the culture has survived and sustained itself for thousands of years demonstrates that there is a living experience of sustainable business, not just a theory or intellectual speculation of what this could look like. It also suggests a very different trajectory for business education and training, where the student is not a consumer of knowledge in a factory but a spirit and soul who needs to be enlightened in a mindful way about the strong links between ethics, culture and enterprise, and how setting one's own principles clearly can lead to long-term contentment and success (cf. Shah and Rankin 2017). The divorce between the individual student's culture, character, and values and the science of modern business is simply not sustainable. We now examine the role of community and social capital in the growth and success of the Jains.

A Community of Enterprise—Social and Commercial

Business today has become obsessed with profit and wealth creation, but we need to recall that this was not always so, nor is it true across many parts of the world and many different faith and culture traditions. A key base and resource of business that is ignored today in business science is community. Communities are like extended families, where relationships are nurtured, volunteering is common, and trust is shaped and replenished. They can be large banks of social capital and reservoirs of learning, knowledge, and wisdom, where the purpose of life is reflected upon and work or enterprise is undertaken to fulfill it. Internships, training, and mentoring can also happen through these communities, such that the young generation is engaged and nurtured to take on adult responsibilities and bring fresh enthusiasm and ideas to the business.

The history of Jain entrepreneurial growth and prosperity is shaped in such living communities, which are entwined and open-minded at the same time, inclusive yet not exclusive of others.[19] Business schools as important global educational institutions are really only sixty years old—prior to that, business training did happen, often in communities. For Jains, elements of this training and mentoring still happen today all over India, and a new trade organization, Jain International Trade Organisation (JITO), has been set up all over India and internationally to support local and global networks of trade, with a wide remit of community building and enterprise. As a community, throughout their history, Jains have built and funded schools and colleges all over India and even boarding houses like Mahavir Jain Vidyalaya that provide urban accommodation for college students from smaller towns. These boarding houses and hostels have also become breeding grounds for new youth relationships and a springboard for business enterprises, like the famous investment bank, Motilal Oswal.

Viewed in this way, the Jain community can be seen as a lifelong university, where education, mentoring, mutuality, purpose, and creativity are regularly nurtured and replenished. There is a wholeness in the rhythms of the festivals and community meals, and wide methods of learning are applied. The syllabus is not specific but generic and comprises a range of subjects and disciplines, taught through lectures, events, volunteering, and experiences. A holistic approach is practiced where the learner is seen as a recipient, embodiment, and an ambassador of wisdom. A community can also be a host for experimentation, trial and error, where mistakes are tolerated and easily forgiven, and risk-taking is encouraged.

Communities become a springboard for hope and transition over the various phases of life. They can also check greed, avarice, and excess in a subtle but effective way, as belonging is valued and shame is costly.

When the community migrates to a foreign country, with a very different culture and way of life, the challenges of assimilation can be tough, and the identity crisis significant. Given the diversity of India, Jains have experienced these challenges throughout their history, and through this also instinctively learned to adapt and fit into different environments and cultures. In an era of globalization, such skills have proved to be a huge asset, as trade requires a high level of cultural intelligence and Jain success shows that the community has honed these skills carefully and creatively. Cross-cultural skills are rarely taught in the modern business school, as they are complex and also not an easy fit for a functionalist and transactional business paradigm.[20] The Jains' field of learning has been in the world of travel and experience, requiring cultural openness and respect for different perspectives and viewpoints.

Community provides grounding to leaders and helps them get a pulse of what is happening and how people are affected by events and circumstances. This is very rare in modern corporate life, where leaders are detached from living societies and autocratically allocate resources without this intimacy.[21] Unlike modern globalization and outsourcing of work and labor, in communities people experience wholeness and meet others who are different from them, rich or poor, men and women, children and young people. Community also helps keep leaders humble and grounded, rather than egoistic and status obsessed. Belonging to community fades the borders between social and commercial enterprise, and while there may be some purely commercially focused, they would provide funds to the needs of the community—whether they are education, housing, or temple construction—and the volunteers who manage these projects provide the time and the skills needed to make them succeed. There would still be some members of the community who love *seva*, or selfless service, like my late father Mr. Keshavji Rupshi Shah, and devote all their time to it. He was very well respected by the entrepreneurs, many of whom became his friends and fellow trustees.

A range of skills and motivations are required to run community enterprises. In contrast, today businesses need separate "corporate social responsibility" divisions, which often end up washing the greedy image of the business and are tokenistic acts.[22] Leadership is one of the most important subjects in business—yet so little is known about Jain business leadership and the accountability and responsibility practiced by them.

Responsible and Accountable Leadership

A Jain doctor in Nairobi, Madhusudan Shah, grew up around a family business, regularly helping in the shop on weekends and holidays.[23] Through this he came to enjoy business and customer service and saw how important it was to protect the brand name and provide quality service. If customers wanted to return goods, then this was not refused, and the product weaknesses were noted so that it would not happen again. After qualifying as a medical doctor, and seeing his parents aging, Dr. Madhusudan decided to play a bigger role in the business and saw a market gap for children's clothing at that time. A neighbor introduced him to a quality manufacturer of children's clothing, who by coincidence was also looking for a retailer and distributor. The rest is history—the business grew manifold, and so did the profits and reputation of the business, Prakash Stores. Dr. Madhusudan's life story shows how professional skills are transferrable, and how entrepreneurial and multitalented Jain leaders are today. They are versatile, dynamic, open-minded, and multifaceted in their ability to lead an enterprise and make it grow and flourish. The African workers in the business were treated like family and highly respected and helped if they had sudden financial needs like illness or death in the family.

Conclusion

In summary, this chapter has introduced a holistic perspective on Jain business and enterprise, which draws from a profound and timeless Jain culture and philosophy of ethical responsibility. This culture and the related values are reinforced by community institutions and religious practices, which become a forum for personal growth and reflexivity, and check greed and excess. Business leaders directly experience a cross-section of society—poor, educated, illiterate, and disabled—and see in their ownership of enterprise a strong sense of social and environmental responsibility that is beyond any laws or regulations. Networks of trust and relationships help generate valuable social and knowledge capital about markets and opportunities that have assisted in the globalization of Jain businesses and their migration to new lands of opportunity. Training, recruitment, and mentoring also happens through these community relationships, informally but constructively. The modern world has seen a rise in networking events and clubs, but here is an example of a group with traditions of integrity, loyalty, and trust that cannot be grown or nurtured easily in a club.

Pluralism and *anekānta* principles have helped Jains to assimilate culturally and work in very different national and international environments and still succeed and prosper. This chapter shows that the Jains make an interesting case study and resource bank for research on sustainable development and enterprise. Given the power of commerce, and its huge influence in global society, Jain wisdom needs to be studied in much more detail to help educate future generations of students about the possibilities of ethical capitalism grounded in values and community.

Notes

1. See Shugan Jain et al. (2023) for a wide perspective on the history, business traditions, and ethical principles and practices of this diaspora.

2. Shah (2020) elaborates on my personal experiences of growing up as a Jain and becoming an academic. Shah and Rankin (2018) express the relevance of Jain business ethics in modern society.

3. Shah (2018) discusses the problems of contemporary accounting and finance education within the wider business academy.

4. Among the rare exceptions in this literature are Laidlaw (1996); Jain et al. (2023); Babb (2013).

5. Shah (2017) elaborates on my critical role in shaping a Western youth renaissance in Jain culture and engagement.

6. For more on Western comprehension of the Jain tradition, see Cort (2001); Dundas (2002); Flügel (2006); Mardia and Rankin (2013); Rankin (2006); Tobias (1991).

7. *Economist* (2015) explains that the Gujaratis are the world's most successful business diaspora. Sheikh (2010) charts the early history of Gujarat trade and commerce in the Middle Ages.

8. Zarwan (1977) studied the East African migration history of the Jains examining particular Jain family business histories and their success stories.

9. Jain et al. (2023) chaps. 5, 6, and 7 are helpful in understanding the Indian social and collective history of Jain business pioneers.

10. Dundas (2002) discusses the critical importance of *abru* or honour in business life, and Jain et al. (2023) elaborate on a range of virtues and case histories of eminent Jain entrepreneurs who established global businesses.

11. This history also applies to European capitalism, where religion and community networks played a central role. These could be Christian, Jewish, or Islamic, but faith was a major motivator and regulator of enterprise. Graeber (2014) exposes how intricately faith and finance have been related throughout human history. Michalos (2008) elaborates on the Middle Eastern heritage. Sacks (1990; 2002) explains the persistence of faith in human society in spite of materialism.

12. Laidlaw (2000) studies the Jains to unravel the theory of a "free" gift.

13. Thomas and Inkson (2009) elaborate on the critical role of cultural intelligence to business success in a diverse world.

14. Shah (2020) elaborates on the science of *aparigraha* and its practical manifestation in enterprise.

15. To understand the role of knowledge in Jain life, see Dundas (2002); Jaini (1998); or Cort (2001).

16. See Bakan (2004), which demonstrates how corporations have become psychopathic. Friedman (1970) emphasized business focus on profit as central to social responsibility. Hertz (2001) laments on the huge political power and unaccountability of multinational corporations.

17. Jaini (2002) elaborates on the role of Jain principles and ethics in sustainable development.

18. See Jain et al. (2023) chap. 11 by Manuel Gomez, which elaborates on the dispute resolution processes in the diamond industry.

19. Rankin (2006) and Rankin (2010) elaborate on the significant contemporary relevance of Jain principles in a vacuous and materialistic West, which has lost touch with spirituality and community.

20. See Thomas and Inkson (2009) for an elaboration of the importance and complexity of cultural intelligence.

21. Piety (2004) laments on the urgency of cultural reform. Luyendijk (2015) elaborates on the cannibalistic culture in international banking and Kay (2015) exposes the greed and avarice of finance. Ruskin (1985) emphasized long ago that "there is no wealth but life." Tett (2010) reflects on the impact of unrestrained greed on the 2008 global financial crash.

22. See Fleming and Jones (2013), which is highly critical of the corporate social responsibility industry and its spin factory.

23. M. S. Shah (2022) is a detailed autobiography of his life and business activities.

References

Babb, Lawrence. 2013. *Emerald City: The Birth and Evolution of an Indian Gemstone Industry*. Aditya Prakashan.

Bakan, J. 2004. *The Corporation: The Pathological Pursuit of Profit and Power*. Free Press.

Brooks, C., E. Fenton, L. Schopohl, and J. Walker. 2019. "Why Does Research in Finance Have So Little Impact?" *Critical Perspectives on Accounting*, no. 58: 24–52.

Cort, J. E. 2001. *Jains in the World: Religious Values and Ideology in India*. Oxford University Press.

———. 1990. "Models of and for the Study of the Jains." *Method & Theory in the Study of Religion* 2 (1): 42–71.

Daly, H., and J. Cobb. 1994. *For the Common Good: Redirecting the Economy Toward Community, Environment and a Sustainable Future*. 2nd ed. Beacon Press.

Dundas, P. 2002. *The Jains*. Routledge.

Economist. 2015. "Going Global: Secrets of the World's Best Business People." December 16. https://www.economist.com/christmas-specials/2015/12/19/going-global.

Ekins, P., M. Hillman, and R. Hutchison. 1992. *Wealth Beyond Measure: An Atlas of New Economics*. Gaia Books.

Elkington, J. 1999. *Cannibals with Forks: The Triple Bottom Line of 21st Century Business*. Capstone.

Fleming, P., and M. Jones. 2013. *The End of Corporate Social Responsibility: Crisis and Critique*. Sage Publications.

Flügel, Peter. 2006. "Jainism and Society." *Bulletin of the School of Oriental and African Studies* 69 (1): 91–112.

Friedman, M. 1970. "The Social Responsibility of Business is to Increase its Profits." *New York Times Magazine,* September 13.

Graeber, D. 2014. *Debt: The First 5000 Years.* Melvin House.

Hare, R. D. 1996. *Without Conscience: The Disturbing World of the Psychopaths Among Us.* Guilford Press.

Hertz, N. 2001. *The Silent Takeover: Global Capitalism and The Death of Democracy.* William Heinemann.

Jain, S., P. Jain, and M. Patel Eds. 2023. *Jain Business Engagement and Ethics: An Overview.* D. K. Publishers.

Jaini, P. S. 1998. *The Jaina Path of Purification.* Motilal Banarsidass.

———. 2002. "Ecology, Economics and Development in Jainism." In *Jainism and Ecology,* edited by Christopher Key Chapple. Harvard University Press.

Kay, J. 2015. *Other People's Money: Masters of the Universe or Servants of the People?* Profile Books.

Kets, de Vries M. 2012. "The Psychopath in the C Suite: Redefining the SOB." *Insead Working Paper no. 119.*

Korten, D. C. 1995. *When Corporations Rule the World.* Earthscan.

Laidlaw. 2000. 1996. *Riches and Renunciation: Religion, Economy and Society Among the Jains.* Oxford University Press.

———. "A Free Gift Makes No Friends." *Journal of Royal Anthropological Institute* 6:617–634.

Lum, Kathryn. 2014. "The Rise and Rise of Belgium's Indian Diamond Dynasties." *The Conversation,* October 19. https://theconversation.com/the-rise-and-rise-of-belgiums-indian-diamond-dynasties-32332.

Luyendijk, J. 2015. *Swimming with Sharks: My Journey Into the World of Bankers.* Faber & Faber.

Mardia, K., and A. Rankin. 2013. *Living Jainism: An Ethical Science.* Mantra Books.

Michalos. 2008. "Ancient Observations on Business Ethics: Middle East Meets West." *Journal of Business Ethics* 79:9–19.

Piety, M. G. 2004. "The Long Term: Capitalism and Culture in the New Millennium." *Journal of Business Ethics* 51 (May): 103–118.

Rankin, A. 2006. *The Jain Path: Ancient Wisdom for the West.* O Books.

———. 2010. *Many-Sided Wisdom: A New Politics of the Spirit.* O Books.

———. 2018. *Jainism and Environmental Philosophy: Karma and the Web of Life.* Routledge Focus on Environment and Sustainability. Routledge.

Ruskin, J. 1985. *Unto This Last and Other Writings.* Penguin Classics.

Sacks J. 1990. *The Persistence of Faith.* BBC Reith Lectures. BBC.

———. 2002. *The Dignity of Difference.* Continuum.

Shah, A. 2018. *Reinventing Accounting and Finance Education: For a Caring, Inclusive and Sustainable Planet.* Routledge.

Shah, A., and A. Rankin. 2017. *Jainism and Ethical Finance*. Routledge.

Shah, B. 2017. "Religion, Ethnicity, and Citizenship: The Role of Jain Institutions in the Social Incorporation of Young Jains in Britain and USA." *Journal of Contemporary Religion* 32 (2): 299–314.

Shah, M. S. 2022. *Madhu's Memories*. Private publication, madhukundan@gmail.com.

Shaxson, N. 2018. *The Finance Curse: How Global Finance is Making Us All Poorer*. Bodley Head.

Sheikh, S. 2010. *Forging a Region: Sultans, Traders, and Pilgrims in Gujarat 1200–1500*. Oxford University Press.

Tett, G. 2010. *Fool's Gold: How Unrestrained Greed Corrupted a Dream, Shattered Global Markets and Unleashed a Catastrophe*. Abacus.

Thomas, D., K. and Inkson. 2009. *Cultural Intelligence: Living and Working Globally*. B. K. Publishers.

Tobias, M. 1991. *Life Force: The World of Jainism*. Asian Humanities Press.

Whyte, D., and J. Wiegratz, eds. 2016. *Neoliberalism and the Moral Economy of Fraud*. Routledge.

Zarwan, J. 1977. *Indian Businessmen in Kenya During the Twentieth Century: A Case Study*. PhD diss., Yale University.

Zwan, N. 2014. "Making Sense of Financialisation." *Socio-Economic Review* 12:99–129.

Part IV

Engaging to Protect Animals and the Environment

8

Jain Virtue Ethics Engaging with Animal Rights

COGEN BOHANEC

One might ask what the role of theory is in the context of *engaged* studies. Is the parameter of inquiry for "engaged studies" to be restricted to the practical rather than the theoretical?[1] At least to some extent, the theoretical is a higher order function of engagement than the practical in that often we act based on our beliefs. As William James puts it, in lectures from 1906 to 1907, our individual philosophies are "the most interesting and important thing" about us since it "determines [our] perspective" that we have on life and therefore guides our actions (James 1987, 487). Without a theoretical understanding, practices (such as ethics) lose their meaning and diminish in their value and may fail to compel behavior. When we discover that we are acting without sufficient reason, our impulse to engage in action diminishes. Moreover, our theoretical understanding of actions creates our value for those actions.

Theoretical "engagement" can involve cross-cultural interactions between intellectual traditions. For example, the Animal Rights and Vegan Movement(s) have increasingly taken notice of the distinctive focus on nonviolence within the Jain tradition. Conversely, many Jains have taken notice of a similar centrality of an ethos of nonviolence in the Animal Rights / Vegan Movement(s) and have been increasingly adopting a vegan lifestyle, which is perceived as consistent with Jain philosophy (cf. Miller and Dickstein 2021). This amounts to a cross-cultural "engagement," which has prominent theoretical dimensions.

But it is important that when cross-cultural theoretical models interact that they don't distort each other, particularly when there is a power differential that can lead to intellectual colonialism. For example, where many intellectuals in the field of animal advocacy have tended to employ utilitarianism (e.g., Peter Singer) or deontology (e.g., Tom Regan) to substantiate their positions, these models seem discordant with traditional Jain ethical frameworks given their contextual uniqueness in European thought after the Enlightenment. For a more fruitful engagement between Jain ethics and modern animal advocacy, we should seek a model with a greater analogous relationship between these traditions. This chapter will explore how the virtue ethics of the Jain tradition can be engaged as an ethical framework (e.g., the virtue ethics of MacIntyre) that is most consistent with Jain philosophy, and how animal advocacy and veganism follow naturally from Jain virtue ethics.

Nietzsche *or* Jainism?

We should not be satisfied with merely presupposing the content of ethical language, for example, that it is "wrong" to commit senseless violence, or it is "right" to help others in need, as if these statements are self-evident and require little more than arbitrary assent to provide adequate impulse for individual and collective ethical action. If we cannot adequately win hearts and minds over to the truth of moral statements as being objectively factual, they will forever remain a matter of opinion. And left to subjective opinion, we should not be surprised when people knowingly or subconsciously fashion their morality to their own self-interest, contrary to the most basic dictates of morality as having a strong altruistic component.

Moreover, we should not be surprised when even the intelligent among us rejects morality as merely a means of social control, and instead chooses "will to power" over the will to morality, as was the compelling reasoning proffered by Nietzsche, resonances of which we can hear in reasoning of those in power who rather choose to aggrandize their own supremacy at the expense of the collective good and the individual good of others. For many powerholders, or those who aspire to greater power in contemporary times, "good" is a matter of mere opinion, not an objectively real quality of a class of actions (such as "charity," for example). The seduction of Nietzsche is alluring to the self-interested capitalist, the power-hungry politician, and the countless citizens who would likewise prefer personal expedience over collective good and who would rationalize their prioritization of self-interest with Nietzsche's claim that moral virtue itself is a self-contradiction:

> A man's virtues are called *good* depending on their probable consequences not for him but for us and society: the praise of virtues has always been far from "selfless," far from "unegoistic." Otherwise one would have had to notice that virtues . . . are usually harmful for those who possess them . . . when you have a virtue, a real, whole virtue . . . you are its *victim*. But your neighbor praises your virtue precisely on that account . . . The "neighbor" praises selflessness *because it brings him advantages* . . . This indicates the fundamental contradiction in the morality that is very prestigious nowadays: the *motives* of this morality stand opposed to its *principle*. What this morality considers its proof is refuted by its criterion of what is moral." (Nietzsche 2022 [orig. 1882], 80–83; passage 21)

Nietzsche would tell us that there is a necessary antagonism with altruistic virtue and self-interest, and morality itself is ultimately based on egoism and self-interest of those who stand to benefit from the self-effacing nature of those who practice moral virtues. According to Nietzsche, the question remains if one is going to act in one's own interest or the self-interest of those who have deceived us with the language of morality and virtue to operate in their interest. Either way, moral virtue is based on egoism and is therefore a self-contradiction.

It is all too easy to underestimate the influence of a Nietzschean approach to ethics in our contemporary society, but most scholars would agree with Ashley Woodward that Nietzsche is certainly "one of the most influential of all modern philosophers" given the "staggering number of books on Nietzsche" that have been published on him and the influential role that he has played in the main thinkers of the Western philosophical canon since he "first began to receive attention in the mid-1880s" (Woodward 2011, 1).

Granting the persuasiveness (and pervasiveness!) of Nietzschean ethical egoism, we can conclude that without a compelling rational basis for morality we should not be surprised when politicians and corporate executives alike would bring ruin to even their own countries for the sake of increasing their own power, and when the populace pursues actions that go against what are normally considered to be fundamental moral virtues based on altruism and care for others. Without a rational basis for morality, we cannot argue that their actions are "wrong," and neither will those who perpetuate violence believe that there is any other dictate (other than legal) to govern their personal action other than what they determine to be in their *own* best interests based largely on material and worldly desires for power and enjoyment.

In *After Virtue*, Alasdair MacIntyre's much acclaimed work on virtue ethics (2015 [1981]), MacIntyre composes a poignant chapter entitled "Nietzsche or Aristotle?" where he juxtaposes Nietzscheanism against Aristotelean-like virtue ethics as the only two persuasive moral theories in modern times:

> Yet it is not of course just that Nietzsche's moral philosophy is false if Aristotle's is true and *vice versa*. In a much stronger sense Nietzsche's moral philosophy is matched specifically against Aristotle's by virtue of the historical role which each plays . . . [I]t was because a moral tradition of which Aristotle's thought was the intellectual core was repudiated during the transitions of the fifteenth to seventeenth centuries that the Enlightenment project of discovering new rational secular foundations for morality had to be undertaken [resulting in deontology and utilitarianism, for example]. And it was because *that project failed* [emphasis added], because the view advanced by its most intellectually powerful protagonists . . . could not be sustained in the face of

> rational criticism that Nietzsche and all his existentialist and emotivist[2] successors were able to mount their apparently successful critique of all previous morality. Hence the defensibility of the Nietzschean position turns *in the end* on the answer to the question: was it right in the first place to reject Aristotle? For if Aristotle's position in ethics and politics—or something very like it—could be sustained, the whole Nietzschean enterprise would be pointless . . . My own argument obliges me to agree with Nietzsche that the philosophers of the Enlightenment never succeeded in providing grounds for doubting his central thesis . . . But . . . that failure itself was nothing other than an historical sequel to the rejection of the Aristotelian tradition. And thus the key question does indeed become: can Aristotle's ethics, *or something very like it* [emphasis added], after all be vindicated? (MacIntyre 2015 [1981], 117–118)

Of course, MacIntyre would answer "yes" to his rhetorical question, and he proceeds to vindicate the Aristotelian tradition. I too would answer "yes" that "something very like" the Aristotelean tradition of ethics can be "vindicated" from the modern onslaught of Nietzsche and his legacy, and this vindication is critical to creating social engagement with various issues of individual, social, and structural violence—including animal advocacy. I would also add that an Aristotelean-like system of virtue ethics does occur in most premodern South Asian traditions,[3] including the Jain tradition.

The Failure of Modern Ethics

So what was lost with the Enlightenment rejection about Aristotelianism that made premodern ethical systems coherent and later ones incoherent? In short, Aristotelianism saw moral statements as objectively real factual statements—rather than subjective opinions of preference—based on a realist appraisal of the teleological structures of reality and the affirmation of metaphysically real essences. When the idea of non-material structures of reality such as essences and teleologies were called into question with the Enlightenment, the factual status of non-material, moral qualities of classes of actions that depended on these structures were also sacrificed. This would lead to materialism, nihilism, postmodernism, and positivism—all of which purported to refute essences, teleologies, and the realism of moral qualities that allowed the content of ethical language to be both factual and meaningful. For MacIntyre, moral language in the absence of essences and teleologies has been decontextualized, causing "the language of morality [to have] passed from a state of order to a state of disorder" (MacIntyre 2015 [1981], 11).

In the absence of a widespread cultural belief in essences and teleologies, we "possess indeed simulacra of morality, we continue to use many of the key expressions. But we have—very largely, if not entirely—lost our comprehension, both theoretical and partial, [of] morality" (ibid., 2). MacIntyre proposes that a "catastrophe sufficient to throw the language and practice of morality into grave disorder" has occurred with the Enlightenment (ibid., 3) but from the "value-neutral viewpoint" of modern academic history "moral disorder must remain largely invisible" since academic value-neutrality only sees successive versions of the history of morality (Puritanism, Victorianism, etc.) "but the very language of order and disorder" is not available to such an academic history due to value-neutrality (ibid., 4). This failure on the part of academic value-neutrality to make sense of moral language and articulate coherent systematic (meta)ethical systems is inherently connected to our social understanding of ethics (ibid., 36).

For MacIntyre, if ethicists agree that there can be first principles from which ethical decisions can be inferred but do not agree on what those first principles might be (e.g., either "utility" or "duties") thereby making moral debate "interminable," then that is a good sign that ethics itself is a failing system (ibid., 6, 21). Without a common metaphysical basis for morality, opposing positions are equally rational but favor different premises (e.g., "utility" or "duties"). Therefore, argument is not rational in absence of shared objective claims, and moral argumentation is reduced to interminable assertion and counter assertion since "we possess no unassailable criteria, no set of compelling reasons by means of which we may convince our opponent" and our own moral standards may become grounded on "some non-rational decision" as a sort of "disquieting private arbitrariness" (ibid., 8).

Functional Concepts

MacIntyre points out that this Enlightenment movement against teleologies also entails a rejection of what he calls "functional concepts," namely that certain ontological statements about what a thing *is* contain an implicit evaluative (containing value) understanding of what it *ought* to do based on its function. Enlightenment value-neutrality is ontological, commonly known as a "fact/value" divide. But premodern ontology saw a reality that was value-ladened, as a "fact/value" synthesis where value is implicit in a reality where the essence of all things implies their teleological ends and their resultant value. In a value-ladened reality, concepts are functional in that they function toward a teleology in relationship to which they derive their essential value. For example, the ontic statement of fact "He is a sea-captain" is functional in that it carries the valid inference that "He ought to do whatever a sea-captain ought to do" since the very thing called a "sea-captain" implies a function that can be performed either well or poorly, and allows one to evaluate a specific sea-captain. Thus sea-captain, like other functional concepts, are ontologically evaluatively commensurate to their ends, their purpose, their *telos*. Likewise, the ontic fact of what a watch *is* necessarily implies that it *ought* to keep time; the ontic fact of what a farmer *is* necessarily implies that the farmer *ought* to maximize efficiency of crop yields, etc. (MacIntyre 2015 [1981], 58).

Thus, when ontology is understood functionally—and therefore teleologically—value, as "evaluative," is implicit in the basic definition of things and we have a basis to argue for what is "right" and what is "wrong" based on their development or attenuation of their value. By this, moral qualities, as evaluative statements about the human condition—as virtues—can be considered as factual statements based on the implicit function of concepts, contrary to emotivism, nihilism, positivism, or other forms of anti-realism about non-material qualities such as essences, teleologies, values, ideals, meanings, and of course, virtues.

Specifically, for Jainism, what a soul *is* consists of who we *should* aspire to be—ethical beings oriented toward the eradication of karma—to meet the soteriological goal of freedom from the suffering inherent in the material world. The term "soul" is understood to be at once functional and evaluative, teleological, and value-ladened, and that implies the inherent value of all living beings, providing a coherent metaphysical basis for animal advocacy. When the self or the soul is understood as a functional concept—and therefore possessing a non-material essence and teleology—the basis and grounding for affording ethical consideration to all living entities, and the commensurate inducement for us to behave ethically as an expression of our proper, healthy functioning, is coherent.

Toward a Jain Virtue Ethic of Animal "Rights"

MacIntyre concisely articulates the basic requirements for ethical language to be coherent and the source of the incoherent nature of modern ethical language:

> The moral scheme which forms the historical background [of Western moral thought as virtue ethics] . . . required three elements: [1] untutored human nature, [2] man-as-he-could-be-if-he-realized-his-*telos* and [3] moral precepts which enable him to pass from one state to the other. But the joint effect of the secular rejection of both Protestant and Catholic theology and scientific and philosophical rejection of Aristotelianism was to eliminate any notion of "man-as-he-could-be-if-he-realized-his-*telos*" [which also implies an essence that must be developed teleologically toward that ends]. Since the whole point of ethics—both as a theoretical and a practical discipline—is to enable man to pass from his present state [item 1] to his true end [item 2], the elimination of any notion of essential human nature, and with it the abandonment of any notion of a *telos*, leaves behind a moral scheme composed of two remaining elements [1 untutored human nature and 3 moral percepts] whose relationship becomes quite unclear. (MacIntyre 2015 [1981], 53–55)

Since, for the most part, premodern Indian thought did not reject essences (with the exception of some Buddhists), teleologies, or the functional nature of things, there was no fact/value divide to contend with in premodern Asian traditions. Therefore, the burden of articulating a Jain virtue ethic is only a matter of showing how it address these three elements that are required for a coherent ethical system, as articulated by MacIntyre: (1) untutored human nature, (2) person-as-they-could-be-if-they-realized-their-*telos*, and (3) the moral precepts which enable one to pass form one to the other.

As a position in favor of animal advocacy, MacIntyre's three-part configuration implies inherent valuation of animals who exist for their own teleological ends insofar as it is believed that animals have a metaphysical essence that is equal to that of humans, which is affirmed by the Jain tradition. That equality is the basis for speaking about "rights" from the perspective of virtue ethics. This is perhaps only marginally similar to how "rights" are related to Kantian "Kingdom of Ends"[4] as a sort of Kantian mild teleological overtone. But one key difference is where Kant's system attempts a universalizable rule-based ethic (as does utilitarianism/consequentialism), virtue ethics proposes a developmental model of human behavior where virtues represent our real, essential "potentials" that will be developed toward our fully realized ends, which are generally denied in deontological and utilitarian systems, rendering those as incoherent as per MacIntyre's critique. Thus, as I am using the term, the virtue ethicist argument for animal rights is not based on universalizable rule-based ethical systems such as the usual relationship between rights and deontology, but rather from the perspective that virtue ethics' animal rights (if we can use this designation) implies the realism of the essences, teleologies, and therefore inherent value and worth, of living beings, animals in particular.

1: Jain Concept of "Untutored Human Nature"

The starting point of a Jain teleological scheme, that accounts for who we "happen-to-be" in our "untutored natural state" (paraphrasing MacIntyre's first requirement for a coherent ethical system, above) is, as the *Ācārāṅga-sūtra* (*ĀS*) tells us, a state "of human (*māṇavāṇaṃ*) suffering (*dukkhaṃ*)." We are to "inquire about (*paveditam*) this world (*iha*)" and "that suffering (*tassa dukkhassa*)" from "virtuous ones (*kusalā*) who teach (*udāharati*) [us] wisdom (*pariṇṇam*)"[5] (*ĀS* 2.6.171). We might say that these "virtuous ones (*kusalā*)" represent who we "could-be-if-we-realized-our-essential nature" (MacIntyre's second requirement). Assumedly these "virtuous ones" will teach us the virtue that has allowed them to advance toward the telos of self-actualized potential (MacIntyre's third requirement), and taken together we can see a coherent MacIntyrean virtue ethic already in this earliest of Jain scriptures.

Related to our suffering, the state of who we "happen-to-be" as our "untutored" human nature (requirement 1) is characterized by the karmic burden that embodied souls carry that prevents us from making the transition from how we "happen-to-be" (requirement 1) to "who-we-could-be" in terms of our realized potential (requirement 2). The *ĀS* tells, "It is because of karmas (*kammuṇā*) that the soul becomes conditioned (*uvāhī*) by extraneous impositions (*jāyai*)"[6] (*ĀS* 3.1.19) and "this is (*iti*) the karma [that] must be completely understood (*pariṇṇāya*) and removed (*savaso*)"[7] (*ĀS* 2.6.172). That is to say that karma creates "impositions (*jāyai, ĀS* 3.1.19)" that prevent the full actualization of one's potential. In the words of the *Yoga-śāstra* (*YŚ*), we can "realize that (*viditam*) karma/actions (*karmāṇi*) produce only suffering (*api duḥka-kṛte*)"[8] (*YŚ* 12.50) since they restrict the full expression of our essential qualities of happiness, consciousness, and energy.

2: Moral Precepts Which Enable One to Pass from Untutored to Essential State

In terms of the virtues that we must cultivate, for Jains wisdom (*prajñā*) and nonviolence (*ahiṃsā*) are inextricably connected to all virtues, similar to Aristotle's "unity of virtue." MacIntyre disagreed with the Aristotelean and Thomistic idea of the unity of virtue, which he explains thusly:

> Suppose it is claimed that someone whose aims and purposes were generally evil, a devoted and intelligent Nazi, for example, possessed the virtue of courage. We ought to reply [as per Aristotle and Aquinas, citing P. T. Geach's problematization of the issue] that either it was not courage that he possessed or that in that kind of case courage is not a virtue. This kind of reply is clearly one that must be made by anyone who holds anything like Aquinas' view of the unity of virtues. (MacIntyre 2015 [1981], 179)

MacIntyre proceeds to argue that moral education would not be possible if such a Nazi were considered to be devoid of virtue (as the "unity of virtue" theory would hold) since there would be no initial virtues from which one could build on, upon which one might further elaborate and educate. Invoking Jain *Anekānta-vāda,* I do not believe that the two propositions are mutually exclusive, and I would affirm some degree of the "unity" idea, but arguing this is beyond the current scope. Suffice it to say, for Jains nonviolence (*ahiṃsā*) provides the unifying element of all other virtues; no other "virtues" (*puṇya*) can be properly considered as such in the absence of *ahiṃsā,* and the presence of *ahiṃsā* is the functional element that makes any behavior virtuous.

To actualize our potential (per item 2), we must first realize that "that the root of karma (*kamma-mūlam*) is violence (*chaṇam*)"[9] (*ĀS* 3.1.21), that is to say that all karma is characterized by some degree of violence that occurs whenever we commit any action. And the principal purpose for any virtuous behavior for Jains is the mitigation of karma. Thus, all virtue must be characterized by nonviolence, the principle that brings unity to all other virtues. This seems consistent with modern notions of intersectionality, for example, where one cannot properly combat any social justice issue without understanding the interrelationship between all forms of systematic violence. For example, we cannot understand the exploitation of animals apart from understanding the exploitation of humans and nature, which are mutually reinforcing systems and paradigms of violence. If one is more prone to harm people or nature, one is more prone to harm animals, and vice versa. Thus, as per intersectionality and similar to both Jain and Aristotelian concepts of "unity of virtue," a holistic account of animal advocacy must include or cohere with a feminist critique, a decolonial critique, an anti-caste discrimination critique, and a critique based on environmental ethics, etc.

In terms of a Jain unity of virtues, non-consumption (*aparigraha*) is a central Jain virtue that follows immediately from the unifying virtue of *ahiṃsā*. As an analogy, we can see that any time we consume, our demand inspires producers to create a supply, and in any supply chain, even of the most ethically produced goods, there is at least some violence. As the *ĀS* tells us, "All those, in this world, who are prone to possession of things, be they few or many, subtle or gross, sentient or insentient, try to acquire and accumulate them. They are prone to possession" because of their attachment to worldly objects[10] (*ĀS* 5.2.31).

All of our actions, our karmas, similarly have some degree of violence associated with them. This acquisitiveness and consumption not only hurts those who are on the receiving end of our karmic activity but also "spells disaster for those who are attached" to worldly consumption. For evidence we can just "see the state of the world!"[11] (*ĀS* 5.2.32) where "that participation in violence is as harmful to those who engage in violence to living beings" as it is to the living beings that are directly harmed. As the perpetrator inflicts violence, and derives worldly benefit from that violence, they also accumulate the karma that restricts their the full expression of their internal goodness, inhibiting MacIntyre's "who-one-could-be-if-one-realized-one's-potential." Thus, that participation in violence "deprives one of spiritual wisdom (*se abohīe*)"[12] (*ĀS* 1.2.23), where wisdom is one of the inherent qualities that one possesses and is one of the virtues by which one might actualize those potentials.

We can see that "one who lacks such wisdom of spiritual insight (*apariṇṇātā*)" as a principle virtue is in "violent" (*vihiṃsai*, from *ĀS* 1.1.1.27) pursuit of their "desires (*icchaete*)" and therefore "employ[s] as weapons (*satthaṃ*)" that which "causes harm even when they are one's own internal conditions (*māṇassa*)" that can be used as weapons upon even the tiniest of elemental beings[13] (*ĀS* 1.2.31). To achieve the Jain spiritual ideal, one cultivates wisdom (*pariṇṇātā*) as one reverses the process. Here "on the other hand (*ettha*), one comes to desire (*icchete*) not to use (*asamāraṃbha*) weapons or other such instruments that cause harm (*satthaṃ*) such as one's own internal [weaponized] conditions (*māṇassa*) upon even the tiniest of elemental beings." And through the absence of violence, even in one's own mind (*māṇassa*) one "develops (*bhavaṃti*) wisdom and spiritual insight (*pariṇṇātā*)"[14] (*ĀS* 1.2.32).

Thus, there is an inherent connection between the virtue of wisdom (*pariṇṇātā*) and that of the practice of nonviolence. Moreover, "having attained such insight (*taṃ pariṇṇāya*), a wise person should never allow for any instrument of harm, internally[15] or externally (*sattaṃ*)" against even the tiniest "beings in the earth, neither should they cause others to do so, nor should they approve of the engagement of anything, internally or externally that causes harm"[16] (*ĀS* 1.2.33). We see this attentiveness toward nonviolence in the behavior of the "monks (*ṇiggaṃṭhāṇa*) and nuns (*ṇiggaṃṭhīṇa*)" in the *Kalpa-sūtra* (*KS*), who "in the course of the Paryuṣaṇa during their monsoon sojourn"[17] are not permitted to partake in these "nine items that cause disorder:[18] milk, curd, fresh butter, clarified butter, oil, jagghery, honey, wine, and meat"[19] (*KS* 7.17). These are listed as problematic in part because they lead to violence through harming or exploiting animals, or the excessive loss of life that is due to consuming items that have been fermented. This type of "constant, incessant (*abhikkhaṇaṃ abhikkhaṇaṃ*) considering (*jāṇiyavvā*), envisioning (*pāsiyavvā*), and sensing (*paḍīlehiyavvā*)" the lives of even the tiniest, minute beings "by monks and nuns" is an essential virtue to cultivate for spiritual progress[20] (*KS* 7.44–45).

Thus, the greatest wisdom is nonviolence, and both wisdom and nonviolence are the principal unifying virtues that are to be pursued where all other virtues are instruments to these ends. This accounts for why the *aṇuvrata*s (lay vows) and *mahāvrata*s (mendicant vows) list of fivefold virtues, here as "vows," always begins with *ahiṃsā*. Interestingly, the language of the *Yoga-śāstra* speaks of these (and other) virtues as not only vows (*vṛata*s) but also as "cultivations" (*bhāvana*s; see Rodríguez in this volume), which justifies why we might liken them to Aristotelean "potentials" (*dunamis*) as teleologies and essences of virtue ethics, where virtues themselves are potentials to be cultivated. This also demonstrates the interrelationship between ethical theory and practice since theory is defined in terms of vows (*vrata*s) and cultivation (*bhāvana*). For Jains, ethical theory is necessarily *engaged*, solving what is often referred to as the "theory/praxis divide" in ethical theory.

Thus, "the one who is disciplined is liberated by the fivefold *bhāvanā*-contemplations" (non-violence, pleasant and true speech, non-stealing, continence, and non-consumption,[21] *YŚ* 1.19). Hemacandra also cites another list of common pan-dharmic *bhāvana*s that are virtues for "cultivation" (*bhāvana*). These are loving kindness (*maitrī*), the joy of completeness (*pramoda*), compassion (*kāruṇya*), and equipoise (*mādhyastha*). But rather than speaking of these as cultivations (*bhāvana*s), as this list is commonly known by Buddhists and Hindu texts, he speaks of these virtues as meditative objects that are to be combined like an "elixir" (*rasāyanam*)" for "proper meditation (*dharmya-dhyānam*)"[22] (*YŚ* 4.117), where meditation on these virtues may contribute to what Aristotle likened to as a "moral habit," underscoring that virtue ethics are a developmental rather than a rule-based approach to ethics.

Of course, Jain texts contain a plethora of other ethical precepts that can be taken as virtues to be cultivated. Collectively, these vows/cultivations are roughly akin to MacIntyre's "conception of the precepts of rational ethics" that lead one from untutored human nature to "the conception of human-nature-as-it-could-be-if-it-realized-its-*telos*" (as above, paraphrasing MacIntyre, 53–53). These are required to actualize oneself "because the gradual cultivation of the five *mahāvratas* by *bhāvanā*-contemplation" allows one to "attain the eternal platform (*avyayam padam*)"[23] as the spiritual telos (*YŚ* 1.25).

3: Jain Concept of "Personhood-as-One-Might-Be-If-They-Realized-Their-*Telos*"

The primary intention of the exercise of Jain virtues is to remove one's karma by the practice of nonviolence to realize one's potential. To remove the obstructions to the actualization of our full potential caused by karma and resulting in our suffering, one must follow the path of "non-karma/action (*niṣkarmatvam*) [that] produces happiness (*sukhāya*)." This can be done by "ceasing to endeavor" (*na . . . prayateta*) toward worldly pursuits that cause karma so that one can achieve a "state of non-action/non-karma (*niṣkarmatve*)" where "liberation is easily attained (*sulabha-mokṣe*)"[24] (*YŚ* 12.50).

If our successful enactment of the cultivation of virtues wisely mitigates our contribution to the suffering of other beings, then our karma will diminish and we will realize our true essential goodness, which includes the full expression of the soul's qualities of happiness (*sukha*, per *YŚ* 12.50), consciousness (*caitanya*), and energy (*vīrya*). If, through our lack of wisdom, we attempt to reach our ends, such as being happy, through incorrect means, then we will not be successful in the actualizing of these potentials, and the result is that we will feel frustrated and incomplete, and we will suffer. Thus, "After gaining knowledge, the *muṇī* should shake to its root their karma-body," that is to say, they should act in ways that mitigate and eradicate karma[25] (*ĀS* 5.3.59).

By this model, worldly desires are a sort of faux telos that entices us, and we must be cautious to rather discern between their temptation and the allure of spiritual realization—both of which *promise* the realization of the happiness that is our potential, but only one of which can actually deliver. Thus, as one becomes "vigilant (*appamatto*) against worldly desires (*kāmehiṃ*)" one thereupon "ceases from (*uvarato*) delinquent behavior (*pāvakammehiṃ*)" and becomes increasingly "energetic and self-secured (*āyagutte*)." Again, wisdom is both the realized potential and the virtue that one practices since "such a person" who has mitigated worldly desire comes to "know the essence of things (*kheyaṇṇe*)"[26] (*ĀS* 3.1.16), including the essential nature of one's soul—the universal telos of all living beings to which the practitioner aspires.

Thus, it is important that our secondary intentions to achieve happiness align with our primary intentions to realize our potential through nonviolence, wisdom, and the concomitant attenuation of karma (as inherently violent)—and wisdom is the primary virtue that allows us to discern between the two. We can do this by being like the "sage who is devoted to the Teachings (or Knowledge)" by contemplating upon the inner self, as one's essence, and thereby "become completely free from attachment."[27] This will help eradicate one's passions for the material acquisition as a false telos, a false happiness, and thereupon help us eradicate our karma (*ĀS* 4.3.32).

When one focuses on the allure of the true telos that exists as a potential in the essential self, one can discern the true telos from the faux telos of worldly happiness. This helps remove karma and actualize that potential, since "Just as fire quickly reduces the decayed wood to ashes, so does a *sādhaka* who is absorbed in the (inner) Self, and (completely) unattached" to all external objects of desire "attenuate and wither away" their karma-body[28] (*ĀS* 4.3.33).

It seems that the practice of the Jain virtues are intended to allow one to "meditate on one's essential, transcendental nature (*paramātmatva*) from meditation on the self (*ātma-dhyānāt*)" in a way that is "transformative like the iron that becomes gold from touching quicksilver"[29] (*YŚ* 12.12). This transformation is the result of the actualization of our true potential as "the highest bliss (*paramānanda*) realized when happiness is complete and nothing else," no material desire or other karmic activity, "seems as brilliant" as our spiritual telos and essence[30] (*YŚ* 12.51).

This telos is described with respect to each Tīrthaṅkara in the *Kalpa-sūtra* as an intensely expanded state of consciousness and seemingly boundless awareness without "a sense of strict delimitations"[31] between "substances (*davvao*), space, time, and psychological conditions (*bhāvao*)." Apart from these ontological categories, the lack of a sense of delimitations between psychological conditions is interesting since they include a lack of "delimitations between anger, pride, attachment, greed, fear, laughter, affection, hatred, quarrel, defamation, harsh words, meanness, gossiping, pleasure and pain, deceitful falsehood and the pain of having misplaced faith"[32] (*KS* 118 for Mahāvīra, 159 for Pārśvānātha). With a unity of virtues comes a unity of consciousness, and psychological vices lack true quiddity and are rather a function of "delimitation," or fragmentation of the inherent goodness of the soul obstructed by karma. Thus, with the full actuality of one's internal, essential potentials there is a commensurate attenuation of mental vices and afflictions characterized by a unity of virtues unified by nonviolence (*ahiṃsā*) itself, and the wisdom to recognize the centrality of *ahiṃsā* to our own true state of happiness. With Jain virtue ethics, care is dialogical: To care for others is to care for ourselves and vice versa—and among these "others" are animals.

Notes

1. Research for this work has been made possible by support from the Arihanta Institute. All translations are my own unless otherwise noted.

2. "Emotivism is the doctrine that all evaluative judgements and more specifically all moral judgements are *nothing but* expressions of preference, expressions of attitude or feeling, insofar as they are moral or evaluative in character . . . But moral judgements [by emotivism], being expressions of attitude or feeling, are neither true nor false; and agreement in moral judgement is not to be secured by any rational method, for there are none [according to emotivists]" (MacIntyre 2007, 11–12).

3. Both Hindu and Buddhist ethical systems have been likened to Aristotelean virtue ethics. When speaking in the context of Patañjali's *Yoga Sūtra*, Perrett and Pettigrove write, "The classical Yoga texts, however, do not explicitly discuss a rather different issue about the nature of the virtue ethics they present: namely, whether Yoga ethics is an *agent-based* virtue ethics or, like Aristotelean ethics, merely an *agent-focused* virtue ethics" (2015, 59; this is a distinction that I hesitate to attribute to Aristotle given his concept of "unity of virtues" but that is beyond the current scope).

In the context of Buddhist ethics, Goodman has written, "In a famous book, Damien Keown (1992) argued that the best theoretical model we have for the structure of Theravāda Buddhist normative thought comes from an analogy with Aristotelian virtue ethics." Goodman proceeds to make several analogies between Buddhist and Aristotelean thought with regard to virtue ethics (2015, 92ff.).

4. For Kant, the "Kingdom of Ends" is only to say that, ethically speaking, we should not treat anyone as a means toward our own ends, but to treat others as having their own ends in-themselves; it did not imply metaphysically real essences or teleologies. Kant argued for this system to be coherent; everyone "ought" to treat everyone else as we ourselves would seek to be treated, otherwise we are inconsistent and incoherent with our ethics, and that becomes the basis for our modern notions of "rights." We can also note the teleological overtone of consequentialism/utilitarianism as well since it is concerned with outcomes, but without metaphysically real essences concepts such as "utility" or "maximum happiness" become arbitrary at best and hegemonic at worst. Neither utilitarianism nor Kantian ethics allows for functional concepts as an inherent fact/value synthesis, thus rendering those systems to be incoherent.

5. *ĀS* 2.6.171: *jaṃ dukkhaṃ paveditaṃ iha māṇavāṇaṃ, tassa dukkhassa kusalā pariṇṇam udāharati* |

6. Translation by Muni Mahendra Kumar (MMK, *Āyāro, Ācārāṅga Sūtra,* 1981), *ĀS* 3.1.19: *kammuṇā uvāhī jāyai* |

7. *ĀS* 2.6.172: *iti kamma pariṇṇāya savvaso* | (savaso, Skt. √*so*).

8. *YŚ* 12.50: *karmāṇy api duḥkhakṛte niṣkarmatvaṃ sukhāya viditaṃ tu* |

9. *ĀS* 3.1.21: *kamma-mūlaṃ ca jaṃ chaṇaṃ* |

10. Translation by MMK, *ĀS* 5.2.31: *āvatī keāvaṃtī logasi pariggahāvatī—se appaṃ vā, bahuṃ vā, aṇuṃ vā, thūlaṃ vā, cittamataṃ vā, acittamataṃ vā, etesu ceva pariggahāvatī* |

11. Translation by MMK, *ĀS* 5.2.32: *etade vegesiṃ mahabbhayaṃ bhavati, logavittaṃ ca ṇaṃ uvehāe* |

12. *ĀS* 1.2.23: *taṃ se ahiyāe, taṃ se abohīe* | "That (*taṃ*) [participation in violence] is as harmful to those (se) [who engage in violence to living beings]. That (*taṃ*) [participation in violence] deprives one of spiritual wisdom (*se abohīe*)."

13. *ĀS* 1.2.31: *ettha satthaṃ samāraṃbhamāṇassa icchete āraṃbhā apariṇṇātā bhavaṃti*|| "Now (*ettha*) the [violent *vihiṃsai,* from 1.1.1.27] one who desires (*icchaete*) to use (*samāraṃbhamāṇassa*) a weapons or instruments that cause harm even when they are one's own internal conditions that can be used as weapons (*satthaṃ,* Sanskrit *śastra*) [upon even the tiniest of elemental beings, from previous verses] becomes (*bhavaṃti*) one who lacks the wisdom of spiritual insight (*apariṇṇātā,* Sanskrit: *aparijñātā*)."

14. *ĀS* 1.2.32: *ettha satthaṃ asamāraṃbhamāṇassa icchete āraṃbhā pariṇṇātā bhavaṃti* ||

15. "Internally" as per *māṇassa* from the previous verses.

16. *ĀS* 1.2.33: *taṃ pariṇṇāya mehāvī neva sayaṃ puḍhavi—satthaṃ samāraṃbhejjā, nevaṇṇehiṃ puḍhavi—satthaṃ samāraṃbhāvejjā, nevaṇṇe puḍhavi—satthaṃ samāraṃbhaṃte samaṇujāṇejjā* ||

17. *KS* 7.17: *vāsāvāsaṃ pajjosaviyāṇaṃ ṇo kappai*

18. *KS* 7.17: *imāo ṇava-rasa-vigaīo abhikkhaṇaṃ āhāriṭṭae*

19. *KS* 7.17: *vāsāvāsaṃ pajjosaviyāṇaṃ ṇo kappai ṇiggaṃṭhāṇa vā ṇiggaṃṭhīṇa vā haṭṭhāṇaṃ āroggāṇaṃ valīya-sarīrāṇaṃ imāo ṇava-rasa-vigaīo abhikkhaṇaṃ āhāriṭṭae* | *taṃ jahāḥ khīraṃ dahiṃ ṇavaṇīyaṃ sappiṃ tellaṃ guḍaṃ macchaṃ majjaṃ maṃsaṃ* |

20. *KS* 7.44–45 (refrain applied to various minute beings): . . . *ṇiggaṃtheṇa vā ṇiggaṃthīe vā abhikkhaṇaṃ abhikkhaṇaṃ jāṇiyavvā pāsiyavvā paḍīlehiyavvā bavae* |"

21. *YŚ* 1.19: *ahiṃsāsūnṛtāsteya-brahmacaryāparigrahāḥ* | *pañcabhiḥ pañcabhir yuktā bhāvanābhir vimuktaye* ||

22. *YŚ* 4.117: *maitrī-pramoda-kāruṇya-mādhyasthāni niyojayet* | *dharmya-dhyānam upaskartuṃ tad dhi tasya rasāyanam* ||

23. *YŚ* 1.25: *bhāvanābhir bhāvitāni pañcabhiḥ pañcabhiḥ kramāt* | *mahāvratāni no kasya sādhayanty avyayaṃ padam* ||

24. *YŚ* 12.50: *karmāṇy api duḥkha-kṛte niṣkarmatvaṃ sukhāya viditaṃ tu* | *na tataḥ prayateta kathaṃ niṣkarmatve sulabhamokṣe* ||

25. Translation by MMK, *ĀS* 5.3.59: *muṇī moṇaṃ samāyāe, dhuṇe kamma-sarīragaṃ* |

26. Ibid. MMK, *ĀS* 3.1.16: *appamatto kāmehiṃ, uvarato pāvakammehiṃ, vīre āyagutte je kheyaṇṇe* |

27. Ibid. MMK, *ĀS* 4.3.32: *iha āṇākaṃkhī paṃḍie aṇīhe egamappāṇaṃ saṃpehāe dhuṇe sarīraṃ, kasehi appāṇaṃ, jarehi appāṇaṃ* ||

28. Ibid. MMK, *ĀS* 4.3.33: *jahā juṇṇāiṃ kaṭṭhāiṃ, havvavāho pamatthati, evaṃ attasamāhie aṇihe* |

29. *YŚ* 12.12: *śrayate suvarṇa-bhāvaṃ siddha-rasa-sparśato yathā loham* | *ātma-dhyānād ātmā paramātmatvaṃ tathāpnoti* ||

30. *YŚ* 12.51: *mokṣo 'stu māstu yadi vā paramānandas tu vidyate sa khalu* | *yasmin nikhila-sukhāni pratibhāsante na kiñcid iva* ||

31. *KS* 118 for Mahāvīra, 159 for Pārśvānātha: *ṇatthi ṇaṃ . . . katthai paḍibaṃdhe*

32. *KS* 118 (Mahāvīra), 159 (Pārśva): *ṇatthi ṇaṃ tassa bhagavaṃtassa katthai paḍibaṃdhe* | *se ya cauvvihe paṇṇatte* | *taṃ jahā—davvao khittao* | *kālao, bhāvao davvao—sacittācita-mīsaesu davvesu* | *khittao—game vā ṇagare vā araṇṇe vā khitte vākhale vā aṃgaṇe vā* | *kālao—samae vā āvaliyāe vā āṇā-pāṇue vā thove vā khaṇe vā lave vā muhutte vā ahoratte vā pakkhe vā māse vā uūe vā*

ayaṇe vā saṃvacchare vā aṇṇayare vā dīh-kāl-saṃjoe | bhāvao — kohe vā māṇe vā māyāe vā lobhe vā bhaye vā hāse vā pijje vā dose vā kalahe vā ababhakkhāṇe vā pesuṇṇe vā par-parivāe vā arai-raī vā māyā-mose vā micchā-daṃsaṇa-salle vā | tassa naṃ bhagavaṃtassa ṇo evaṃ bhavai |

References

Āyāro, Ācārāṅga Sūtra. 1981. Translated by Muni Mahendra Kumar. Today and Tomorrow's Printers & Publishers.

Goodman, Charles. 2015. "Virtue in Buddhist Ethical Traditions." In *The Routledge Companion to Virtue Ethics*, edited by Lorraine Besser-Jones and Michael Slote. Routledge Philosophy Companions. Routledge.

Hemacandra. 2002. *The Yogaśāstra of Hemacandra: A Twelfth Century Handbook on Śvetāmbara Jainism*. Translated by Olle Quarnström. Department of Sanskrit and Indian Studies, Harvard University.

James, William. 1987. "Pragmatism." In *William James: Writings 1902–1910*. Based on lectures at Columbia University, 1906–1907. Library of America.

MacIntyre, Alasdair. 2015 [1981]. *After Virtue: Third Edition*. University of Notre Dame Press.

Miller, Christopher Jain, and Jonathan Dickstein. 2021. "Jain Veganism: Ancient Wisdom, New Opportunities." *Religions* 12:512. https://doi.org/10.3390/rel12070512.

Nietzsche, Friedrich. 2022. *The Gay Science*. Kindle edition. Grapevine India Publishers. First published in 1882.

Goodman, Charles. 2015. "Virtue in Buddhist Ethical Traditions." In Besser-Jones and Slote, eds., *The Routledge Companion to Virtue Ethics*.

Perrett, Roy W., and Glen Pettigrove. 2015. "Hindu Virtue Ethics." In Besser-Jones and Slote, eds., *The Routledge Companion to Virtue Ethics*.

Woodward, Ashley. 2011. "Whose Nietzsche?" In *Interpreting Nietzsche: Reception and Influence*, edited by Ashley Woodward. Bloomsbury. ProQuest Ebook Central, https://ebookcentral-proquest-com.dtl.idm.oclc.org/lib/dtl/detail.action?docID=730008.

[illegible]

References

Āyāro, Āyāraṅga Sutta. 1981. Translated by Muni Mahendra Kumar. Today and Tomorrow's Printers & Publishers.

Goodman, Charles. 2015. "Virtue in Buddhist Ethical Traditions." In *The Routledge Companion to Virtue Ethics*, edited by Lorraine Besser-Jones and Michael Slote. Routledge Philosophy Companions. Routledge.

Hemacandra. 2002. *The Yogaśāstra of Hemacandra: A Twelfth Century Handbook on Śvetāmbara Jainism*. Translated by Olle Qvarnström. Department of Sanskrit and Indian Studies, Harvard University.

James, William. 1987. "Pragmatism." In *William James: Writings 1902–1910*. Based on lectures at Columbia University, 1906–1907. Library of America.

MacIntyre, Alasdair. 2015 [1981]. *After Virtue*. Third Edition. University of Notre Dame Press.

Miller, Christopher Jain, and Jonathan Dickstein. 2021. "Jain Veganism: Ancient Wisdom, New Opportunities." *Religions* 12:512. https://doi.org/10.3390/rel12070512.

Nietzsche, Friedrich. 2022. *The Gay Science*. Kindle edition. Grapevine India Publishers. First published in 1882.

Goodman, Charles. 2015. "Virtue in Buddhist Ethical Traditions." In Besser-Jones and Slote, eds., *The Routledge Companion to Virtue Ethics*.

Perrett, Roy W., and Glen Pettigrove. 2015. "Hindu Virtue Ethics." In Besser-Jones and Slote, eds., *The Routledge Companion to Virtue Ethics*.

Woodward, Ashley. 2011. "Whose Nietzsche?" In *Interpreting Nietzsche: Reception and Influence*, edited by Ashley Woodward. Bloomsbury. ProQuest Ebook Central, https://ebookcentral-proquest-com.[illegible]/lib/du/detail.action?docID=730063.

9

Ahiṃsā, Anekānta, and Animal Rights

Engaging Plurality in Our Planetary Context

ANDREW BRIDGES

The Promise Jain Concepts Hold for the Ethical Understanding of Animal Rights

Humanity's treatment of animals appears to defy rationality in manifold ways. Collectively speaking, humanity does not hold a unified coherent opinion on the moral status of animals, nor do many of us, as individuals, reach reflective equilibrium (Morrow 2018, 97)[1] in our moral decision-making involving animal rights and animal well-being. A person may acknowledge that chickens, pigs, and cows feel pain and express purposiveness as significantly as dogs and cats, while at the same time regularly consuming the former but being horrified to consume the latter (ibid., 96).[2] Animals unwillingly serve as society's food, clothing, jewelry, furniture, entertainment, experiments, and pets. The moral reactions humans have to the cruelty, slaughter, and commodification of animals is, likewise, manifold—from understanding such actions as morally forbidden to morally permissible, and even at times, morally praiseworthy.

What would happen if we engaged these relevant contemporary ethical issues surrounding animal well-being and rights that are so well known to scholars of animal studies and the Anthropocene[3] with principles in the Jain tradition? To answer this question, in this chapter I explore three Jain concepts: *anekānta* (many-sidedness), *ahiṃsā* (non-harming), and the Jain concept of life, as a way of approaching the moral status of animals, given the myriad perspectives held by individuals regarding animals. I argue that the Jain principle of *ahiṃsā*, the Jain concept of life, and the Jain ontology of *anekānta* provide a dynamic and robust philosophical framework for determining the moral status of animals within our contemporary situation. In the sections that follow, I share how each of these Jain concepts engage with contemporary questions of the moral status of animals, and how each of these three concepts mutually inform and support one another. Before presenting the philosophical richness and ethical importance of these concepts, I turn to the most significant difference between humans and animals and explain what this difference suggests for ethical engagement concerning animal rights and well-being.

What Our Contemporary Experience of the Anthropocene Suggests About the Difference Between Humans and Animals

In his work *Homo Deus: A Brief History of Tomorrow*, Yuval Noah Harari elaborates on the most distinctive characteristic that separates humans from animals, and, consequently, has allowed humans to dominate both the planet and every other animal species. This distinctive characteristic we humans have is our profoundly powerful imaginations, which produce elaborate shared intersubjective realities among members of our species. Harari explains,

> During the last 70,000 years the intersubjective realities that Sapiens invented became ever more powerful, so that today they dominate the world. Will the chimpanzees, the elephants, the Amazon rainforests and the Arctic glaciers survive the twenty-first century? This depends on the wishes and decisions of intersubjective entities such as the European Union and the World Bank; entities that exist only in our shared imagination. No other animal

> can stand up to us, not because they lack a soul or a mind, but because they lack the necessary imagination. Lions can run, jump, claw and bite. Yet they cannot open a bank account or file a lawsuit. And in the twenty-first century, a banker who knows how to file a lawsuit is far more powerful than the most ferocious lion in the savannah. (Harari 2017, 151)

An important aspect of this distinction between humans and animals that Harari mentions concerns how religions have prioritized the place of the human being as more significant than that of the animal. Ethics and understandings of the moral status of animals vary widely both among and within religious traditions (ibid., 95). Harari correctly identifies the Jain religion as emphasizing *ahiṃsā,* and therefore, seeking to inflict the least amount of harm upon animals, insects, plant life, and the ecosystems of the planet, writing, "Jain monks are particularly careful in this regard [with respect to not harming life]. They always cover their mouths with a white cloth, lest they inhale an insect, and whenever they walk they carry a broom to gently sweep any ant or beetle from their path" (ibid., 94–95). He also nevertheless points out that despite the emphasis on *ahiṃsā,* "all agricultural religions—Jainism, Buddhism and Hinduism included—found ways to justify human superiority and the exploitation of animals (if not for meat, then for milk and muscle power)" (ibid., 95).

This prioritization of the power and privilege of the human being present in varying degrees within and throughout the religious traditions of the world is a phenomenon this chapter addresses. The gravity of this prioritization within the Anthropocene and facilitated by the powerful intersubjective imaginations of human being means that improvements in animal rights and well-being will have to begin with humans reconceptualizing their understanding of the moral status of animals. This chapter aims to show that the emphasis of Jain ethics is not on the superiority of the human being vis-à-vis animal life, but rather the tradition's emphasis is placed on *ahiṃsā* and on *parasparopagraho jīvānām* (the interdependence of all life)[4] in a way that checks the abuses of human anthropocentricism during the Anthropocene. The Jain principles of *ahiṃsā, anekānta,* and the Jain concept of life can morally enrich our collective intersubjective imaginations concerning the moral status of animals and provide us with adequate views, knowledge, and moral conduct to understand the moral significance of preventing harm to these living beings—both collectively as a species and individually as life-forms.

Anekānta and the Elephant in the Room: An Ethically Structured Approach to Plurality

By titling this section "*Anekānta* and the Elephant in the Room: An Ethically Structured Approach to Plurality," one feature of Jain metaphysics I wish to emphasize is its matrix for nurturing and acknowledging the plurality of life to its fullest potential. The most common illustration used by scholars for the explanation of *anekānta* is the blind individuals who encounter an elephant (see figure 9.1). This illustration of *anekānta* correctly and powerfully

Figure 9.1. A Jain rendition of seven blind men making limited truth claims based on their one-sided (*ekānta*) viewpoints about what they perceive as they feel different parts of an elephant. Following Cort's arguments (2000), note that only the Jinas who have a complete, many-sided (*anekānta*) view of reality pictured in the upper corners are able to perceive the entire elephant for what it actually is. *Source:* Romana Klee, CC BY-SA 2.0.

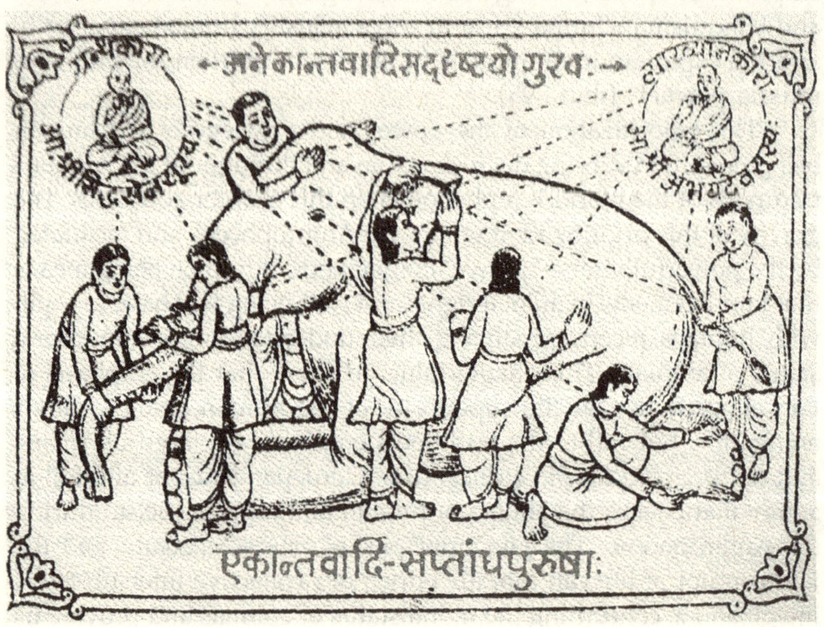

illustrates the reality and situatedness of the view of the individual human, while expressing the larger, much more expansive and yet inclusive nature of reality. This illustration is thereby quite effective in promoting understanding of the non-absolutism of any one perspective, as well as the appreciation of the myriad true perspectives informed by the particularity of their situatedness. Being a description of the metaphysical nature of reality, *anekānta* is not only an ontological space where peaceful epistemological inquiry can be undertaken among individuals with disparate viewpoints. *Anekānta* is also the ontological space for sustaining a variety of disparate perspectives through nonviolence.[5] *Anekānta* not only proposes that value is a metaphysically real quality of souls (*jīva*), but its ontology also negates *ekānta*. It is the ontology abating all attempts at absolutism. As John Cort has pointed out, *anekānta* was not historically used in this way as a form of "intellectual *ahiṃsā*" in the Jain tradition (see Cort 2000), though in more recent times, Jains have adapted *anekānta* as a form of "intellectual *ahiṃsā*" as I am also proposing we can constructively do in this chapter (also see Long in this volume).

One particular Jain scholar who I find quite ably elucidating this metaphysical aspect of *anekānta* within the lived structure of our contemporary society is Kamla Jain, who identifies *anekānta* with secularism in the article "Anekanta in Present Day Social Life." In this article Jain equates *anekānta* with secularism in the context of the secular government of India.[6] Through this comparison, Kamla Jain stresses that "a secular state protects all religions equally and favors none at the expense of others . . . It does not mean indifference to religion nor does it mean opposition to religion. It only means that the state as such does not identify itself with any particular religion and not only tolerates but appreciates every religion" (Kamla Jain 2004, 118–119). With this comparison Kamla Jain emphasizes that secularism means that government supports and appreciates all religions. In practice this is an extremely difficult aim to achieve, particularly in a secular democracy where votes can change or maintain policies and laws, and where people's values are at least in part informed by their religious beliefs. In such cases, the function of the government for maintaining equitable plurality is extremely important. The apprehension of what plurality means in the minds of a government's citizens is of equal importance. *Anekānta,* as Jain correctly acknowledges, provides a structure that can be concretized in varying degrees in secular governments, such as in the secular government of India. Religious truths are not simply attested to by declaration; in many cases, they are also lived. In expressions of lived truth, truth has existence that can be experienced. *Anekānta* is not merely the belief that multiple perspectives exist, it is the ontology of their expression. In appreciating every religion, secularism expresses the truth of the ontology of *anekānta.*

I suggest that this same ontological feature of *anekānta,* which Jain correctly explains is comparable to the ideal aims of the secular state, is also appropriate for engaging in conversations concerning the complexity of animal rights in our planetary context. Within this context, the appropriate utilization of *anekānta,* I suggest, is twofold. The first is the use of the ontological space for the peaceful epistemological inquiry by human beings with ostensibly disparate points of view concerning the moral status of nonhuman animals that simultaneously incorporates the viewpoints of nonhuman animals as much as possible. Here I have in mind John Koller's reflection on the ontology of *anekānta,* when he explains, "The *anekāntavāda* philosophy can be seen as providing an ontological basis for the principle of non-violence . . . This has important ecological implications, for it legitimizes considerations from nonhuman perspectives, enabling us to consider the effects of our actions on nonhuman life-forms and environments" (Koller 2002, 20). As the ontological space is utilized in this way, we must acknowledge an important fact that Christopher Key Chapple brings to our attention in his article "Animal Ethics": "One fact stands true: animals generally have no voice through which to advocate for themselves" (Chapple 2018, 69). When considering the utilization of *anekānta* for peaceful epistemological inquiry, it appears that robust participation on the part of the animal is, at best, extremely limited. *Anekānta* is not a concept that allows animal participation in as robust and sophisticated a manner as humans who utilize the anthropocentric structures available to them—e.g., secular democracy or in interreligious dialogue—to either understand or appreciate plurality or to peacefully debate the viewpoints of nonhuman animals. The nonhuman animal, it appears, lacks the powerful intersubjective imagination that we humans possess and utilize to argue our positions regarding what we believe ourselves and nonhuman animals to be. The nonhuman animal lacks robust conceptual awareness—at least as far as current science can conclude—to fully comprehend the varieties of commodities humans aim to transform them into. Nor can animals make elaborate presentations concerning what they would certainly *not* like to be, that is, food, clothing, jewelry, entertainment, furniture, etc. This one degree of difference between human and nonhuman animals should in no way be viewed as a diminishment of animals' complex emotional lives, desire for life, and expression, but only as a realization that humans must advocate for animal well-being and remain sensitive to the perspectives of animals. This dimension of animal advocacy is exemplified perfectly in the story of Parsvanatha advocating for the animals not to be slaughtered for his wedding. Parsvanatha's articulation of the animals' tantamount value and perspective to humans is understood in our contemporary context as a role of *anekāntavāda* (see Barbato 2017, 174–176).

The existential condition that the nonhuman animal inhabits brings us to the second constructive utilization of *anekānta*. This second utilization is of the metaphysical structure of *anekānta* itself as a nonviolent matrix for the perseveration and nurturing of particular perspectives, which includes the perspectives of nonhuman animal life. Although nonhuman animals are unable to participate as fully in the intersubjective realities being discussed and debated by their human counterparts, the pluralistic structure of *anekānta* would insist that the intersubjective realities of the animals still exist as they are. Animals should not be harmfully destroyed and transformed into that which humans would tenaciously declare them to be. As life-forms capable of liberation in a future lifetime, their ontological status is not that of commodity or material resource. The most appropriate utilization of *anekānta* to the moral status of animals becomes the imperative that they be allowed to exist in-themselves and for-themselves, and free from harm.

We need look no further than the story of the blind men and the elephant itself to understand the issue of failing to see the intersubjective realities and viewpoints of nonhuman animals in our current uses of *anekānta*. We can add here to Harari's aforementioned observation that even Jains have "found ways to justify human superiority and the exploitation of animals (if not for meat, then for milk and muscle power)" by adding that animals' perspectives have also been unintentionally overlooked for the purposes of human philosophical discourse (Harari 2017, 95). Elephants, like many other animals, have been shown to have complex emotional lives (McCarthy 1995), and yet they have no recognized perspective in the story of the blind men so often used to illustrate *anekānta* in Jain philosophical discourse. Direct consideration of what we do indeed know about the perspectives of nonhuman animals from science and animal studies (e.g., Bekoff 2000), along with diminishing human selfish behavior, appears to be emphasized as a contemporary role of *anekānta* in, for example, the Jain Declaration of Nature. Singhvi elucidates *anekānta*'s role in diminishing the tendency toward privileging human viewpoints at the expense of animals (which Harari points out) when he writes, "Because it is rooted in the doctrine of *anekāntavāda* and *syādvāda*, Jainism does not look upon the universe from an anthropocentric, ethnocentric or egocentric viewpoint. It takes into account the viewpoints of other species, other communities and nations and other human beings" (Singhvi 1990, 8). Considering the perspectives of manifold other nonhuman animals, especially those billions of land animals who are routinely farmed, tortured, and slaughtered for human consumption, and yet who want to live, is facilitated by the ontology of *anekānta* and is, of course, how *anekānta* has generally been understood by Jains in ancient history.

Further Considerations Concerning the Validity of the Ontological Structure of *Anekānta*

Humanity holds myriad philosophical interpretations concerning the ultimate nature of reality. For those who hold a differing ontological understanding than what *anekānta* propounds, what additional arguments can make *anekānta*'s ontology compelling? For those who seem convinced that it is morally permissible to engage in the commodification of animals without any ethical concern for their well-being, what might change their mind? With respect to further philosophical arguments, Joseph Prabhu provides an idea concerning how to utilize practical reason in a similar way that

Kant did to demonstrate the practical necessity of particular ideas for the ongoing existence of life as we know it. When Prabhu aims to argue for the cogency of reincarnation, he does so in Kantian fashion, explaining,

> It is the concrete texture of our moral lives that suggests the need to go beyond the parameters of a single earthly life. The seriousness of our endeavor to shape our lives according to ideals of truth, wisdom, love and compassion, and all that they entail in terms of the development of virtue, together with the sense of inadequacy in our actual achievements, warrant the presumption that a single life cannot be all that we are destined to have. To grant that would make a mockery of our moral experience. (Prabhu 1989, 66)

Prabhu utilizes both practical reasoning and the development of the virtues of truth, wisdom, love, and compassion to reason for the cogency of the ontological truth of reincarnation. The seriousness of our moral experience vis-à-vis our particular finite moral insufficiencies suggests to Prabhu the practical truth of reincarnation. Similarly, I find that in our contemporary planetary context of the Anthropocene, the pattern of reasoning that Prabhu has demonstrated to suggest the ontological reality of reincarnation can also be utilized to suggest the ontological reality of *anekānta.*

In our contemporary experience of the Anthropocene, where anthropocentrism and human hegemony toward ecosystems and animals is catastrophic, I find it can be effectively demonstrated that the ontological reality of *anekānta* possesses universal relevance. For those who do not already hold the ontological structure of *anekānta* to be an accurate depiction of reality (as, at the very least the negation of *ekānta*), *anekānta* moves from an imagined ideal—one that often conflicts with human desires to radically transform aspects of the planet and the attachment of absolutism (*ekānta*)—to a practical necessity, without which contemporary life as we know it will not be possible. This is because one realizes that to disregard or destroy the perspective of other life-forms is not only an act of *hiṃsā* but a moral error of *ekānta.* This realization conflicts with our moral duties and sensibilities to ensure that life (for all life-forms) as we know it remains a viable possibility for future generations.

In the article "Parenting the Planet," Sarah Krakoff utilizes the metaphor of adulthood to explain the qualitatively different sense of power and relationship the human species has with the planet. She describes this with a metaphor of parenting that suggests that humans as a species during our contemporary time in the Anthropocene have reached adulthood, and that the responsibility we collectively have to other species and the environment—given our immense power—should be one analogous to parenting. Krakoff states, "In the Anthropocene, the implications of attitudes and actions toward the environment are quite different than in previous eras, when human activity was capable of only the most ephemeral effects on the world" (2018, 548). However, during the last century, and in our current one, our abilities to reshape the environments of the planet have increased exponentially, and with this increase in our collective power has come an increase in the destructive consequences and devastation for animals and their ecosystems.

Harari, in his chapter "The Anthropocene" in his work *Homo Deus: A Brief History of Tomorrow,* cites one such example of the power humanity has exerted over animals in changing the ratio of wild and domesticated animals. Harari summarizes some of these effects stating, "The world contains 40,000 lions compared to 600 million house cats; 900,000 African buffalo versus 1.5 billion domesticated cows; 50 million penguins and 20 billion chickens. Since 1970, despite growing ecological awareness, wildlife populations have halved (not that they were prospering in 1970) . . . At present, more than 90 per cent of the large animals of the world (i.e., those weighing more than a few pounds) are either humans or domesticated animals" (71–72). When this new quality and scale of collective human effort and enterprise are put into practice without care given to the collective consequences such actions will have, the future well-being of life on this planet is placed in jeopardy. Life as we know it becomes unsustainable. Put another way: Collectively, our way of life and our interrelatedness to other species no longer becomes possible.

With such novel and powerful abilities that allow humanity to either nurture or destroy entire species, ecosystems, or the planet itself, different truths demonstrated through practical reasoning related to ethical human behavior must be brought into consideration. We, collectively, are not able to sustain (i.e., continue to make possible) our current collective way of life with our continued behavior toward other species and ecosystems. This existential condition came into being during the latter half of the twentieth century and demonstrates the futility of humanity's behavior toward other species and ecosystems as well as the futility of the ontologies that inform them and inform moral value. Practical reasoning suggests an ontology in support of plurality as opposed to ones justifying *hiṃsā* and *ekānta.*

The ontological structure of *anekānta* appears an appropriate truth to hold given both humanity's collective power that has come to fruition in our current time and humanity's role-based obligation (i.e., metaphorically role-based obligation of parent, as Krakoff suggest) to future generations and to other species. This role-based obligation to other species derives from the awareness that if human collective destructive behavior continues unabated, the lives and the perspectives of myriad species will perish. Without the belief in *anekānta*—or a similar ontological truth with peaceful epistemological implications—it seems unlikely that there will be the required manifestation of the moral behavior collectively required by humans for interspecies life on this planet to continue. Such a catastrophe would make a tantamount mockery of our moral experience (as the one Prabhu suggests if reincarnation were not true), and I suggest offers compelling evidence (via practical reasoning) for the ontological validity of *anekānta.*

Ahiṃsā, the Jain Concept of Life, and the Ideology of Infinite Mutability

I now aim to provide the reader with a contrast between, on the one hand, the Jain principle of *ahiṃsā* and the Jain concept of life and, on the other hand, the ideology of infinite mutability[7] with respect to the manner in which we view the moral status of animals and animal well-being. The ideology of infinite mutability is described with the term "ideology" because I wish to express an incompleteness that the view propounds. Ideologies often confuse what is contingent with what is universal, and after this error is embraced and experienced it can be difficult to see past this error. This particular ideology, when applied to animals (as well as to the earth's ecosystems) views animals as material objects that humans are able to transform into other objects.[8] This ideology holds that there is no essential value in the particularity of an animal in-itself as a particular unique living being, nor is there necessarily any unique value in the animal being alive as opposed to being slaughtered and having its body be transformed into any number of objects of humans' desire.

Ahiṃsā, which I suggest is a corrective to the harmful ideology of infinite mutability, often translated as "nonviolence," is one of the five vows of the Jain religion and is also an essential aim of most all Jains. In the book *An Ahimsa Crisis: You Decide*, Sulekh C. Jain explains from an emic perspective, "In Jainism, ahimsa is the basis for the fundamental right of the existence of all life forms (jiva)" (2016, 73). This principle of nonviolence is understood within the context of the Jain karmic system and is understood to apply to all forms of life: human, animal, insect, plant, and even microbial life. All life has the potential for liberation from the cycle of *saṃsāra* once it is in human form, and much of nonhuman life has the ability to be reincarnated in human form. Ideally, all thoughts, speech, and actions should be considered and performed in the spirit of *ahiṃsā*. While existing and moving about in the world, Jains acknowledge that some harm (particularly to plant and insect life) is unavoidable, but the aim is to reduce harm as much as possible to all living beings. Sulekh Jain further explains "The Two Types of Ahimsa," stating, "The practice of ahimsa can be either passive, which is manifested by not causing harm to others in any shape or form . . . or active, proactive or positive, which is evidenced in the principle of helping to alleviate the suffering of others to the best of one's ability . . . In this sense, ahimsa means that when an act of himsa ["harm"] is being committed, one cannot be a mere bystander or spectator" (ibid., 76). Both of these types of *ahiṃsā* are, for example, present in the Jain Declaration on the Climate Crisis. The first type of passive *ahiṃsā* is found in the Jain Declaration's request for Jain communities to commit to a variety of actions to reduce harm, such as "Serve only vegan food and use only vegan items in rituals such as aartis and pujas in temple."[9] The second type of active *ahiṃsā* is exemplified in the Jain Declaration's suggestions to business and government leaders, such as the proposal to "Remove subsidies for the meat and dairy industries, eliminate favorable treatment for fertilizer and pesticide companies and incentivize the research and development of agricultural practices that use no chemical pollutants or byproducts of animal cruelty" (ibid.). If we accept this emic understanding of *ahiṃsā* as both passively not harming and actively preventing harm, *ahiṃsā* also has the practical dimension in our complex world of understanding and supporting the actions and policies that will do the least amount of harm. This practical dimension is particularly important concerning how to promote the path of least violence when understanding the interrelatedness of humans, animals, and the environment.

In the article "Ecology, Economics, and Development in Jainism," Padmanabh S. Jaini considers the practice of *ahiṃsā* as a "balanced approach," which Jains have adopted historically in daily life and practical activities. This balanced approach, Jaini also finds, is related to Gandhi's explanation of any activity's relationship to violence. In this article, Jaini quotes Gandhi's explanation, "Strictly speaking, no activity is possible without a certain amount of violence, no matter how little. Even the process of living is impossible without a certain amount of violence. What we need to do is to minimize it to the greatest extent possible" (Jaini 2002, 150–151). Jaini also provides the malaria control project as an example of a situation where a balanced approach to reducing harm necessarily requires careful evaluation, explaining,

> Controlling the spread of malaria has, in the past involved the killing of millions of mosquitoes by spraying insecticides that are harmful to the environment. Although this project still involves killing, there is an effort to reduce harm to insects and the environment by emphasizing multiple means of intervention with a decrease in the use of insecticides, more focused spraying with less environmentally harmful chemicals, and the increased use of medicated mosquito nets. The degree to which killing and environmental harm is reduced in comparison to past projects could be an indicator in evaluating a project such as this. (ibid., 152)

The Jain principle of *ahiṃsā* when understood within the context of the Jain concept of life provides a robust philosophical framework for the moral status of animals in our contemporary situation. This contemporary situation is one that contains unprecedented challenges, complexities, and responsibilities related to animal well-being. *Ahiṃsā,* in the context of the Jain concept of life, asserts that every life form whether it is human, animal, insect, or plant has value and has a soul (*jīva*) that undergoes reincarnation and in human form is able to achieve liberation. The role of the human being in the Jain tradition is one of assistance to all life-forms in achieving this goal. Life forms, conceptually understood in Jain ethics, should not be harmed because of the inherent value of their soul, but rather assisted or supported in order to allow other life forms to live free from harm. Elaborating on *ahiṃsā* and the Jain concept of life, Sulekh C. Jain writes,

> All around in this universe (irrespective of what life form/shape one is), every single living being, big and small, human and nonhuman, plant and organism, has a soul just like me. All souls are eternal . . . All souls are spiritually equal to each other . . . No soul wants or desires suffering. All souls have the same rights to live peacefully and undisturbed as I do. Since all souls are just like me and have the same rights and privileges as I do, I have no right to harm, kill, torture, disturb or interfere in any way in the life and existence of another soul. (2016, 73–74)

With respect to the inherent value of the animal's soul, and their desire for their own well-being, we observe that *ahiṃsā,* in the context of the emic Jain concept of life, seeks the well-being of each individual life form.

In contrast to the principle of *ahiṃsā* and the Jain concept of life, the ideology of infinite mutability can be used with respect to the way in which nonhuman animals are actually viewed and treated in most everyday circumstances. Again, our extremely powerful intersubjective imagination creates myriad potential objects we imagine transforming the animal body into, and then we transform these animals into these objects of human consumption and commodity. Through these practices, humans make the animals appear infinitely mutable, and prior centuries of success in transforming bodies of animals into the commodities and resources humans desire them to be only appears to support the views of this ideology further. This ideology promotes metaphorical blindness to the reality of the animal as an individual living being that is neither mutable material nor a variety of commodities. In the Anthropocene, particularly, the ideology of infinite mutability is ostensibly experienced by humans with respect to animals at alarming frequency—so much so that people often experience the objects and commodities animals' bodies have been transformed into before they ever experience the particular animal, or even experience a member the species of this animal. The phenomenological prevalence of the mutability of the nonhuman animal body, unfortunately, adds cogency to this ideology, and in doing so it does detriment to the concept of the animal as a living being. With greater amounts of large-scale violence toward animals and greater systematic restructuring of animals into artificial harmful environments, such as in the case of factory farming, the metaphoric and literal sightlessness humans experience concerning the truth of animals as living beings only increases.

From such destructive acts, humans as consumers may not experience the animal as a living being at all; they only ostensibly experience the ideology of infinite mutability when interacting with the commodities that were produced by the life and death of the animal they never met or knew. The Jain principles of *ahiṃsā* and *anekāntavāda* call infinite mutability into question, asking us to consider both the desire of all animals to live and not be harmed for human consumption, and, furthermore, the particular perspectives each of these types of animals possess and the corresponding implication of dignity and respect afforded to them.

Conclusion: *Ahiṃsā, Anekānta,* and the Jain Concept of Life Gaining Prevalence of Practice

In this chapter, I have engaged three inter-related subjects of discussion pertaining to animal rights and well-being with principles gleaned from the Jain philosophical tradition. The first subject of discussion was the qualitative differences of our contemporary situation in the Anthropocene itself. When compared to any previous geological epoch, I argued that in the Anthropocene, different ethical and metaphysical frameworks than those we are currently accustomed to are more clearly understood (through practical reason) as appropriate for the ethical situation we collectively find ourselves in.

The second subject of discussion was the ethical and metaphysical frameworks themselves, their robust and dynamic interrelated components as well as their coherence in our planetary context. The features of the Jain ethical and philosophical systems that I examined were the principle of *ahiṃsā,* the Jain concept of life, and the Jain ontology of *anekānta.* The Jain philosophical concept of *anekānta* was presented as having manifold significance for engagement in issues involving animal rights and well-being. *Anekānta* gives us new tools to engage with contemporary moral issues and questions involving animal rights both as a metaphysic and as a groundwork for nonviolent, epistemological inquiry among individuals holding disparate views on animals' moral status. To avoid privileging the perspectives of humans alone, *anekānta*'s coherence and pragmatic value for the preservation of the perspective of animals was also demonstrated. The robust and interrelated features of *ahiṃsā* and the Jain concept of life were also presented as an alternative to the destructive and prevalent ideology of infinite mutability.

The third interrelated subject of discussion concerning engagement on moral issues pertaining to animal rights and well-being was the argument that animals have the right to embody their perspective. This argument was based not only on the implications of Jain ethics and the Jain concept of life but also on the inadequacy of the ideology that holds the view that animals are commodities that can be rendered infinitely mutable. Greater prevalence of the practice of *ahiṃsā* toward animals will lead to their experiences of harm being greatly reduced, and in cases of greater freedom for existence being experienced. As the perspective of the animal as a living being, existing for itself, is experienced with as great a frequency or greater frequency than their commodification, their perspective can be further understood and appreciated. As engagement in ethical issues involving the moral status of animals through *anekānta, ahiṃsā,* and the Jain concept of life increases, the prevalence allows humanity in our contemporary context to understand the philosophical view and ethical conduct to promote peace and reduce harm to all forms of life, both human and nonhuman.

Notes

1. Reflective equilibrium refers both to "the process of eliminating the inconsistencies in your moral belief" and to the state in which "all of your moral beliefs 'fit together' well, which means—at a minimum—that they do not conflict with one another" (Morrow 2018, 97).

2. This example of reflective equilibrium is taken from David Morrow's *Moral Reasoning* text as an example against factory farming (though it can also serve as an example against the utilization of animals for food consumption and products) (Morrow 2018, 96).

3. Here the term "Anthropocene" is utilized to express "the era of ubiquitous human influence on the Earth's geological systems." This definition of the term is taken from Sarah Krakoff's article "Parenting the Planet" (2011). Krakoff, when rendering the definition of the Anthropocene, refers to the contribution of Nobel Prize winner Paul Crutzen, who popularized the term "The Anthropocene" (Crutzen and Stoermer 2000, 17–18). This ubiquitous human influence has grown tremendously over roughly the past hundred years, and so this nuanced use of the term "Anthropocene" refers particularly to the collective contemporary abilities and potentials humanity has to reshape seemingly every aspect of the planet.

4. This phrase is from chap. 5.21 of the *Tattvārthasūtra,* and I find quite a profound translation of this phrase to be by the Jain scholar and practitioner Shugan C. Jain—in his translation of the *Tattvārthasūtra*—which reads, "(The function) of Souls is to help one another" (Umāsvāti 2011, 184).

5. This feature is extremely important for various engagements in nonviolent dialogue in a host of arenas, and *anekānta* provides the ontological groundwork for these engagements. Elaborating on these ideas, Jeffery D. Long writes, "Because of the metaphysical realism that underlies them [differing worldviews], the Jain doctrines do not relegate any experience to the realm of illusion. The experience at the core of all world's religions can thus be affirmed as authentic perception of reality" (2009, 171).

6. Refer to King 1999, 51.

7. Krakoff (2018, 558) describes a similar view of Earth as "an infinitely malleable resource," which she asserts is "maladaptive optimism."

8. Aspects of this ideology conceptually go back to at least Descartes, who recklessly posits animals to merely be machines (automata) made of flesh. Avenues for the expression of this ideology have only expanded as our manipulation of the material world and of animal anatomy has exponentially increased in sophistication.

9. Jain Declaration on the Climate Crisis, October 2019, available at https://veganjains.com/jain-declaration-on-the-climate-crisis-oct-2019/#_ftn17.

References

Barbato, Melanie. 2017. *Jain Approaches to Plurality: Identity as Dialogue.* Brill Rodopi.

Bekoff, Marc. 2000. "Animal Emotions: Exploring Passionate Natures." *BioScience* 50:861–870.

Chapple, Christopher Key. 2018. "Animal Ethics." *Sophia* (Springer), 57: 69–83.

Cort, John E. 2000. "Intellectual Ahiṃsā Revisited: Jain Tolerance and Intolerance of Others." *Philosophy East and West* 50:324–347.

Crutzen, Paul, and Eugene F. Stoermer. 2000. "The Anthropocene." *Global Change Newsletter* 41.

Harari, Yuval Noah. 2017. *Homo Deus: A Brief History of Tomorrow.* Harper Perennial.

Jain, Kamla. 2004. "Anekanta in Present Day Social Life." In *Ahimsa, Anekanta, and Jainism,* edited by Tara Sethia. Motilal Banarsidass Publishers.

Jain, Sulekh C. 2016. *An Ahimsa Crisis: You Decide.* Prakrit Bharati Academy.

Jaini, Padmanabh S. 2002. "Ecology, Economics, and Development in Jainism." In *Jainism and Ecology: Nonviolence in the Web of Life,* edited by Christopher Key Chapple. Harvard University Press.

King, Richard. 1999. *Orientalism and Religion: Postcolonial Theory, India, and "The Mystic East."* Routledge.

Koller, John M. 2002. "Jain Ecological Perspectives." In Chapple, ed., *Jainism and Ecology.*

Krakoff, Sarah. 2011. "Parenting the Planet." In *The Ethics of Global Climate Change,* edited by Denis G. Arnold. Cambridge University Press.

———. 2018. "Parenting the Planet." In Morrow, ed., *Moral Reasoning.*

Long, Jeffery, D. 2009. *Jainism: An Introduction.* I. B. Tauris.

McCarthy, Susan, and Jeffery M. Masson. 1995. *When Elephants Weep: The Emotional Lives of Animals*. Dell.

Morrow, David R. 2018. *Moral Reasoning*. Oxford University Press.

Prabhu, Joseph. 1989. "The Idea of Reincarnation." In *Death and Afterlife*, edited by Stephen T. Davis. Palgrave Macmillan.

Singhvi, L. M. 1990. *The Jain Declaration on Nature*. Federation of Jain Associations.

Jain Declaration on the Climate Crisis. October 2019. https://veganjains.com/jain-declaration-on-the-climate-crisis-oct-2019/#_ftn17.

Umāsvāti. 2011. *Jainism, Key to Reality (Tattvārthasūtra)*. Edited and translated by Shugan C. Jain, Digamar. 2nd ed. Jain Trilok Shodh Sansthan.

10

An American Panjrapole

Engaging Tradition and Innovation at Luvin Arms Animal Sanctuary

JONATHAN DICKSTEIN

Felix doesn't remember me but it's my own fault. I first met Felix at his home in Lafayette in the spring of 2016. Four months later I moved hundreds of miles away to Santa Barbara to pursue my doctorate. I visit him whenever I travel to Colorado, but that is rarely more than once each year and, sadly, I sense that our time is running out. Felix is nine and that is quite old for a pig who was bred for size and destined for slaughter shortly after his first birthday. A nonindustrialized pig might live between fifteen and twenty years, but it is nearly impossible to imagine a pig of Felix's size surviving, not to mention thriving, that long, even if debilitating arthritis from selective genetic breeding were his only significant medical problem. My regrets and forebodings aside, on this frigid morning in January 2024 I am overjoyed to see him and feel him, this massive black and white spotted softie. I scratch his floppy ear as he nuzzles through a pile of hay. He doesn't remember me but I consider him my friend and I always will.

Ever since finding his "forever home" in October 2015, Felix has met thousands of other humans as one of the earliest residents of Luvin Arms, a Jain-founded farmed animal sanctuary now occupying forty acres in Erie, Colorado. In this chapter I highlight how animal rescue, care, and hospice are social engagements that Indian Jain communities have practiced long before the twenty-first century, and long before the modern farmed animal sanctuary movement (Abrell 2021; Donaldson and Kymlicka 2015; Pachirat 2018). However, to my knowledge Luvin Arms is the only Jain-founded panjrapole[1] ("animal sanctuary") in North America and perhaps anywhere outside of India. Even more significant than its mere presence is how Luvin Arms is a site of contemporary diasporic "engaged Jainism" (see Miller's introduction in this volume), marked by a complex convergence of old and new, traditional and unorthodox, native and diasporic, religious and secular, and conservative and progressive. This chapter introduces these various elements through historical research; personal experience with the sanctuary; interviews with the co-founder, staff, and volunteers; and reflections on how Luvin Arms, while continuing the practice of animal caregiving in the Jain tradition, also shoulders the concerns of contemporary mainstream animal and vegan advocacy.

Farm and Sanctuary in Colorado

The town of Erie, located in Weld and Boulder counties in Colorado, has a population of a little over thirty thousand. Luvin Arms Animal Sanctuary is located on Colorado Road 7, accessible from Denver by Weld County Road 8/Erie Parkway, right off Interstate 25. Taking the right turn onto Road 7, one drives a short distance before spotting a small farm-like property on the right. This is a private residence of the owners of Cleland's Dairy. A small number of cows and other animals are kept at this location, and veal crates and miscellaneous functional and formerly functional structures and equipment are visible without obstruction from the road. Cleland's primary dairy operation is situated a half mile away, where, according to a 2015 *Denver Post* story, 1,100 animals are confined and exploited for their milk (Jaffe 2015). The same article lists approximately 160 dairies operating in Colorado, yet from a cursory search on the US Farm Data website in March 2024, there are now between 245 and 303 dairies (or at least dairy farmers) active in the state.

To anyone driving by this satellite location and then approaching Luvin Arms, the animal sanctuary might appear—by contrast, and ironically so—significantly more farm-like than Cleland's modest lot. The sanctuary's sprawling fenced pastures and impressive, red-painted structures conjure up the traditional American childhood image of Old MacDonald's farm. If one is lucky, they will spot pigs, goats, and cows strolling and socializing in the open air, and up until his recent passing, perhaps even Tony the llama. Yet crucially unlike conventional farms, animal sanctuaries exist to serve their residents' interests rather than the owner's financial ends. However, this fact does not change the dissonant feeling I have when processing Luvin Arms' resemblance to the idyllic farm of storybooks. Its visual, architectural, and organizational similarities to the idealized farm—its red barns, pastures, and species-determined pens—are not what disturb me, at least not personally (Donaldson and Kymlicka 2015, 54–55). Rather, I am haunted by how the image of "the farm" continues to generate a cozy feeling in me, even when I know what lurks behind it.

Fortunately, my conflicting experience upon arrival at Luvin Arms never really surprises me. It is impossible to overemphasize how firmly the "the farm" has been ontologized—and topographized—in the American imaginary. We think and speak as if farms have always existed and always will exist, as if the "natural" landscape is incomplete (even "uncivilized"; Kim 2015, 43–52) in the absence of farmed animals and "farmland." As a scholar of ancient Indian religions, I am routinely hurtled back to the famous creation story of the *Ṛg Veda* in which the Cosmic Man is sacrificed and dismembered to become the world: "It [the sacrifice] was made into the animals: those of the air (and both) those that belong to the wilderness and those that belong to the village" (*RV* 10.90.8, in Jamison and Brereton 2017, 539). "Village animals" (Skt. *grāmya*)—otherwise translatable as "domesticated animals" or "farm animals"—issue immediately from this primordial sacrifice, emerging at the very start of cosmic organization. Animal exploitation appears, at least according to this verse from the *Ṛg Veda*, predetermined. The cow, for example, is a dairy cow from the instant the world begins. Her dharma is to be milked. She belongs on the farm and to the farm (Jain 2014; Narayanan 2019).

The enduring assumption of the ontological fixity of the farm is palpable to anyone working in animal advocacy. While the public may nominally oppose "factory farming," only a small minority decry "small," "local," and so-called "humane" animal operations (Anthis 2017; Bohanec 2023). The dominant thinking holds that the problem is not *that* humans use animals, but rather only *how* humans use animals. Once this viewpoint is coupled with the uncritical claim that humans treated animals "well" or "right" sometime in the forever undatable past, the fall from the (farm) land of Eden narrative is complete (even if there was no animal consumption in Eden, per Genesis 1.29–30) (Stanescu 2019). To paraphrase the widespread sentiment: Yes, things are bad now, but not everywhere and certainly not before. We simply need to reclaim the earlier way of using animals the right way. Admittedly, I both despise and fall prey to this fantasy of cozy human-farmed animal relations. But, to repeat, I am not surprised by the conflict in experience. Prior to 2015 I had never stepped foot on an animal sanctuary and therefore had no other lived context for farmed animals other than farms and zoos, places where exploitation isn't just normal, but is also *right*.

"We Need YOU!"

Let's step back nearly a decade. It was August 2015 and I had just finished two years of coursework for my master's degree in religious studies at the University of Colorado, Boulder. I was a seasoned student of classical yoga philosophy and yoga ethics and had adopted a vegetarian—and eventually vegan—diet several years earlier from exposure to the ethic of *ahiṃsā* (and a solid dose of yoga conformity). In July, out of curiosity I joined the Boulder (and Beyond!) Vegan Meetup Group (BVMG) a group mostly populated by middle-to-upper-class Boulderites connected by a mission "to educate people about the powerful effects of our food choices and the many benefits of a plant-based diet for humane, environmental and health reasons" (BVMG n.d.). On August 8 I received an email through the group advertising a volunteer opportunity—happening that very day—at a new animal sanctuary. The email attachment read:

> We need YOU!
>
> Luvin Arms is a small group of people that decided to make a difference for animals in need. We want to be their voice and give them the happy life they so much deserve. We would like to create a place where they can be safe, loved and well cared for. Right now, we are in the process of forming a 501c3 and we have secured a 23-acre property in the heart of Boulder County, where we hope to be able to give a safe and loving place for many animals in need. (BVMG, email to author, Aug. 8, 2015)

The email asked volunteers to bring and donate almost anything that could be put to use: hammers, nails, gloves, glasses, trash cans, "assorted types of tools"—basically anything with carrying, cleansing, constructive, and deconstructive utility. This made sense. The founders of the sanctuary, Shaleen and Shilpi Shah, admit that they knew absolutely nothing about clearing land or building structures, and were equally ignorant about caring for farmed animals. The Shahs had never even had a pet.

At the time I was focused on my thesis and regrettably missed this volunteer day, which in retrospect was *the* pivotal moment for the eventual trajectory of the sanctuary. Shaleen and Shilpi's original idea for animal rescue, no matter how fresh and undeveloped at the time, was small in scale. They envisioned rescue primarily as a family endeavor, a way for them and their young children to have an "experience together." However, as Shaleen reminisced about the day that changed everything, "The very first workday . . . that shifted completely. Thirty-plus strangers show up to help us clean and fix and build that place . . . and then *they kept coming*. That experience, you know . . . reassured us like, okay, no, this is not just us . . . this is something . . . it is a community that really wants this, and in bringing a larger vision we can really benefit animals in a much bigger way" (Shaleen Shah, interview, Nov. 8, 2023).

I submitted my thesis that winter. The following spring, with animal and vegan advocacy gaining traction on my ethical radar, I joined the community of staff and volunteers on this humble lot in Lafayette. This is where I met Felix, his brother Franklin, and the other inaugural rescues. A few of the original residents—Felix, goats Alfie and Arya, horses Jale and Niblet—still live and thrive at Luvin Arms, now located at the larger site in Erie.

The Not-So-Jain Jain Founding of Luvin Arms

Shaleen and Shilpi Shah are a Gujarati Jain couple who never imagined founding an animal refuge that, in under nine years, would save over 850 farmed animals from abuse, neglect, abandonment, and slaughter. The mission of the sanctuary, as advertised on its website and in nearly all its literature and videos, is "Ahimsa: Nonviolence Toward All Living Beings" (Luvin Arms n.d.). In a remarkable monograph dedicated to "animal homes" in India, Deryck Lodrick notes how "inscribed in some prominent position over a door or in all pinjrapoles [*sic*] can be found the words *ahiṃsā parāmo dharma* (*ahiṃsā* is the greatest of religions)" (1981, 16). The website of Luvin Arms is its twenty-first-century gateway, and the guiding principle of *ahiṃsā* is equally prominent therein.

Over Zoom in November 2023, I asked Shaleen Shah about his upbringing in India and the United States, especially his religious upbringing. Shaleen was raised in Ahmedabad, Gujarat, until the age of ten, at which point his family moved to Jacksonville, Florida. Shaleen recounted the marked differences between the two sides of his family. His father's family, from Ahmedabad, are Derāvāsī Jains (lit. "temple-dweller"), also known as Mūrtipūjaka Jains (lit. "image-worshiper"; Long 2009, 20; Wiley 2009, 152). His mother's family, from Rajkot and Wankaner in western Gujarat, are Sthānakavāsī Jains (lit. "lodging house-dweller"; Dundas 2002, 251–54). While these two sects both belong to the Śvetāmbara (lit. "white-clad") wing of Jainism, they differ greatly in terms of orientation and practice. Derāvāsī Jains, the largest Śvetāmbara sect, engage in image worship of Mahāvīra and the other Tīrthaṅkaras ("ford-makers"), those extraordinary individuals (otherwise known as *jina*s or "conquerors") who have achieved liberation (*mokṣa*) and thereby have conquered the cycle of birth and death (*saṃsāra*). Lay Derāvāsī Jains venerate material images (*dravya pūjā*) in both temples and at home shrines, and perform mental worship (*bhāva pūjā*), while Derāvāsī ascetics only perform the mental worship of images. Sthānakavāsī Jains, by contrast, a sect that developed between the fifteenth and seventeenth centuries CE, reject material image worship for both laypeople and ascetics, attributing its practice to the moral decrepitude of the present age. Accordingly, Sthānakavāsīs only practice mental worship of Mahāvīra and the other Tīrthaṅkaras. Consistent with this general distinction, Shaleen contrasted the formalism and ritualism of his father's family with the emphasis on "philosophy and culture" of his mother's, expressing how, even at a very young age, he resonated immensely more with the latter.

In 1993, as a sixth-grade student at Ridgeview Elementary School in Orange Park, Shaleen was confronted with the myriad challenges of otherness, assimilation, and integration. He was the sole Indian and sole vegetarian at his school. At all times he was encircled by a white American community that perceived Indians as "backward" and India as a land of "snake charmers, yogis, and fakirs." In the years that followed, owing to an inescapable pressure to fit in and a personal impulse toward self-exploration, Shaleen investigated other philosophies and religions, ranging from Buddhism to Wicca. Distancing himself from Jainism and seemingly any formal religiosity, throughout high school and college Shaleen self-identified as "born Jain" but otherwise independently philosophical and spiritual. A "borderline atheist and borderline agnostic," Shaleen practiced vegetarianism and believed in the values of nonviolence and compassion, but he no longer tied his diet or values to Jainism. This general orientation continued for years, even during and beyond the founding of the sanctuary.

The birth of Luvin Arms is equal parts sad and magical. In July 2014, the Shahs adopted their first animal, Jale, an Arabian mare acquired more so as a pet than as a rescue. Shaleen absolutely adored horses, having ridden them as a child in India, and he envisioned riding Jale while also imparting the skill to his two young sons, Aarav and Avi. In the process of learning novel riding techniques from a "Kung Fu master," techniques that demanded keen attentiveness to Jale's own will, Shaleen experienced a "moment of inspiration": "I could see that she [Jale] is this incredible being, so in tune with her surroundings that she can connect at a profound level. How could I continue to bend her to my will for my desire to ride? She, and all other living beings, deserve to live their own lives on their own terms" (Shah 2023). This revelation about Jale's sophisticated individuality prompted the Shahs to learn about the harms, injuries, and fatalities pervading horse racing, and this knowledge quickly instigated a family pivot from animal *use* to animal *rescue,* yet still with a focus on horses. Coincidentally, Shilpi Shah had adopted a vegan diet a few years prior, eschewing dairy products shortly after the birth of their first son Aarav. Her decision stemmed from health concerns for herself and her child, as well as from newly acquired information about the harms intrinsic to the dairy industry, specifically regarding the standard separation of mother and calf (Gillespie 2018; Narayanan 2023). However, during that time, *ahiṃsā* for the Shahs manifested exclusively as a dietary restraint and had not yet motivated proactive measures to help living animals. Their second horse, Niblet, adopted in July 2015, would be the first animal saved under their new—albeit still emerging—value of "*ahiṃsā* in action."

Only one month after rehoming Niblet at Luvin Arms, the Shahs learned about a mare, later named Belle, who was being sold with her two babies at a slaughter auction not far from their home. They rushed out to save the entire family. While waiting for Belle and her children to be presented for sale, Shaleen witnessed—for over six hours—cows, sheep, goats, and pigs, all being "pulled, pushed, or kicked into the auction floor, sold by the pound" (Shah 2023). It was the first time Shaleen saw, truly saw, other farmed animals as individuals, no different than their beloved Jale. He and Shilpi soon realized that their plan to rescue horses, and only horses, no longer made sense. Feeling helpless at the sight of so many animals in pain and need, the Shahs returned home, devastated.

That very night the Shahs' phone rang. Twenty-three acres of land located only two miles from their home in Lafayette had suddenly become available to lease. Their friend, who casually conveyed this information with no cognizance whatsoever of the Shahs' exhausting day at the auction and the revelation that followed, asked if they knew anyone who might be interested. Shaleen and Shilpi were stunned. And excited. And nervous. They talked all night. Ultimately, they could not deny this "clear sign from the universe that they needed to act." They signed the lease the following day. Not long thereafter I received the email asking for volunteers to pitch in at a new sanctuary situated just outside of Boulder.

Jainism, Jain-*specific* values, and any thought of strategically publicizing the sanctuary to the American Jain community were absent during the early thinking and decision-making of Luvin Arms. It was not until years later, partially owing to the encouragement of Shaleen's father, that the Shahs embraced expanding the sanctuary project in this direction. With a smile confessing a thick slice of irony, Shaleen admitted that since doing so, he, the skeptic, the one who only saw the "hypocrisy in religion," began to experience a "new rediscovery of Jainism" (Shaleen Shah, interview, Nov. 8, 2023).

Panjrapoles of the Past and Present

Luvin Arms was founded on the principles of *ahiṃsā* (non-harming) and *karuṇā* (compassion), yet the Shahs interpreted these not as Jain-specific values but rather "universal values."[2] Upon hearing this interpretation, I shared with Shaleen that I, for one, did not grow up with any of these values, at least not explicitly, and cannot recall "nonviolence" ever being spoken in my home or among my family members. This is not to say that I was encouraged to harm others, or that harming was tolerated, but rather only that a *duty* to be nonviolent, to follow an *ethic* of nonviolence that implicated my familial, cultural, and religious identity and community, was completely nonexistent. I confess that it is from this position, of being an outsider to the Jain tradition and the founding of Luvin Arms, that I connect the genesis of the sanctuary to Jain values and the traditional Jain panjrapole. However, I am clearly not the only one making this connection. In fact, I trail several years behind members of the global Jain community who, from the outset, received the sanctuary as an American panjrapole. Luvin Arms is a nonprofit organization funded entirely by private donors, including wealthy Jain donors, and lay Jains have always been the primary benefactors of Indian animal sanctuaries. Hence, while Shaleen may not have intended to start or operate a "Jain" animal sanctuary, inescapable is the fact that centuries ago and today, in India and elsewhere, Jains interpret animal rescue as a very Jain issue. Accordingly, for many

Jains, Luvin Arms Animal Sanctuary, founded by a Jain family from Gujarat, is merely a panjrapole on another continent.

Unfortunately, literature on the ancient history of panjrapoles is thin. Most secondary sources direct readers to the major English-language monograph on the subject, Lodrick's *Sacred Cows and Sacred Place* from 1981 (Burgat 2004; Chapple 2006; Cort 2002; Evans 2014; Narayanan 2023). Lodrick states that "the earliest documentary evidence for the existence of animal homes in India occurs with the reign of Ashoka (ca. 269–232 B.C.)" (Lodrick 1981, 81). This "documentary evidence" for "animal homes" is Aśoka's Rock Edict II:

> Everywhere . . . King Piyadasi [Aśoka] has established two kinds of medical services: medical services for humans and medical services for domestic animals. Wherever medicinal herbs beneficial to humans and domestic animals were not found, he had them brought in and planted everywhere. Likewise wherever root vegetables and fruit trees were not found, he had them brought in and planted everywhere. Along roads he had trees planted and wells dug for the benefit of domestic animals and human beings. (Olivelle 2024, 282–83; also see Pillar Edict VII [iii], 317–18)

The edict from the third century BCE describes medical facilities and watering holes for both humans and nonhumans. Lodrick lists Bhandarkar, Smith, and Sinh Jee as those "accept[ing] this to mean that pinjrapoles [*sic*] were in existence during Ashoka's reign" (Lodrick 1981, 57; Bhandarkar 1955; Sinh Jee 1896; Smith 1920). However, the extension of veterinary and watering services to domestic animals is distinct from the establishment of "animal homes" for animals to live out the remainders of their lives free from human use and premature death. In addition, this evidence survives in a Buddhist context rather than in a Jain one—Aśoka was a Buddhist convert—so while Lodrick adds that "the institutions could well have existed among the Jains at an earlier time" (Lodrick 1981, 59), there is no clear evidence, at least to this author's knowledge, of the operation of panjrapoles during such an early period.

Formal prohibitions against killing cows (and other animals) and measures for the protection of "useless" cows exist through the Common Era, especially in Hindu sources (e.g., in the *Arthaśāstra* and *Mānava Dharmaśāstra*), yet even the establishment of cow-specific shelters is different from multispecies animal sanctuaries that rescue animals from harmful, and typically extractive, human-animal relations. Moreover, as Yamini Narayanan has most recently emphasized, most modern and contemporary Indian *gaushala*s operate more so as dairies than as sanctuaries, engaging in the same exploitative processes from which contemporary "Western" animal sanctuaries seek to liberate their animals (Narayanan 2023, chap. 4).

By the middle of the second millennium CE, European accounts show that Jain panjrapoles had been in operation for some time. As but one example, English merchant Ralph Fitch wrote upon visiting Cambay (in present-day Gujarat) in 1591: "In Cambaia [*sic*] they will kill nothing, nor have any thing killed: in the Towne they have Hospitals to keepe [*sic*] lame Dogs and Cats, and for birds. They will give meate [*sic*] to the Ants" (Purchas 1905, 170). Fitch's reporting echoes the veterinary focus from the much earlier inscription, yet the inclusion of "wild" animals such as birds, as well as the mention of ants (*jīvat khan* or "insect room"; Lodrick 1981, 19), indicates an expansion beyond "cow protection" to consider other animals and to provide lifelong care for them without any expectation of "return." The existence of similar institutions all over India is corroborated by additional accounts from European witnesses (Lodrick 1981, 68–70). The salient point is that while evidence for the antiquity of the Jain panjrapole is wanting, the operation of animal sanctuaries by Jains in India has at least endured for centuries. Today, all lay Jains are aware of the existence of the sanctuaries and understand how the ethic of nonviolence impels positive acts of rescue and caregiving.[3]

Technically speaking, discussions of *ahiṃsā* in Jain texts such as the *Ācārāṅga Sūtra* (1.1.1.5 in Jacobi 1884), *Tattvārtha Sūtra* (6.9 in Tatia 2011), and *Ratnakaraṇḍa Śrāvakācāra* (53 and 72 in Jain 2022) extend a threefold test for the vow. *Ahiṃsā* requires refraining from (1) performing acts of harm oneself (*kṛta*), (2) causing others to perform acts of harm on one's behalf (*kārita*), and (3) consenting to acts of harm to be performed in one's presence or vicinity (*anumata*). This most serious vow derives from a recognition of the capacity for suffering (*duḥkha*) in all sentient organisms, a recognition that generates a feeling of compassion (*karuṇā*) for their experiences of suffering. Comprehensive nonviolence requires that one not only avoid direct (*kṛta*) and indirect (*kārita*) participation in the production of others' suffering, but also that one intervene in ways that prevent and alleviate others' suffering (*anumata*) and potentially even foster their experiences of enjoyment. Decades ago, anthropologist James Laidlaw referred to Jain *ahiṃsā* as an "ethic of quarantine" (Laidlaw 1995, 159). While this label conceivably—even if not convincingly—accounts for Jain vegetarianism and other exercises of restraint, it fails to enfold active *ahiṃsā* that includes gestures of prevention, rescue, and caregiving customary in the Jain tradition. A framed quotation at Luvin Arms, attributed to Shaleen and Shilpi, speaks loudly: "The promise of a safe, loving home for life made to each rescued individual is a bond we cannot break. It warms our hearts to spread Ahimsa and compassion for generations to come, and a forever home is a promise kept."

Active *ahiṃsā,* which I understand as positive intervention for the sake of another's well-being (contrasted with the negative character—the "not"—of a restraint), motivates the "forever homing" of Luvin Arms' residents. Their forever home is made "safe" and "loving" not only by eliminating the sources of harm to which they were previously subjected, but also by enriching their lives through personal attention, stimulation, and the development of positive human-animal and animal-animal relationships.

Figuring It Out

When Shaleen professed to having universal values rather than Jain values in mind when founding the sanctuary, I wondered about how the global enculturation of Jains into *the* "religion of nonviolence" might generate the assumption of *ahiṃsā*'s timeless validity and universal application. While this phenomenon may have had some influence on Shaleen's thinking, from speaking with him it appeared that two other factors played equal if not greater roles. The first factor is his healthy and enduring skepticism about organized religion that motivated his early quest for more personal, universal, and secular values. The second and much more pragmatic factor relates to the audience envisioned by Luvin Arms, a sanctuary physically located in northern Colorado in the United States of America, operating digitally as an exclusively English-language institution with mostly North American visitors. Shaleen reflected on how his upbringing in Florida directly influenced how Luvin Arms initially presented itself:

> Going back to how I grew up in Florida, I recognized that I'm different. We're different skin, different culture, different perspective, and what I did not want to get in the way was that when people come for tours and we're asking them to be inspired to compassion and giving up eating whatever they eat and choosing plant based, choosing compassion, what I didn't want to be in that mix, very consciously, was the fact that we were not like them, Shilpi and I. (Shaleen Shah, interview, Nov. 8, 2023)

Shaleen and Shilpi made a conscious decision to take a cautious, behind-the-scenes approach to reduce the likelihood that physical or digital guests would construe vegetarianism, veganism, or animal rescue as especially Jain (or even Indian) practices. Provided the routine ethno-religio-centric disavowal of nonwhite and non-Christian lifeways in the United States, as well as the dogged conception of Indian religions as "exotic" and "extreme," this decision is far from unreasonable. Accordingly, the *ahiṃsā*-centric messaging that appears boldly in Luvin Arms' current literature, videos, educational materials, and tours, was almost entirely absent at the outset.

Shaleen described how it was their first executive director, Shartrina (a non-Jain and non-Indian), who, after seeing burgeoning discourses with Jain communities about the sanctuary stressing *ahiṃsā, karuṇā,* and *jivdayā* (compassion for all beings), strongly suggested that these Jain values also feature prominently in Luvin Arms' mission statement, informational materials, and overall content. Interestingly, rather than deculturizing or "de-Jainizing" the sanctuary for the sake of more secular or "popular" branding,

Shartrina pushed to foreground the convergence and entanglement of Jain values, the Jain panjrapole, and the Western animal sanctuary movement at Luvin Arms. The Shahs consented to this modification in messaging insofar as they themselves would not be Luvin Arms' face, rather preferring its messengers to be the non-Jains and non-Indians constituting the majority of staff and volunteers at the sanctuary. Since then, while Shaleen and Shilpi continue to delegate the bulk of Luvin Arms' public-facing content to the animals, staff, and volunteers, they now—with greater clarity, financial stability, and social acceptance—publicly celebrate *ahiṃsā,* the Jain *ahiṃsā,* as the sanctuary's guiding principle.[4]

Fast-forward to 2024. While visiting the sanctuary, I asked staff and volunteers about how much they knew, if anything, about the Jain tradition and the ethic of *ahiṃsā*. Unsurprisingly, most knew almost nothing about Jainism as a religion other than its emphasis on nonviolence and compassion, and how these values presumably motivate Jains to rescue animals in need. Longstanding Jain vegetarianism and Jain *karma* theory were mentioned by a few individuals, although they admitted that they had first been exposed to Jainism through a college course or some other outlet besides the sanctuary.

Most importantly, it soon became apparent that nonviolence as *ahiṃsā*—the Jain *ahiṃsā*—comfortably cooperates with more ecumenical, if not also to say "secular," understandings of nonviolence and compassion. Staff members shared how Shaleen has given presentations to staff and volunteers about the basics of Jainism, the ethic of *ahiṃsā,* and Jain karma theory. Now somewhat more informed about the religious background of the founders—as well as many visitors, supporters, and donors—staff members seem both confident and happy about participating in a community with shared universal values, even if their starting points and personal affiliations vary. Jolene, the resident care director, captured the overall spirit:

> When Shaleen came to speak to us about being Jain and coming from that . . . to me I can't relate with like a God or, you know, organized religion in that way because that's just not where I come from or what I believe. But I can definitely get behind compassion for all beings

> and nonviolence towards all beings . . . We're not like preaching a religion to people. It's really just nonviolence for all animals. And to me, I think that's something that's universal and people can get behind more than like . . . "It's a religion." (Jolene Wells, interview, Jan. 10, 2024)

This sentiment resonates with Shaleen's original feeling about nonviolence and compassion being universal values *rather* than unique features of the Jain religion. Yet I would argue that the injection of any such "rather" is unwarranted, for there is no need to pit a universal secular value against a particular Jain value (and let us not omit the historical relationship between the two). The validity of nonviolence as a broad, flexible, and thereby universal concept need not de-Jainize the uniqueness of *ahiṃsā* as understood within the tradition. The Venn diagrams simply converge, expressing a "both / and" situation rather than an "either / or."

On the ground level, one tangible way that the Luvin Arms community unites "universally" is through its unanimous support for the vegan messaging of the sanctuary coupled with the personal adoption of a vegan lifestyle.[5] While being vegan is not a strict requirement for staff members or volunteers, the practice is certainly encouraged. The acceptance and practice of veganism among Luvin Arms' staff aligns with what the Shahs (and other Jains) regard as a significant ethical oversight in Jain lacto-vegetarianism—its neglect of the numerous injuries inflicted upon dairy animals, eventually culminating in their slaughter. The "dairy question" represents one of the new opportunities available to twenty-first-century Jains to adapt their values and diets to the current circumstances of farmed animals in India and abroad (Miller and Dickstein 2021; Vallely 2002; 2004). Notably, Jain veganism is not only a lay, diasporic phenomenon, but also one developing among Jains in India, including among prominent ascetics (Miller and Dickstein 2021, 12–13).

The shared values of nonviolence and compassion also cooperate in the sanctuary's dedication to promoting animals' experiences of enjoyment. This dedication manifests in Luvin Arms' adherence to the "key commitments" (Donaldson and Kymlicka

2015, 51–52) of all modern farmed animal sanctuaries, and through its continuation-with-innovation of the spirit of the traditional Jain panjrapole. All Luvin Arms staff interpret active compassion not only as saving animals from further experiences of human-inflicted harm—a core value of any panjrapole—but also as demanding sustained efforts to foster animals' thriving. In short: Survival isn't enough. Shaleen described the prospect of saving, feeding, and housing animals, but then doing little else: "When we save them from one harm, but essentially then ignore their needs, and treat them as caged lives . . . that in itself is *hiṃsā*" (Shaleen Shah, interview, Nov. 8, 2023). Jolene echoed the same feeling: "Sure, housing them and rescuing them initially is great, but it comes with so much more . . . [otherwise] it's basically just like sticking a human in a jail cell without anything to do. They get food and water, but they need more" (Jolene Wells, interview, Jan. 10, 2024).

This "more" is initially addressed by providing animals with medical attention, including routine checkups, preventative care, surgical interventions, and alternative, noninvasive therapies (e.g., acupuncture, massage, and physical therapy). These services help the animals cope with their specific physical, psychological, and emotional traumas, alongside the hardships of basic biological existence. The animals' needs are also respected by gradually increasing the "animal-centered design" of the sanctuary (Hess 2020; Piedmont Farm Animal Refuge n.d.). At Luvin Arms, this approach currently involves rotating pens and pastures, carefully intermingling species to facilitate a greater diversity of animal-animal interactions and friendships, and introducing stimulating structures and toys appropriate to individual species and individual personalities. Animal-centered design contributes to what could more generally be referred to as the *enrichment* focus of Luvin Arms.

A key component of the enrichment focus—one lauded by all staff and volunteers—is a practice called "clicker play" (elsewhere referred to as "clicker training"). The aim of clicker play is to use a tool (a clicker) to establish a "shared language, a shared communication, that they [the animals] can then ask what they need and we can ask them for things we need from them" (Vegan Jains 2023). Typically, what is "needed from them" is the animal's consent to participate in an activity that is genuinely in their best interest, even if they are not yet (or will ever be) aware of that fact. Such activities include having their hooves clipped, receiving a medical exam or medication, ascending into a trailer to be taken to the veterinarian, or simply moving to a different area of the sanctuary. Nearly all the animals at Luvin Arms have experienced severe human-inflicted traumas, so callously performing acts in their best interests without accounting for their individual feelings of fear, stress, anger, and sadness falls short of *ahiṃsā* in action. Clicker play helps develop the ease, confidence, and trust required for holistic rehabilitation and more affirmative interactions with human caregivers and visitors.

Conclusion: Zooming Out

> Kindness towards all living beings, no matter what species they are, if they are alive and have a heartbeat, then they deserve to live out the rest of their lives and not be used as commodities.
>
> —Interview with Katya Rasmussen, Luvin Arms resident care specialist, Jan. 9, 2023

Unfortunately, there is a tendency to mark beliefs, values, and practices as "authentic" or "essential" to a group insofar as they map onto the marker's conception of the key characteristics of that group. The simplistic framing of veganism, for example, as *essentially* a contemporary Euro-American, white, middle-class "lifestyle" obscures the global history of vegan and vegan-adjacent thought and practice of the past three millennia. Moreover, elsewhere my co-authors and I have asserted that "as praxis, veganism does not require establishing abstract metaphysical principles or a fixed playbook for animal liberation that ignores local contexts" (Dickstein et al. 2022). Similarly, animal rescue and caregiving need not establish and depend upon unanimously accepted "abstract metaphysical principles," Jain or otherwise, nor do these practices require minimizing "local" religious and historical contexts. In this chapter I have not asserted that Luvin Arms Animal Sanctuary is *in essence* a Jain panjrapole or *in essence* a modern, secular, farmed animal sanctuary, for what is to be gained by asserting either? Rather I have illustrated how Luvin Arms emerged, developed, and operates at an ever-evolving nexus of religious, cultural, historical, and regional sensibilities, including Jain ones. Luvin Arms is deeply engaged with animals' lives and humans' lives, and this engagement is motivated by a broader project to transform perspectives and practices regarding the global exploitation of nonhuman life. This multifaceted intervention in the world requires neither the secularization of Jain values into universal values nor a "Jainization" of the secular values of the farmed animal sanctuary movement. In this instantiation, engaged Jainism expresses itself in dialogue with the people, institutions, and movements of the world that share its core values, and even welcomes self-reflection and self-redefinition when the ever-changing world requires an ever-adaptive Jainism.

Perhaps Shaleen Shah's "new discovery of Jainism" stems from a recognition that Jain thought and practice is alive and dynamic and porous, thereby open to ongoing reinterpretation and redefinition. The three popular guiding lights of the tradition—*ahiṃsā* (nonviolence), *aparigraha* (non-attachment), and *anekāntavāda* (non-one-sidedness)—gesture to an openness of mind and heart for the sake of our own betterment and that of everyone around us. While Luvin Arms may not have been consciously founded on Jain values, its birth and life cannot be fully disentangled from Jain philosophy or history. Fortunately, there is no religious or secular mandate to isolate or harmonize all the elements operating at the sanctuary. Their fluidity and complexity only add to their allure, and to the enchantment of Luvin Arms as a whole, or at least that is what I tell myself to justify another trip to see Felix.

Notes

1. "Panjrapole" (alternatively "pinjrapole," and less frequently "panjarapole" and "pinjarapole") are English language renderings of the Gujarati word *piñjrāpoḷ* (also see the Marathi *pāñjarapōḷā*). The Gujarati term derives from the Sanskrit word *pāñjara,* meaning a cage or enclosure. While the etymology of the remainder of *piñjrāpoḷ* is uncertain, a "panjrapole" in virtually any context refers to a site at which old, infirm, and needy animals of various kinds receive daily care for the remainder their natural lives. In this chapter, following convention I use "panjrapole," although "pinjrapole" would be equally suitable.

2. In Jainism, *ahiṃsā* (nonviolence) is the principal vow (*vrata*) of the five vows for ascetics and laypeople. *Karuṇā* (compassion) is not a vow but rather one of the four "contemplations" (*bhāvanās*) that strengthen one's vows. For a summary, see Wiley 2009.

3. On Gandhi's Jain-informed perspective on *ahiṃsā*, cow-protection, and panjrapoles, see Burgat 2004.

4. Regarding the current presence of Jainism at the sanctuary, consider how in 2024 Luvin Arms offers four "Jain Summer Retreats" (Luvin Arms n.d.).

5. On perceiving the sanctuary as an end in itself or as a means for vegan advocacy, see Abrell 2021, 138–141.

References

Abrell, Elan. 2021. *Saving Animals: Multispecies Ecologies of Rescue and Care.* University of Minnesota Press.

Anthis, Jacy Reese. 2017. "Animals, Food, and Technology (AFT) Survey 2017." Sentience Institute, November 20. https://www.sentienceinstitute.org/animal-farming-attitudes-survey-2017.

Bhandarkar, D. R. 1955. *Aśoka (The Carmichael Lectures).* University of Calcutta Press.

Bohanec, Hope, ed. 2023. *The Humane Hoax: Essays Exposing the Myth of Happy Meat, Humane Dairy, and Ethical Eggs.* Lantern Publishing and Media.

Burgat, Florence. 2004. "Non-Violence Towards Animals in the Thinking of Gandhi: The Problem of Animal Husbandry." *Journal of Agricultural and Environmental Ethics* 17 (3): 223–248.

BVMG (Boulder Vegan Meetup Group). n.d. "*Boulder (and Beyond!) Vegan Meetup Group.*" Accessed January 12, 2024. https://www.meetup.com/coloradovegans/.

Chapple, Christopher Key. 2006. "Inherent Value Without Nostalgia: Animals and the Jaina Tradition." In *A Communion of Subjects: Animals in Religion, Science, and Ethics,* edited by Paul Waldau and Kimberly Patton. Columbia University Press.

Cort, John E. 2001. *Jains in the World: Religious Values and Ideology in India.* Oxford University Press.

Dickstein, Jonathan, Jan Dutkiewicz, Jishnu Guha-Majumdar, and Drew Robert Winter. 2022. "Veganism as Left Praxis." *Capitalism Nature Socialism* 33 (3): 56–75.

Donaldson, Sue, and Will Kymlicka. 2015. "Farmed Animal Sanctuaries: The Heart of the Movement?" *Politics and Animals* 1 (1): 50–74.

Dundas, Paul. 2002. *The Jains*. Routledge.

Evans, Brett. 2014. "Engaged Jain Traditions and Social Nonviolence: Ethnographic Case Studies of Lay Animal Activists and Service Oriented Nuns." *CrossCurrents* 84 (2): 201–218.

Gillespie, Kathryn. 2018. *The Cow with Ear Tag #1389*. University of Chicago Press.

Hess, Tara. 2020. "Breaking the Mold: How Animal-Centered Design Can Transform Sanctuaries." Open Sanctuary, March 6. https://opensanctuary.org/breaking-the-mold-how-animal-centered-design-can-transform-sanctuaries.

Jacobi, Hermann. 1884. *Jaina Sūtras, Part 1*. Oxford University Press.

Jaffe, Mark. 2015. "Colorado Dairies, Farms Trying to Cut Consumption of Electricity Benefit from Energy Subsidy." *Denver Post*, August 3, 2015. https://www.denverpost.com/2015/08/03/colorado-dairies-farms-trying-to-cut-consumption-of-electricity-benefit-from-energy-subsidy.

Jain, Champat Rai. 2022. *Ratnakaranda Shravakachara of Samantabhadra: The Spiritual Life of the Householder*. Kaveri Books.

Jain, Pankaj. 2014. "Bovine Dharma: Nonhuman Animals and the Swadhyaya Parivar." In *Asian Perspectives on Animal Ethics: Rethinking the Nonhuman*, edited by Neil Dalal and Chloe Taylor. Routledge.

Jamison, Stephanie W., and Joel P. Brereton. 2017. *The Rigveda: The Earliest Religious Poetry of India*. Oxford University Press.

Kim, Claire Jean. 2015. *Dangerous Crossings: Race, Species, and Nature in a Multicultural Age*. Cambridge University Press.

Laidlaw, James. 1995. *Riches and Renunciation: Religion, Economy and Society Among the Jains*. Clarendon Press.

Lodrick, Deryck. 1981. *Sacred Cows, Sacred Places: Origins and Survivals of Animal Homes in India*. University of California Press.

Long, Jeffrey D. 2009. *Jainism: An Introduction*. I. B. Tauris.

Luvin Arms. n.d. "About." Accessed November 5, 2023. https://luvinarms.org/about.

———. n.d. "Camps & Activities." Accessed February 10, 2024. https://luvinarms.org/camps-activities.

Miller, Christopher Jain, and Jonathan Dickstein. 2021. "Jain Veganism: Ancient Wisdom, New Opportunities." *Religions* 12 (7): 512. https://doi.org/10.3390/rel12070512.

Narayanan, Yamini. 2019. "'Cow Is a Mother, Mothers Can Do Anything for Their Children!' Gaushalas as Landscapes of Anthropatriarchy and Hindu Patriarchy." *Hypatia* 34 (2): 195–221.

———. 2023. *Mother Cow, Mother India: A Multispecies Politics of Dairy in India*. Stanford University Press.

Olivelle, Patrick. 2024. *Ashoka: Portrait of a Philosopher King*. Yale University Press.

Pachirat, Timothy. 2018. "Sanctuary." In *Critical Terms for Animal Studies,* edited by Lori Gruen. University of Chicago Press.

Piedmont Farm Animal Refuge. n.d. "Animal-Centered Design." Accessed February 20, 2024. https://www.piedmontrefuge.org/animal-centered-design.

Purchas, Samuel. 1905. *Haklutyus Posthumus, or, Purchas His Pilgrimes, Vol. 10*. James MacLehose and Sons.

Shah, Shaleen. 2023. "Ahimsa in Action: The Story of Luvin Arms Animal Sanctuary." YouTube. October 2. https://www.youtube.com/watch?v=nMWzfO7vwhc.

Sinh Jee, H. H. Sir Bhagavat. 1896. *A Short History of Aryan Medical Science*. Macmillan and Co.

Smith, V. A. *Asoka*. 1920. Clarendon Press.

Stanescu, Vasile. 2019. "Selling Eden: Environmentalism, Local Meat, and the Postcommodity Fetish." *American Behavioral Scientist* 63 (8): 1120–36.

Tatia, Nathmal, translator. 2011. *That Which Is: Tattvārtha Sūtra*. Umāsvāti/Umāsvāmi. Yale University Press.

Vallely, Anne. 2002. "From Liberation to Ecology: Ethical Discourses Among Orthodox and Diaspora Jains." In *Jainism and Ecology: Nonviolence in the Web of Life*. Harvard University Press.

———. 2004. "The Jain Plate: The Semiotics of the Diaspora Diet." In *South Asians in the Diaspora*. Brill.

Vegan Jains. 2023. "Explaining Clicker Play." YouTube. November 22. https://www.youtube.com/watch?v=Oj0WEjHAsXs.

Wiley, Kristi L. 2006. "Ahiṃsā and Compassion in Jainism." In *Studies in Jaina History and Culture,* edited by Peter Flügel. Routledge.

———. 2009. *The A to Z of Jainism*. Scarecrow Press.

11

A Jain Perspective on Faux Meat

Engaging Jain Philosophy with Contemporary Debates

JOEY TUMINELLO

While the production and popularity of plant-based ("faux") meat that closely resembles animal flesh is promising in terms of reducing support for industrial animal agriculture and its associated environmental harms, some philosophers have argued that it poses another ethical issue through the symbolic endorsement of animals as "edible." In this chapter, I discuss the relationship between these views and Jain teachings on violence through thought. In so doing, this work contributes to the development of a critical-constructive model of engaged Jain studies (see Miller's introduction in this volume). Specifically, I aim to demonstrate the value of taking Jain philosophy seriously in general and its implications for the production and consumption of the latest generation of faux meat. At the same time, rather than championing a strictly emic perspective of Jain thought, I hope to further demonstrate its value by putting Jain philosophy in critical conversation with other contemporary philosophical perspectives on this topic.

Susan M. Turner argues that "by producing and selling tofu which has the taste, texture and appearance of regular nonhuman animal meat, we are participating in the nonartistic representation of nonhuman animals as mere resources. Assuming vegetarianism is morally correct on deontological grounds, such acts must be morally wrong" (2005, 6). Rebekah Sinclair defends a perspective that resonates with Turner's exposition of deontological concerns, arguing that "plant-based meats are never really free of the animal they intend to substitute, and they therefore reproduce certain frameworks of intelligibility that keep animals edible even if they are not eaten" (2016, 230).

Beyond denouncing the physical actions of killing and eating animals, I also examine Jain teachings warning against the symbolic representation of animals in food, as well as contemporary Jain perspectives on faux meat. I argue that Jainism's triadic ontology of violence (i.e., Jainism's emphasis on avoiding violence through thought, word, and action, rather than merely focusing on physical action alone) provides further support for taking faux meat's ethical concerns seriously. At the same time, I do not think that Jainism provides grounding for the total cessation of production or consumption of faux meat for the following reasons:

1. While consuming faux meat may generate more negative karma than foods that are unaccompanied (or less accompanied) by violence in thought, it also is ethically superior to the consumption of foods that entail violence through thought *and* physical violence.
2. Even if Jains do not generally consume faux meat themselves, or see such consumption as violent, it can also be plausibly interpreted as an imperfect and perhaps temporary solution leading to potentially great reductions in animal and environmental harm.
3. It is debatable whether the replication of the aesthetic experience of flesh can ever be fully disentangled from the "real thing," or from the intentions embedded in the production process, but the possibility of some degree of disentanglement merits serious consideration.

Faux Meat and the Promise of Flesh Resemblance

While people have rendered plant-based proteins and other ingredients to resemble and replace animal flesh since at least as early as 965 CE (Shurtleff and Aoyagi 2013, 5), the degree to which meat substitutes bear a likeness to their counterparts has increased exponentially in the late twentieth and early twenty-first centuries. Over the last few years alone, companies such as Beyond Meat and Impossible Foods have created, refined, and mass-produced vegan hamburger patties that "bleed," using ingredients such as beet juice or leghemoglobin (derived from soy) in an attempt to replicate the aesthetic experience of consuming actual flesh. Reflecting on the Impossible Patty's likeness to meat, Oregon restaurateur Matt Adams has claimed that "It's actually confusing people. They'll send it back thinking it's meat" (Odegard 2019). Burger King's chief marketing officer Fernando Machado made a similar observation regarding the fast-food chain's testing of an Impossible Whopper in limited markets, prior to its current widespread availability: "People on my team who know the Whopper inside and out, they try it and they struggle to differentiate which one is which" (Popper 2019). Even Nestle has developed an Awesome Burger to compete with the Beyond and Impossible Burgers, and the company's recent statement on this topic recognizes the increasing demand for plant-based burgers as well as the recent shift away from faux meat's previous inadequacies in terms of its resemblance to animal products, captured well by Koltrowitz (2019), who writes, "Many consumers recognize that less meat in their diet is good for them and for the planet, but plant-based meat alternatives often do not live up to their expectations."

Rather than merely creating products that strongly resemble meat, entrepreneurs such as Ethan Brown, CEO of Beyond Meat, are explicitly questioning ontological assumptions regarding what meat *is*:

> Our obligation is to provide the consumer with a better meat, one that is freed from the animal and capable of delivering more of what consumers want – taste, protein, nutrients, convenience – with less of the downside. Just

> as few people (perhaps none?) railed passionately for or against preserving the land-line and embraced mobile phones, if we are successful, we will see consumers – in a relatively short period of time and with less controversy than one might expect – welcome a better meat, one that is made from plants. (Brown 2016, 5)

Brown's comment on shifting consumer expectations has proven to be prescient, as his company has become wildly successful since the Beyond Burger's 2016 debut. At the time of this writing, Beyond Meat products are available in about 130,000 stores and restaurants around the world, including chains such as TGI Friday's and Carl's Jr.

Given the well-established negative impacts of industrial animal agriculture, or "factory farming," on humans, animals, and the environment, this all seems to bode especially well. In a 2015 nationally representative survey, two-thirds of respondents reported reductions in meat intake over a three-year period, especially regarding red and processed meat (Neff et al. 2018, 1841). To some extent, these dietary changes map on to a growing concern regarding health impacts of meat-eating, as evinced by the World Health Organization's recent report showing positive associations between red meat consumption and colorectal cancer (WHO 2015). A University of Michigan Life Cycle Assessment comparing the production of a quarter-pound Beyond Burger patty with a conventionally produced beef patty of the same size found that "the Beyond Burger generates 90% less greenhouse gas emissions, requires 46% less energy, has >99% less impact on water scarcity and 93% less impact on land use than a 1/4 pound of U.S. beef" (Heller and Keoleian 2018, 7).

By multiple metrics, it seems readily apparent that the production and consumption of the latest generation of plant-based faux meat is good, and perhaps even morally obligatory for many people given the current ecological circumstances coupled with the public's desire for meat. While I am not attempting to refute this view, I do want to call attention to possible ethical concerns regarding faux meat and the representation of animals as food. Though these concerns do not necessarily override the importance of producing and consuming faux meat, I argue that they should be taken seriously, and that a socially engaged Jain perspective provides valuable insight as to why.

Animal Ethics and the Endorsement of Edibility

While some popular discourse has included concerns regarding faux meat consumption, discussion is largely centered on issues of personal health. For example, a side-by-side nutrition comparison in *Men's Journal* indicates that the Impossible Burger has a comparable amount of saturated fat to a beef burger, and both the Beyond and Impossible Burgers have more than five times the sodium of an unseasoned beef patty (Lemonier 2016). Other concerns include the breakdown and limited absorption of nutrients in ultra-processed foods, vegan or not. Further, prior to concluding in January 2019 that Impossible Foods' use of soy leghemoglobin was compliant with food safety regulations (Williams 2019), the US Food and Drug Administration wrote in a 2015 memo that "the arguments presented, individually and collectively, do not establish the safety of soy leghemoglobin for consumption, nor do they point to a general recognition of safety" (Strom 2017). There are, of course, some pertinent responses to some of these concerns (e.g., regarding important differences in *sources* of fat, and the reduced or eliminated need to add more salt to a preseasoned patty), though a detailed critical examination would be beyond the scope of this paper.

Aside from health and nutrition–related concerns, there is a small but growing recognition of the symbolic qualities and possible ideological function of consuming faux meat. After outlining other arguments against this practice, journalist Maria Chiorando briefly remarks on a possible concern with endorsing the representation of animals as food: "Finally, some have questioned whether buying these products perpetuates the idea that animals' bodies are food, hence our need to try and replicate them" (Chiorando 2018). A 2018 piece from *Food & Wine* reiterates the existence of this position, while similarly embedding a brief mention within a long-form article on concerns regarding the processing and sodium content in the latest generation of faux meat: "The question has been posed, however: Are there any downfalls to these cutting-edge plant-based products? Among vegan circles, there's a sort of pride in rejecting animal analogues: 'I just don't crave those anymore,' some will say" (Chandra 2018).

In a blog post titled "Are Animal Crackers Vegan?" sociologist Corey Lee Wrenn brings this concern for the symbolic representation of animals beyond faux meat. Applying Matthew Cole and Kate Stewart's examination of the construction of children's toys and the perpetuation of dominant and speciesist perspectives of animals (Cole and Stewart 2016, 9), Wrenn argues that "consuming animal crackers is ritualistically anti-vegan, as it socializes speciesist sentiments and human supremacy in children" (Wrenn 2016). Connecting the evolution of the artwork on boxes of animal crackers and the perpetuation of the idea of captivity as consensual (on the part of the animals), Wrenn provides important support for cultivating concern regarding the representation of animals in (and in relation to) food products.

In addition to Carol Adams's (2010) exposure of the links between the oppression of women and animals through their representation and objectification as "meat," two key academic papers explicitly focus on ethical concern regarding the representation of animal flesh in faux meat production.

In the article "Beyond Viande: The Ethics of Faux Flesh, Fake Fur and Thriftshop Leather," Susan M. Turner applies utilitarian and deontological ethical theories to examine, among other questions, whether it is ethical to produce, sell, and eat faux meat (2005, 1). Because of utilitarianism's appeal to consequences in determining an action's moral valence, as well as the theory's emphasis on maximizing happiness and minimizing suffering for the greatest number of sentient beings, the ethics of faux meat's production, sale, and consumption depends on the outcomes of engaging in these activities. While Turner observes that the relevant social scientific data was unavailable at the time of writing, she argues that a utilitarian should ideally find out the following information in rendering a moral assessment of this issue:

> We need to know if there is a tendency for vegetarians who eat faux meat to lapse as a result. Also, we would need to know if there is a greater chance a meat eater will consider becoming vegetarian when there are faux meat options available. If the overall result is more

> conversions back to meat than to vegetarianism, then faux meat will be morally problematic according to a utilitarian like [Peter] Singer. If there is no difference or more vegetarian conversions, then faux meat might be off the utilitarian hook. (ibid., 7)

If the necessary data were available, these would be the variables to plug into a utilitarian calculation to determine the moral valence of the production, sale, and consumption of faux meat. This theory may provide a strong case against faux meat if it happens to lead to more overall suffering in comparison with other dietary choices, though Turner thinks the reverse of this is likely true (ibid., 8). However, from a utilitarian perspective, intentions and motives have no direct bearing on whether an action is permissible, impermissible, obligatory, or supererogatory. On this view, the representation of animals as mere resources within faux meat is not morally problematic in and of itself.

On the other hand, Turner illustrates how a deontological ethical framework may lead to different conclusions on this issue. Recall that the philosopher Tom Regan modified Kantian ethics by replacing a being's rational capacity with the quality of being a *subject-of-a-life* as the central criterion that determines moral worth (Regan 1983). Thus, on Regan's deontological approach, any animal that is a subject-of-a-life has intrinsic moral worth such that they should not be treated as if they exist as mere resources, instruments, or tools to be exploited for others' gain. Applying this deontological approach to her ethical examination of faux meat, Turner writes: "By *producing* and *selling* tofu which has the taste, texture and appearance of regular nonhuman animal meat, we are participating in the nonartistic representation of nonhuman animals as mere resources. Assuming vegetarianism is morally correct on deontological grounds, such acts must be morally wrong" (2005, 6). While Turner notes that the ethics of *eating* faux meat is less straightforward than the ethics of producing and selling it from a deontological perspective, she ultimately argues that eating faux meat must be immoral because its consumption relies on the immoral practice of producing it, "even though the consumer may not be endorsing a representation of nonhuman animals as mere resources" (ibid., 6). In addition to its innovative application of normative ethical theories to some undertheorized practices, this article illustrates the need to take seriously the ethical dimensions of faux meat, including those concerning the often-overlooked act of representation itself.

Drawing on Carol Adams's work as well as the philosophy of Jacques Derrida, Rebekah Sinclair defends a perspective that resonates with Turner's exposition of deontological concerns, arguing that "plant-based meats are never really free of the animal they intend to substitute, and they therefore reproduce certain frameworks of intelligibility that keep animals *edible* even if they are not eaten" (2016, 230). Sinclair applies Derrida's concept of the "trace"—the conceptual presence that is inevitably implied by an absence—to illustrate the ways that the success of faux meat (especially those products that intend to perfectly replicate the aesthetic experience of consuming animal flesh) is dependent on interpretations of animals as beings who are okay to kill and eat. While not altogether dismissing the promise of faux meat in reducing animal slaughter, Sinclair importantly shows that focusing on this material consequence is not philosophically or ethically sufficient: "We must also ask whether or not [meatless meats] will alter the intellectual, economic and epistemological conditions that make slaughter and exclusion possible to begin with" (ibid., 233). Because the above conditions will not be satisfactorily altered through meatless meat, and because of the importance of recognizing animals as community members rather than as mere food or instruments for human satisfaction, Sinclair presents her case in hopes that we might eventually move beyond these attempts to reclaim the gustatory experience of animal flesh.

Violence Through Thought in Jainism

Thus, there is a small but growing amount of scholarship on the ethical dimensions of faux meat, and it has also received some attention within popular discourse. Here, I provide an overview of the recognition of and advocacy against violence through thought within Jain teachings. This discussion illustrates the significance and nuance of Jain ethics, as well as the importance of an engaged Jain approach in further substantiating and augmenting debates on the symbolic representation of animal flesh through faux meat.

Jainism entails the strongest and most thorough commitment to nonviolence (*ahiṃsā*) of the major Indic philosophico-religious traditions, and this is due in part to the Jain teaching that violence is not a strictly physical phenomenon. Characterizing this holistic ontological understanding of violence and its negation, Ramakrishna Puligandla writes, "The practice of non-violence in thought, word, and action is the cardinal virtue [in Jain ethics]" (1997, 35). In this way, Jainism recognizes thought and its expression through language as possible avenues toward violence (and subsequently the accrual of negative karma) *alongside* physical action.

This opposition to violence through thought and word goes beyond a strictly instrumental concern. From a narrower consequentialist perspective, it would be reasonable to advocate against harmful thoughts only if there was good reason to believe that those thoughts tended to lead to physical violence. Acknowledging but also moving beyond this concern with the material impact of thought, Jainism's triadic conception of violence[1] additionally entails that violence in word and thought can be karmically binding in itself. Subramania Gopalan clarifies this key distinction: "Non-violence and non-killing are generally associated with 'acts' so that if the individual concerned does not indulge in the prohibited acts he is absolved of the sins that might accrue to him. But though the act itself has to be avoided, the intention also must be pure. Since an act is always preceded by an intention and a will, mere avoidance of the act may not necessarily mean that there was no intention" (1973, 160). Even when one avoids an act of physical violence, this avoidance does not automatically exempt the moral agent from generating negative karma through thoughts or words. The categories of nonphysical violence have a moral valence that overlaps with but is separable from violence in action.

The Jain monk Ācārya Kundakunda's classic text *Pravacanasāra* provides further insight into a Jain ontology of violence: "The ascetic (*muni, śramaṇa*) whose activities are without proper diligence certainly causes injury (*hiṃsā*) to the living beings, whether they die or not. The ascetic who observes diligently the fivefold regulation of activities (*samiti*) does not cause bondage even if he has caused injury to the living beings" (2018, 269). This quote illustrates the ontological and ethical independence of violence in thought from violence in action, as well as the intimate relationship between violence toward others and violence toward oneself. As it is relevant to the theme of this chapter, concern for the karmic consequences of one's actions for oneself is directly tied to the universality of vegetarianism among Jains. Reflecting on his field work with Jain communities in India, Aaron Gross further clarifies this relationship:

> I frequently encountered the notion that one way to be reborn as an animal—or at least transmigrate in their direction—is to eat them. I have no reason to think this has changed recently. This danger of eating animals was only occasionally formally put forward by Jain ascetic leaders in their sermons to laity as a reason to be vigilant in dietary practice, but it was always there in the background. If this possibility of becoming an animal by eating an animal is inquired after, as I sometimes did in interviews, it was invariably affirmed as accurate. (Gross 2018, 100)

On the Jain view, concern for avoiding harm to others is bound up with avoiding harm to oneself by, for example, setting oneself on a path toward a rebirth that brings one further away from liberation (*mokṣa*). In his introduction to the edited volume *Jainism and Ecology*, Christopher Key Chapple astutely foregrounds the ecological dimensions of nonviolence within Jain practice: "The ethics of nonviolence as developed by the Jains looks simultaneously inward and outward. The only path for saving one's own soul requires the protection of all other possible souls" (2002, xxxv). Jainism's deep concern with the avoidance of violence includes but goes beyond concern for human and nonhuman animal welfare, to encapsulate a recognition of the interdependence of all life and the impact of this interdependence on the karma of all living beings. The Jain understanding of karma applies to physical acts such as eating, but also applies to the accrual of negative karma through thought and word. As a result, the Jain commitment to vegetarianism simultaneously entails ethical concern regarding behaviors, objects, and events that incite violent thoughts, in addition to and apart from violent physical actions. This relationship between the Jain ontology of violence, karma, and consumption yields important insights into the ethical dimensions of faux meat's representation of animal flesh.

Jainism on Faux Meat: Contributions to the Discourse

Since Jainism's roots in the sixth century BCE, it has shared fundamental tenets with Hinduism while also diverging in ways that shed light on a Jain perspective on faux meat. One such divergence is Jainism's opposition to the use and killing of animals in sacrificial ritual. This avoidance is undergirded by Jainism's recognition of the shared "existential trajectory" of human and more-than-human animals as five-sensed beings (Vallely 2014, 52). Beyond denouncing the physical actions of killing and eating animals, there are also some instances of Jain teachings warning against the symbolic representation of animals in food. This concern is illustrated in the Jain tale of king Yaśodhara. Spanning a conversation on the soul between a Jain ascetic and a guard, the ascetic recounts the karmic fate and painful deaths and rebirths of two nearby chickens:

> This cock here is the (reborn) king Yaśodhara who in a previous life was the father of our king Yaśomati. And this hen was in a previous existence Candramatī, the crude mother of the same king Yaśodhara. Not being prepared to relinquish (totally) their customary *dharma,* they slaughtered a cock made of flour as sacrifice to the goddess to whom they were devoted. Due to the maturation of that evil deed they have become this pair of chickens whose minds are now at peace, being intent on listening to my discourse on the true religion. (Hardy 1990, 127)

This story illustrates the connection between the Jain conception of rebirth and the construal of animal ethics beyond the moral valence of physical actions alone. In the case of Yaśodhara and Candramatī, substituting the killing of an animal with the sacrificial use of an animal likeness is laden with karmic implications. Though it is acknowledged that this is not morally identical to animal sacrifice, it is still recognized as part of a larger spectrum of violence, as well as potentially contributing to future physical violence. Even if there is not always a one-to-one correlation between a particular thought and a particular action, thoughts exist in a mutually influential feedback loop with physical actions, informing our interpretations of the world and of ourselves.

Elaborating on the Jain concern with self-harm and its relationship to harming others, P. K. Jain reflects on violence in thought and its application to the consumption of animal likenesses: "Violence in thought is as detrimental to the development of character as violence in action. To this extent, candies and chocolates shaped as animals are generally not consumed in Jain families. Imagine a child going around eating the 'head of a rabbit' or 'leg of a man.' What will be his/her psychology and personality? If you want to eat chocolate, just do that. Why lace it with an unappetizing thought of cruelty to animals and/or cannibalism?" (Jain 2000). P. K. Jain takes attitudes toward and interpretations of animals to be vital aspects of human character that people need to cultivate and develop in the right ways. If one continues to develop and embrace interpretations of animals as beings that it is okay to kill and eat (and to generally treat as only instrumentally valuable), this also might indicate a deficiency in one's character. This deficiency of character impacts oneself and others, as "old habits die hard" and it can be difficult to break free from deeply ingrained patterns in thought and behavior instilled over long periods of time. Though P. K. Jain does not directly address the development of faux meats that are intended to (and sometimes *do*) resemble animal flesh in a near-indistinguishable fashion, his discussion indicates a broader application of the concept of violence in thought to a range of edible likenesses of animals including (but not limited to) faux meat.

While a formal sociological study of lay Jain perspectives on, and consumption of, faux meats would make a significant contribution to the available literature on this subject, there is a small amount of popular discourse that shows how some individual Jains engage with the issue of faux meat consumption in light of their position that violence can occur through thought. On the question-and-answer website Quora, one thread explores whether it is a sin to prepare and eat Jain versions of foods that were originally made in ways that violate Jain dietary ethics.[2] A Quora user named Divya offered the following response: "Intentions and thoughts matter the most in Jainism . . . You should not eat non-veg. You should not eat veg thinking it to be non-veg" (Divya 2017). This clearly illustrates the Jain view regarding the moral valence of thought, as well as the notion that avoiding the physical consumption of animal flesh does not automatically exempt one from partaking in violence or generating negative karma. A comment from Sarvarth Jain also resonates with this idea: "Now, intention is the thing that matters whenever an activity is done. If intentions are non-violent, bondage of *shubh* [i.e., 'auspicious'] karma will take place and vice versa. Likewise in our eating habits also, our intention matters" (Jain 2017). Again, this illustrates a Jain perspective on faux meat where thoughts themselves have ethical import, in relation to but also independent from physical actions. Especially regarding the latest generation of meat analogues that "bleed" and that are otherwise engineered into extremely close facsimiles of animal flesh, the possible violence in thought associated with the production and consumption of those products clearly presents ethical issues from a Jain perspective.

Another fascinating popular discussion of the Jain diet and faux meat takes place in the cookbook *Jain Food: Compassionate and Healthy Eating* by Manoj Jain et al. Before describing particular Jain-friendly recipes, the first seven chapters of the book provide a comprehensive overview of Jain teachings and practices related to food (Jain et al. 2005, 11–62). In a chapter on contemporary food choices, the authors briefly remark on the popularity of faux meat: "Meat substitutes such as hot dogs made from soy or 'vegetarian steak' have come into the market. These may be options for non-Jains who have grown up with the taste of hot dogs and seek a nonviolent alternative. However, for Jains, such food may be repulsive and can be avoided" (ibid., 58). Interestingly, the authors omit an explicit discussion of violence through thought, instead appealing to the aesthetic sensibility of Jains who have not grown up eating meat. Rather than advocating an absolutist stance against the consumption of faux meat, the authors acknowledge that it is a comparatively more ethical alternative to the consumption of animal flesh, especially for people who may miss the taste of meat and who might otherwise eat meat if reasonable facsimiles were unavailable.

On this note, while I hope to have provided some clarification regarding a Jain perspective on faux meat as well as the importance of engaging with this perspective in understanding and evaluating faux meat's ethical dimensions, I do not think that Jainism provides grounding for the total cessation of production or consumption of faux meat for the following reasons.

First, a core component of Jain thought is the acknowledgment that life must feed on life to continue to exist, thus survival in all its forms necessarily entails some degree of violence. The emphasis, then, is on cultivating a lifestyle that minimizes harm as much as possible and generating auspicious or positive karma rather than negative. This is especially true regarding the expectations of lay Jains, whose "Lesser Vows" parallel but are less demanding than the "Great Vows" required of Jain ascetics. For example, as Paul Dundas observes, "While the ascetic is required to eschew any act of violence whatsoever, the layman must instead try to the best of his ability to avoid any pointless destruction of life forms" (1992, 163). To use a more extreme example, while some (though a rare few) Jain ascetics attempt to unburden from past karma and cease their generation of karma by fasting to death (*sallekhanā*), lay Jains are instead expected to try their best to practice *ahiṃsā* with the knowledge that they will inevitably be complicit in violence (to different degrees) throughout their lives. While consuming faux meat may generate more negative-karma than foods that are unaccompanied (or less accompanied) by violence in thought, it also is ethically superior to the consumption of foods that entail violence through thought *and* physical violence.

Second, though Jains are not strict consequentialists (or, perhaps more accurately, they are not reductive materialist consequentialists) given their defense of the moral valence of thought, their broader emphasis on *ahiṃsā* would still necessitate some concern for harm reduction. Given the above discussion of the popularity of faux meats such as Beyond and Impossible Burgers, in addition to the increasing numbers of meat-eaters who are incorporating more vegan meals into their diets, the general promotion of faux meat consumption could plausibly be interpreted, from a Jain perspective, as good in certain key ways. This does not obviate underlying concerns such as the violence inherent in the symbolic perpetuation of animals as edible and exploitable. However, industrial animal agriculture is a nexus of extraordinary violence toward so many lives and communities. Even if Jains do not generally consume faux meat themselves, or see such consumption as violent, its production and consumption can also be plausibly interpreted as an imperfect and perhaps temporary solution with potentially great positive impacts for the environment, animals, and public health. This position of compromise (i.e., the tentative acceptance of the violence through thought generated by faux meat because it is comparatively preferable to the mass consumption of animal flesh), which I find to be consistent with Jainism's strong emphasis on *ahiṃsā*, is an important illustration of the potential for Jain thought to transform and to be transformed through engagement with contemporary social issues.

Third, though this may be far off given the ubiquity of meat consumption in so many places, a Jain perspective can also recognize that it is possible to experience faux meat with something in mind besides its resemblance to flesh. Further, those who have never consumed meat may even lack a proper frame of reference to elicit violence in thought through the consumption of faux meat. While at a systemic level faux meat production may be deeply linked with the imitation of a product that resulted from physical violence, at the individual level faux meats can be evaluated in reference to themselves and/or other plant-based products. For example, there are already many vegan "burger" patties that, while shaped like a burger that might be made from ground beef, are also clearly not trying to bear any strong resemblance to flesh (e.g., patties made from ground or pureed beans, vegetables, and grains without any elaborate processing). It is debatable whether the replication of the aesthetic experience of flesh can ever be fully disentangled from the "real thing," or from the intentions embedded in the production process, but the possibility of some degree of disentanglement merits serious consideration. If such disentanglement did prove to be possible, this could provide further support for the ethical acceptance of faux meat consumption from a Jain perspective, at least within certain contexts.

Conclusion

To conclude, I hope to have provided further support for recognizing and seriously considering the ethical dimensions of faux meat, which are undertheorized in comparison to adjacent areas of food, animal, and environmental ethics. Complementing the emerging Western scholarship from philosophers such as Turner and Sinclair, Jain philosophy offers important insights into this subject, grounded in Jainism's conception of violence through thought, word, and physical action. While the study of Jainism is a humbling experience in itself, Jain theory and practice also deserves a place at the table in elucidating matters of ethics that are often dismissed or taken for granted. This inclusivity does not simply consist of advocating for Jain positions from an emic perspective, but of taking Jainism seriously enough to put it in critical dialogue with other philosophical positions. I hope to have made some headway toward such engagement here.

Notes

1. Note that I am introducing the term "triadic" here. This is not, to my knowledge, a preexistent way of describing the Jain conception of violence, but I use it as a shorthand to refer to the Jain view that violence can occur through word and thought in addition to physical acts of violence as conventionally conceived.

2. In addition to abstaining from the consumption of animal flesh, Jainism also has a complex and nuanced set of *abhakṣya* ("not to be eaten") foods, including some root vegetables and other plant life. For further discussion of Jain dietary restrictions, see Cort 2001, 128–129.

References

Adams, Carol. 2010. *The Sexual Politics of Meat: A Feminist-Vegetarian Critical Theory.* Continuum.

Brown, Ethan. 2016. "Beyond Meat." In *The Future of Meat Without Animals,* edited by Brianne Donaldson and Christopher Carter. Rowman & Littlefield.

Chandra, Gowri. 2018. "The Great Veggie Burger Debate: Are They Actually Good For You?" *Food & Wine,* March 1. https://www.foodandwine.com/news/great-veggie-burger-debate-are-they-actually-good-you.

Chapple, Christopher Key. 2002. Introduction to *Jainism and Ecology,* edited by Christopher Key Chapple. Harvard University Press.

Chiorando, Maria. 2018. "Should Vegans and Vegetarians Eat 'Fake Meat?' " *Plant Based News*, May 14. https://www.plantbasednews.org/post/should-vegans-and-vegetarians-eat-fake-meat.

Cole, Matthew, and Kate Stewart. 2016. *Our Children and Other Animals: The Cultural Construction of Human-Animal Relations in Childhood.* Routledge.

Cort, John E. 2001. *Jains in the World: Religious Values and Ideology in India.* Oxford University Press.

Divya. 2017. "Divya's Answer to 'as per Jainism . . .' " Quora, September 21. https://www.quora.com/As-per-Jainism-I-have-heard-that-a-person-went-to-hell-because-he-made-hen-from-flour-to-sacrifice-so-if-we-prepare-eat-eggless-cake-Jain-biryani-or-any-other-Jain-version-of-food-which-originally-is-made-in-non-Jain-way-isnt-this-a-sin/answer/Divya-1033.

Dundas, Paul. 1992. *The Jains.* Routledge.

Gopalan, Subramania. 1973. *Outlines of Jainism.* John Wiley & Sons.

Gross, Aaron S. 2018. "Humane Subjects and Eating Animals: Comparing Implied Anthropologies in Jewish and Jain Dietary Practice." In *Dharma and Halacha: Comparative Studies in Hindu-Jewish Philosophy and Religion,* edited by Ithamar Theodor and Yudit Kornberg Greenberg. Lexington Books.

Hardy, Friedhelm. 1990. "Karmic Retribution: The Story of Yaśodhara from the Brhatkathākośa." In *The Clever Adulteress and Other Stories: A Treasury of Jain Literature,* edited by Phyllis Granoff. Motilal Banarsidass.

Heller, Martin C., and Gregory A. Keoleian. 2018. "Beyond Meat's Beyond Burger Life Cycle Assessment: A Detailed Comparison Between a Plant-Based and an Animal-Based Protein Source." Regents of the University of Michigan. http://css.umich.edu/sites/default/files/publication/CSS18-10.pdf.

Jain, Manoj, Laxmi Jain, and Tarla Dalal. 2005. *Jain Food: Compassionate and Healthy Eating.* MJain.net.

Jain, P. K. 2000. "Dietary Code of Practice Amongst Jains." Paper presented at the thirty-fourth World Vegetarian Congress, July 2000. Toronto, Canada.

Jain, Sarvarth. 2017. "Sarvarth Jain's Answer to "as per Jainism . . .' " Quora, September 18. https://www.quora.com/As-per-Jainism-I-have-heard-that-a-person-went-to-hell-because-he-made-hen-from-flour-to-sacrifice-so-if-we-prepare-eat-eggless-cake-Jain-biryani-or-any-other-Jain-version-of-food-which-originally-is-made-in-non-Jain-way-isnt-this-a-sin/answer/Sarvarth-Jain.

Koltrowitz, Silke. 2019. "Nestle Goes Vegan with Meat-Free Burger Range." Reuters, April 2. https://www.reuters.com/article/us-nestle-burger/nestle-goes-vegan-with-meat-free-burger-range-idUSKCN1RE1A6?feedType=RSS&feedName=lifestyleMolt.

Kundakunda, Ācaryā. 2018. *Pravacanasāra*. Translated by Vijay K. Jain. Vikalp Printers.

Lemonier, Gabrielle. 2016. "Great-Tasting Veggie Burgers Are Here, but Are They Any Healthier?" *Men's Journal*, November 9. https://www.mensjournal.com/food-drink/great-veggie-burgers-are-here-but-are-they-any-healthier-w449490/.

Neff, Roni A., Danielle Edwards, Anne Palmer, Rebecca Ramsing, Allison Righter, and Julia Wolfson. 2018. "Reducing Meat Consumption in the USA: A Nationally Representative Survey of Attitudes and Behaviours." *Public Health Nutrition* 21:1835–1844. https://doi.org/10.1017/S1368980017004190.

Odegard, Kyle. 2019. "Bo & Vine, New Corvallis Restaurant, Brings Foodie Approach to Burgers." *Corvallis Gazette-Times*, January 21. https://www.gazettetimes.com/business/bo-vine-new-corvallis-restaurant-brings-foodie-approach-to-burgers/article_9da52333-e9e9-5569-9edc-5b45d589ed64.html.

Popper, Nathaniel. 2019. "Behold the Beefless 'Impossible Whopper.'" *New York Times*, April 1. https://www.nytimes.com/2019/04/01/technology/burger-king-impossible-whopper.html.

Puligandla, Ramakrishna. 1997. *Fundamentals of Indian Philosophy*. D. K. Printworld.

Regan, Tom. 1983. *The Case for Animal Rights*. University of California.

Shurtleff, William, and Akiko Aoyagi. 2013. *History of Tofu and Tofu Products (965 CE to 2013)*. SoyInfo Center.

Sinclair, Rebekah. 2016. "The Sexual Politics of Meatless Meat: (In)Edible Others and the Myth of Flesh Without Sacrifice." In *The Future of Meat Without Animals*, edited by Brianne Donaldson and Christopher Carter. Rowman & Littlefield.

Strom, Stephanie. 2017. "Impossible Burger's 'Secret Sauce' Highlights Challenges of Food Tech." *New York Times*, August 8. https://www.nytimes.com/2017/08/08/business/impossible-burger-food-meat.html.

Turner, Susan M. 2005. "Beyond Viande: The Ethics of Faux Flesh, Fake Fur and Thriftshop Leather." *Between the Species* 5:1–14. https://digitalcommons.calpoly.edu/cgi/viewcontent.cgi?article=1044&context=bts.

WHO. 2015. "Q&A on the Carcinogenicity of the Consumption of Red Meat and Processed Meat." World Health Organization, October. https://www.who.int/features/qa/cancer-red-meat/en/.

Vallely, Anne. 2014. "Being Sentiently with Others: The Shared Existential Trajectory Among Humans and Nonhumans in Jainism." In *Asian Perspectives on Animal Ethics: Rethinking the Nonhuman*. Routledge.

Williams, Ashley. 2019. "Impossible Foods Ingredient Deemed 'Safe to Eat' by FDA." GlobalMeatNews.com, January 7. https://www.globalmeatnews.com/Article/2019/01/07/FDA-declares-Impossible-Foods-ingredient-safe-to-eat.

Wrenn, Corey Lee. 2016. "Are Animal Crackers Vegan?" December 3. http://www.coreyleewrenn.com/are_animal_crackers_vegan/.

12

Jain Ecotheology Engaging with Ecopsychology

COGEN BOHANEC

An Overview of Ecotheology

As an environmentalist, longtime animal rights activist, and ethicist,[1] I have become less interested in "rule-based" environmental ethics (e.g., deontology, utilitarianism) since human behavior seems to be characterized by resistance to rules at least as much as by adherence to them.[2] Beyond a strictly injunctive approach to conservation, ecotheologians seek to address the impulses governing human behavior through the formation of religious identity and culture. Religious traditions have the potential to construct new paradigms, delegitimate paradigms of oppression and domination, and contribute to a pluralistic approach to addressing social injustices—concerns that are addressed within the textual tradition of Jain Dharma. Ecopsychology proposes that the paradigmatic causes of ecocide are aggregations of the psychology—the *unhealthy* psychological tendencies—of individuals who are in need of healing as a sort of restoration of our individual healthy psychological conditions. Since this proposition is consistent with Jain theology,[3] we can *engage* in a productive interdisciplinary dialogue between ecopsychology and Jain philosophy, and we might therefore speak of Jain ecopsychology as a subset of Jain constructive theology, and Jain ecotheology.

I have elsewhere (Bohanec 2022) proposed that ecotheology may consist of a methodology that employs three main methods: (1) responding to critique, (2) theologizing the secular, and (3) reframing traditional categories. The first method involves addressing concerns that religious traditions uphold paradigms of oppression and domination of the natural world; the second involves showing how secular fields of thought can be interpretive lenses to understand theological traditions, a task I will engage in herein with ecopsychology. The third item conversely shows how aspects of a theological tradition can be expanded to address environmental concerns. I will open with the first method but will not distinguish between the second and third explicitly, although the reader will no doubt be aware that the secular category of ecopsychology is being employed in service of the Jain tradition (2), and that I am citing the Jain textual tradition to address environmental concerns (3).

Possible Critiques of the Jain Tradition

The advent of ecotheology largely followed a lecture that Lynn White Jr. gave in 1966 titled "The Historical Roots of Our Ecologic Crisis" in which White suggested that elements of Christian theology normalized the exploitation of nature. This critique inspired numerous Christian ecotheologians to respond to White's critiques, and the field of ecotheology was born. Tucker notes that White's critiques have underscored the importance of challenging "otherworldly goals" and purported rejection of the world that is present in Christian thought. White's critiques suggest a need for Christian ecotheologians to engage in a "task of revaluing nature so as to prevent its destruction" (Tucker 2006, xxv).

Likewise, perhaps the strongest eco-critique that might be levied against dharmic traditions is that they can be too world denying, and too otherworldly, implying that practitioners therefore may not have sufficient motivation to care for the natural world. When the *śramaṇa* (ascetic) norms that infuse dharmic traditions create excessive disdain for the world, and when the locus of value is otherworldly, then there may be a concomitant devaluation of this world, so the critique goes. For this reason, Nelson believes that the ascetic underpinnings of a tradition (in his case, Advaita Vedānta) "carry the potential to seriously undermine environmental concern" (Nelson 1998, 62). A critic of the Jain tradition might posit that similar ascetic tendencies within the Jain tradition might likewise serve to devalue the natural world (e.g., Dundas 2002).

A response to this critique would be to show where the Jain tradition venerates the natural world despite the other worldly orientation of an ascetic tradition that devalues worldly conditions such as sensory pursuits, etc. This veneration of the natural world is woven into the *śramaṇa*, ascetic norms of the *Ācārāṅga-sūtra* (*ĀS*, fifth–first century BCE) as if the compiler (Kshama-shraman Devardhigani) were aware of the possibility of ascetics becoming too otherworldly and indifferent to the beings of the natural world. The first chapter of the text addresses concerns of violence against living beings in the natural world, such as earth-beings (1.2ff.), water beings (1.3ff.), fire beings (1.4ff.), vegetative life (1.5), animals and mobile beings (1.6), and beings with "air bodies" (1.7). Only after these extensive injunctions against violence to the natural world are thoroughly discussed are the ascetic norms of the tradition examined.

Even in the *Ācārāṅga-sūtra*'s discussions focusing on ascetic disciplines, it is as if one is being enjoined to *not* become so indifferent to the world that one becomes indifferent to the suffering of others since the injunctions of nonviolence are constantly interspersed throughout (e.g., 2.2, 4.2, 5.5, 6.1, and 8.1). The text is clear in terms of firmly establishing a sense of care for the natural world in the context of—rather than being in opposition to (as per the critique of White, Nelson, Dundas, and others)—ascetic norms.

There are a variety of philosophical underpinnings that make Jain philosophy unique among world religions. For example, the Jain tradition proposes a nontheistic, ontological pluralism in contrast to some other dharma traditions that tend to rather favor absolute monism or a form of qualified monism (with the exceptions of the theistic pluralisms of Nyāya-Vaiśeṣika and Madhva's Vedānta and the pluralism of souls in Yoga-Sāṃkhya). By Jain ontological pluralism, all living beings are individual entities, valued intrinsically precisely because of their distinctness. As a "nontheistic" tradition, for Jains, each living entity (*jīva*) contains a divine essence whereby rather than having a monotheistic God as the locus of sanctity, reverence, and veneration—all measures of ultimate valuation—the souls of countless beings serve as the decentralized locus of value. This position has radical ethical implications when the ultimate source of valuation is not removed from living beings no matter how small—and the natural world is infinitely pervaded by these. All living beings have the same ontological status,[4] have souls, and are worthy of life; there is no superior deity from the absolute ontological standpoint, only from a soteriological perspective (as enlightened souls, or Jinas).

Theologizing Ecopsychology and Reframing Jain Psychology

Ecopsychology examines why people engage in behaviors that are environmentally destructive and seeks to understand the psychological factors that might motivate people to be more sustainable. My proposition here is that if we are to "theologize" the otherwise secular field of ecopsychology, one would have to show that the Jain tradition is conceptually aligned with the insights of ecopsychology; that is, the tradition might be understood to assist in, or parallel, the goals of ecopsychology. This would reframe traditional Jain categories in the process, as per the methodology of ecotheology that I've proposed elsewhere (see Bohanec 2022).

One of the topics that ecopsychologists have addressed is the relationship between psychology and modern consumerism where consumption habits observed in the "media and advertising industry" both create and reveal "a vast collective realm of projected desires, fears and aspirations," making consumptive habits "a rich new field of diagnostic material" for ecopsychologists (Kanner and Gomes 1995, 78–79).

Kanner and Gomes ask, "Why is it that when environmentalists speak of the need to reduce consumption they arouse such intense anxiety, depression, rage, and even panic?" (78–79). As if to answer that question the *Tattvārtha-sūtra* (ca. second–fifth century CE) states, "A hellish life is the result of material acquisitiveness and being aggressive with various enterprises"[5] (*TAS* 6.15/6.16). Our consumptive habits, particularly when they are "aggressive" (root *rabh*) indicate—and lead to—a life of unhappiness ("hellish"). We cannot ultimately derive happiness from consumerism because, as the *Uttarādhyayana-sūtra* (*UA*; ca. 500 CE) tells us, "Even at the time of materialistic enjoyment one's desire is still beyond satiation"[6] (*UA* 32.28). As we misunderstand the locus of happiness to be external—mistakenly believing that contentment can be derived from material acquisition—we may react with hostility when it seems that our misplaced sense of happiness is being challenged or threatened.

Moreover, the *Uttarādhyayana-sūtra* tells us that as one advances spiritually in one's meditation practice (*dhyāna*), one abandons mental states of anxiety (*ārta*) and malice (*raudra*) and one's mental state is "purified" (*śukla*)[7] (*UA* 30.35), proposing a tangible relationship between what we might call psychological healing (from *ārta* and *raudra*) to a more "pure" (*śukla*) mental state free from vexation from these maladies. This healing is described in the context of a chapter that directly challenges consumerism with a "Path Towards Austerity" (*tapo-mārga-gati*;[8] *UA* ch. 30), which proposes that through austerity (*tapas*) the consumerist urges of "aversion (*rāga*) and attachment (*dveṣa*)" are removed. This in turn mitigates the negative karmas[9] (*UA* 30.1) that cause our suffering and our misguided desire for material acquisition. This is consistent with links between mental health and consumerism proposed by some writers of ecopsychology (cf. Kanner and Gomes 1995).

The removal of aversion (*rāga*) and attachment (*dveṣa*)—which can be taken to be some of the psychological impulses behind consumerism—is the means by which a living being attains "pure happiness" (*ekānta sukha*), which is characteristic of liberation (*mokṣa*) (*UA* 32.2).[10] Thus, the remedy for the condition of mental dis-ease is to practice austerities that "free one from (*virahita*) the influx of karma (*āśrava*)," including abstentions from a variety of actions that would be related to modern consumerism, especially "violence to living beings" (*prāṇi-vadha*) and "covetousness" (*parigraha*)[11] (*UA* 30.2).

The *Uttarādhyayana-sūtra* provides an analysis of the interrelationship between our consumptive urges and mental states that produce our psychological suffering (*duḥkha*)—states such as material desire (*tṛṣṇa*, *rāga*)—and constrain our psychological abilities (*moha*). There is a mutual relationship between our materialistic desires (*tṛṣṇa*) and the debilitation of our psychological abilities represented by "delusion" (*moha*). The text tells us that "as a crane is produced from an egg and an egg is produced from crane, in the same way the origin of delusion (*moha*) is said to be craving (*tṛṣṇa*) and that of craving (*tṛṣṇa*) is said to be delusion (*moha*)"[12] (*UA* 32.6). We delude (*moha*) ourselves with consumerist desires because we falsely believe that material gain will cause us happiness. But aversion (*dveṣa*) and attachment (*rāga*) to material conditions ultimately are the cause of suffering—represented by the cycle of transmigration—through the process of accruing karma[13] (*UA* 32.7) by the inevitable violence present in any economic supply chain.

Thus, the way to end our psychological afflictions is not to pursue materialistic ends, but rather to be rid of psychological misery by being free of material desires. Material desires (*tṛṣṇa*) cause delusion (*moha*), which in turn causes suffering (*duḥkha*), so removing material desire is the means of freeing oneself from one's afflictions—psychological or otherwise[14] (*UA* 32.8). This amounts to a challenge against the psychological toll of modern consumerism, a challenge that is implicit within the Jain tradition and explicit with authors of ecopsychology.

Kanner and Gomes link the feeling of consumerist entitlement for "endless comfort and convenience" as "part of a syndrome that psychologists call narcissism," "characterized by an inflated, grandiose, entitled, and masterful self-image, or 'false self.' " Narcissists "constantly strive to meet the impossibly high standards of their false self, frequently feeling frustrated and depressed by their inability to do so, but also avoiding at all costs recognizing how empty they truly feel" (Kanner and Gomes 1995, 78–79).

Jain thinkers also deal with issues of consumption as they relate to a false sense of identity, evidenced by Mahāvīra being described as "without ego" (*amama*) when he attained liberation (*Kalpa-sūtra*; *KS* 118). In terms of ego (here as "false self" as per Kanner and Gomes's definition of narcissism), the *Dravya-saṃgraha* (*DS*; ca. tenth century CE) differentiates between "worldly perspectives" (*vyavahāra*) of selfhood based on "material, karmic" (*pudgala-karma*) identities and our essential self, represented by the soul (*jīva*). By the analysis of the *Dravya-saṃgraha,* the features of our psychology (*bhāva-karma*) are the result of interaction between one's soul and the external environment (*dravya-karma*) that occurs when the soul exerts agency (*kartā*). Specifically, "From a worldly perspective (*vyavahāra-naya*), the soul exerts agency over (*kartā*) the material world of karma, etc. (*pudgala-karma*). But from a more precise perspective (*niścaya-naya*), a purer perspective (*śuddha-naya*), the soul is removed from karma exerting agency (*kartā*) over purely psychological conditions (*śuddha-bhāva*)"[15] (*DS* 8). The conditions of the soul's agency here are not that the soul (*jīva*) *directly* affects the material reality of karma (as *dravya-karma*). The soul (*jīva*) only directly affects one's psychological conditions (*bhāva-karmas*) and it is these psychological conditions (*bhāva*) that then in turn affect material reality (*dravya-karma*), such as through the decisions we make based on ideas and conditions that we have. Therefore, generally speaking (*vyavahāra-naya*) we can say that the soul (*jīva*) exerts agency over material reality. But more precisely (*niścaya-naya* or *śuddha-naya*) the soul exerts agency on material reality through the intermediary of psychological conditions (*bhāva*)[16] (Ghoshal 1989, 25–26).

The interaction between the *dravya-karmas* (external karma) and the soul (*jīva*) via the medium of our psychological conditions (*bhāva*) determines our mental condition, or perhaps more germane to ecopsychology, the state of our mental health. The *Dravya-saṃgraha* tells us, "From a worldly perspective (*vyavahāra-naya*), the soul experiences pleasure (*suha*, Skt. *sukha*) and suffering which are the results of material karma (*pudgala-karma*). From a more precise perspective (*niścaya-naya*) the soul only experiences psychological conditions (*bhāva*) that are separate (*cedana*) from external, material karma"[17] (*DS* 9). Thus, whatever suffering and pleasure that one feels due to consumerism is the result of our external engagements, which creates a false sense of identity—similar to the "false self" of Kanner and Gomes—with the objects of those external engagements, leading to the psychological turmoil that is experienced by one's conscious essence, here as the soul (*jīva*), related to the consumerist impulses of aversion and attachment (*dveṣa* and *rāga*/*tṛṣṇa*), which mistakenly (*moha*) seek to satisfy a misguided sense of self (*bhāva-karma* as *mamatva*).

The affinity between ecopsychology and Jain philosophy is telling by the prolific use of the word "soul" by ecopsychology authors, and especially the trope of the soul's return to its "home," which seems to imply a sort of soteriological motif among those authors. For example, Roszak proposes that "exploring the psychological dimensions of our planetary ecology" has a "noble and affirmative project: that of returning the troubled human soul to the harmony and joy that are the only solid basis for an environmentally sustainable standard of living" (1995, 15). Hillman might add that "all psychologies [are] ultimately therapies by definition because of their involvement with soul" (1995, xviii). His presentation of Jung's "psychoid," which is our understanding of self as "partly material, partly psychic, [as] a merging of psyche and matter," sounds strikingly like the model of the interrelatedness of identity between *dravya-karma, bhāva-karma,* and the soul presented above in the *Dravya-saṃgraha.*

Moreover, Hillman notes, "Since the 'discovery of the unconscious,' every sophisticated theory of personality has to admit that whatever I call me to be 'me' has at least a portion of its roots beyond my agency and my awareness" (1995, xviii). Likewise, the karmic patterns that inform the psychology of selfhood of Jain psychology also remain below our immediate awareness and as these latent karmic deposits come to fruition in ways that we do not choose in our decisions, perceptions, etc.

Hillman also posits that "the greater part of the soul lies outside the body," that "we cannot accurately set borders to human identity," and that "in this world soul the human soul has always had its home" (1995, xxi–xiii). Jain philosophy would agree on the inextricable connection between the internal and the external, since "one who knows the inner-self (*antar-ātman*) knows the external world; one who knows the external world (*bahiyā*) knows the inner-self (*antar-ātman*)"[18] (*ĀS* 1.7.147).

However, what Hillman speaks of as "soul" we might rather consider as a broader "selfhood." In agreement, from a Jain perspective, we have aspects of our identity that may be quite external to whatever may be encased within our physical bodies based on our relationships of identity-forming activities with the external world. Where Hillman asserts that we "cannot accurately set borders to the human identity," the Jain tradition proposes that we can in fact employ a classification between what we are in essence versus peripheral features of our identity.[19] These gradations between "external" (*bahir-ātman*), "internal" (*antar-ātman*), and "transcendental" (*paramātman*) degrees of selfhood are described by

Hemacandra in the *Yoga-śāstra* (*YŚ*): "Identity with the body and its external relationships etc. is constructed by perceiving the self as external (*bahir-ātman*). And that which governs over the body and its external relationships is constructed as the internal self (*antar-ātmā*).[20] The transcendental self (*paramātman*) is understood as consisting of the form of consciousness and happiness, completely deprived of mistaken appearances, pure, beyond the purview of sensory perception, and with infinite virtues"[21] (*YŚ* 12.7–8). Where the Jain tradition might disagree with Hillman that "the most profoundly collective and unconscious self is the natural material world," the Jain tradition seems to come to a similar understanding as ecopsychology, based on this graded selfhood that Hillman appears to take as defining of ecopsychology as establishing "an individual's harmony with his or her 'own deep self,'" which "requires not merely a journey to the interior but a harmonizing with the environmental world" (Hillman 1995, xix).

Such "harmonization with the environmental world" is essential to the Jain tradition, evidenced by its many entreaties for nonviolence to the living beings of the natural world. For example, in the *Ācārāṅga-sūtra*:

> The violent one who employs weapons or instruments that cause harm [upon even the tiniest of beings—even when these weapons are one's own internal conditions[22] comes to lack the wisdom of spiritual insight.[23] On the other hand, one who desires *not* to use such mechanisms of harm [upon even the tiniest of elemental beings] develops wisdom and spiritual insight.[24] Having attained such insight, a wise person should never allow for any instrument of harm, internally or externally, against [even the tiniest] beings in the earth, neither should they cause others to do so, nor should they approve of the engagement of anything, internally or externally, that causes harm.[25] (*ĀS* 1.1.1.31–33)

This is because "participation in violence is as harmful to those who engage in violence to living beings" since it "deprives one of spiritual wisdom (*se abohīe*)"[26] (*ĀS* 1.2.23), what some psychologists have called the perpetrator effect.

Ecopsychologists seem to pragmatically employ the term "soul" illustratively (that is to say, perhaps without implying any ontological commitment) to refer to that part of our being that is essential and is not damaged by the psychological wounding that is peripheral to our spiritual essence—the psychological wounding that in turn causes damaged humans to reallocate their own inner wounding upon the external environment. This understanding of the soul-language of ecopsychology is surprisingly consistent with the Jain understanding. For Jains, karma would represent the psychological wounding that is peripheral to the pure, unwounded, soul-essence (*jīva*). Since the *jīva* is without violent tendencies, all destructive actions are a result of either karmic impulses or karmic "wounding" occluding the essential goodness of the soul. The *Tattvārtha-sūtra* further tells us, "The intense karmic consequences that occur because of the arising of materialistic desire (*kaṣāya*), causes one to behave in a way that is deluded"[27] (*TAS* 6.14). When our actions are motivated by material desire it is because we mistakenly feel that we are incomplete, and that psychological sense of incompleteness causes one to engage in "deluded" karmic activities—such as unconscionable pollution, excessive consumption, etc.—that causes pain to others. Where ecopsychology intersects with Jain philosophy, that internal pain is transferred from the psychologically damaged subject (*moha*) onto the living beings of the natural world.

Conclusion

Of course, interdisciplinary dialogues that employ analogies, like any argument by analogy, require that one account for dissimilarities and that one can demonstrate that nonetheless, irrespective of dissimilarities, an analogous relationship can be adduced. Generally, the field of psychology is ambivalent about philosophical claims of ontology and epistemology, and rather prefers the metaphysically neutral position of psycholog*ism*, namely, the idea that philosophies regarding metaphysics, epistemology, meaning, etc. can be explained as revealing psychological conditions without affirming any ontological commitment, as a sort of methodological (*not necessarily* philosophical) relativism. This allows ecopsychologists to engage in soul-language without necessarily affirming or denying a belief in the metaphysical existence of a soul, but rather as a pragmatic tool to explain the human subject's relationship to the natural world or for human subjects to express their feelings about their individual experiences.

Of course, psychologism would be in contrast to the non-relativistic metaphysical commitments of the Jain tradition where, for Jains, soul-language is not merely a description of what one's experiences "are like" subjectively but are rather descriptions of what is real objectively. But by applying a pragmatic maxim to the soul-language of ecopsychologists (e.g., the truth of a statement is evinced by the usefulness of its application), the Jain tradition might argue that the usefulness of soul-language implies that there is at least some degree of objective truth to such language—that is, if we were to accept a parallel between Jain philosophy and pragmatism that I have argued for elsewhere.[28] Thus, the usefulness of "soul"-language on the part of ecopsychologists and the metaphysical belief in the reality of the soul of Jains are insubstantial when considering the shared, overlapping assumptions that I've articulated above, and we can rightfully speak of Jain ecopsychology.

Moreover, there are several other otherwise secular categories of environmental thought that could be "theologized" by the Jain tradition, and conversely the implications of the Jain tradition could be broadened to expand those fields (as per methods 2 and 3). The advantage for ecopsychology is that it moves beyond bare altruism and alter-centricity—although these are certainly present in the tradition—to underscoring the immense potential benefits gained by the individual through the cultivation of ecological awareness and conscientiousness, benefits such as addressing one's psychological health and healing. Thus, despite its transcendental and ascetic focus, for millennia the Jain tradition has been aware of these important connections between human psychology and the natural world by proposing that psychological health and spiritual development necessarily require an intense sensitivity and care toward all of the living beings of the natural world—no matter how minute they may seem to the current state of our senses that have been blunted by the karma accrued through the violence inherent in all material consumption.

Notes

1. Translations herein are my own unless otherwise noted, consulting Mahāprajña 1981; Ghoshal 1989; Lalwani 1999; and Bothara 2011. Some Ardhamāgadhī terms have been Sanskritised for recognizability.

2. This is also part of the rationale of why I have framed the Jain tradition in terms of "virtue ethics"; see "Jain Virtue Ethics Engaging with Animal Rights" in this volume.

3. In this work, I use the term "theology" loosely to refer to the religious philosophy of a tradition, not to be confused with "theism," which proposes a monotheistic God and which is not within Jain teachings.

4. While this may be true largely with the ontological constituency of souls as being conscious / happy / energetic beings (*caitanya* / *sukha* / *vīrya*), this might be a slight overstatement since some souls have the quality of *bhavyatva*, which makes them capable at least of achieving liberation, while other souls, by Wiley, "that lack this quality, called *abhavyas*, are not capable of attaining either proper insight or liberation" (Wiley 2004, 57).

5. *TAS* 6.15/16 (alternate numbering): *bahvārambha-parigrahatvaṃ ca nārakasyāyuṣaḥ* || A hellish life (*nārakasya+āyuṣaḥ*) [is the result of existing in the state of] material acquisitiveness (*parigrahatvaṃ*) and being aggressive with multiple enterprises (*bahu+ārambha*).

6. *UA* 32.28: *saṃbhoga-kāle ya atittilābhe* || Even at the time of materialistic enjoyment (*saṃbhoga-kāle*) one's (*ya*) desire [*rūvāṇuvāeṇa*, glossed as *anurāga* by Bothara] is still beyond satiation (*atittilābhe*).

7. *UA* 30.35: *aṭṭaruddāṇi vajjittā, jhāejjā sumamāhie* | *dhammasukkāiṃ jhāṇāiṃ, jhāṇaṃ taṃ tu buhā vae* || Having abandoned (*vajjitā*) anxiety [*aṭṭa*, Skt. *ārta*] and malice [*ruddāṇi*, Skt. *raudra*] one meditates (*jhāejjā*) upon the good (*sumamāhie*). Indeed (tu) that (taṃ) meditation (*jhāṇam*) becomes (*buhā vae*) meditation (*jhāṇāiṃ*) that is pure (*sukkāiṃ*, Skt. *śukla*) dharma (*dhamma*, Skt. *dharma*).

8. Ardhamāgadhī: *tavamaggagaī*.

9. *UA* 30.1: *jahā u pāvagaṃ kammaṃ, rāga-dvesa-samajjiyaṃ* | *khavei tavasā bhikkhu, tamegaggamaṇo suṇa* || Listen attentively [*suṇa*] to the process through which an ascetic destroys the demerit-karmas acquired due to attachment and aversion [*rāga-dveṣa*]. (Translated by Pravartak Amar Muni.)

10. *UA* 32.2: *nāṇassa savvassa pagāsaṇāe, annāṇa-mohassa vivajjaṇāe* | *rāgassa dosassa ya saṃkhaeṇaṃ, eganta-sokkhaṃ samuvei mokkaṃ* || The soul (living being) attains liberation (*samuvei mokkaṃ*, Skt. *mokṣa*) that is the abode of ultimate bliss (*eganta-sokkhaṃ*, Skt. *ekānta sukha*) through manifestation of all encompassing (right) knowledge (*nāṇassa savvassa pagāsaṇāe*, Skt. *jñānasya sarvasya*), removal (*vivajjaṇāe*, Skt. *vivarjana*) of

ignorance (*annāṇa*, Skt. *ajñāna*), delusion (*mohassa*) and complete destruction of attachment and aversion (*rāgassa dosassa ya saṃkhaeṇaṃ*, Skt. *rāgasya doṣasya*). (Translated by Pravartak Amar Muni.)

11. *UA* 30.2: *pāṇa-vah-musāvāyā, adatta-mehuṇa-pariggahā virao | rāībhoyaṇavirao, jīvo bhavai aṇāsavo* || "A soul (*jīvo*, Skt. *jīva*) becomes (*bhavai*, Skt. *bhavati*) free from (*virao*, Skt. *virahita*) the in-flux of *karmas* (*aṇāsavo*) by abstaining from (*virao*, Skt. *virahita*) violence (*pāṇa-vah*, Skt. *prāṇi-vadha*]), falsehood (*musāvāyā*, Skt. *mṛśāvāda*), stealing (*adatta*), sexual intercourse (*mehuṇa*, Skt. *maithuna*), covetousness (*pariggahā*, Skt. *parigraha*) and food intake during night (*rāībhoyaṇavirao*, Skt. *rātri-bhojana-virati*)."

12. *UA* 32.6: *jahā ya aṇḍappabhavā balāgā, aṇḍaṃ balāgappabhavaṃ jahā ya | emeva mohāyayaṇaṃ khu taṇhā, mohaṃ ca taṇhāyayaṇaṃ vayanti* || As a crane is produced from egg (*jahā ya aṇḍappabhavā balāgā*) and egg is produced from crane (*aṇḍaṃ balāgappabhavaṃ jahā ya*), in the same way (*emeva*) the origin of delusion (*moha*) is said to be craving (*tṛṣṇa*) (*mohāyayaṇaṃ khu taṇhā*) and that of craving (tṛṣṇa) is said to be delusion (moho) (*mohaṃ ca taṇhāyayaṇaṃ vayanti*). (Translated by Pravartak Amar Muni.)

13. *UA* 32.7: *rāgo ya doso vi ya kamma-bīyaṃ, kammaṃ ca mohappa-bhavaṃ vayanti | kammaṃ ca jāī-maraṇassa mūlaṃ, dukkhaṃ ca jāī-maraṇaṃ vayanti* || They say that (*vayanti*) attachment (*rāga*) and aversion (doso, Skt. *dveṣa*) are both (*vi ya*) the seeds of *karmas* (*kamma-bīyaṃ*, Skt. *karma-bīja*) and *karma* (*kammaṃ ca*) is said (*vayanti*) be produced from delusion (*mohappa-bhavaṃ*, Skt. *moha-bhava*). And (ca) they say (*vayanti*) *karma* is the root of (*mūlaṃ*) birth and death (*jāī-maraṇassa mūlaṃ*, Skt. *janā-maraṇa*), and birth and death considered to be (vayanti) suffering (*dukkhaṃ ca jāī-maraṇaṃ vayanti*).

14. *UA* 32.8: *dukkhaṃ hayaṃ jassa na hoi moho, moho hao jassa na hoi taṇhā | taṇhā hayā jassa na hoi loho, loho hao jassa na kiṃcaṇāiṃ* || One who is free of delusion gets rid of misery [*dukkhaṃ hayaṃ jassa na hoi moho*]; one who is free of cravings gets rid of delusion [*moho hao jassa na hoi taṇhā*]; when craving ends greed is destroyed [*hayā jassa na hoi loho*]; and one who is rid of greed has nothing left; he becomes free of possessions [*loho hao jassa na kiṃcaṇāiṃ*]. (Translated by Pravartak Amar Muni.)

15. *DS* 8: *puggalakammādīṇaṃ kattā vavahārado du ṇiccayado | cedaṇakammāṇādā suddhaṇayā suddhabhāvāṇaṃ* || From a worldly perspective (*vavahārado*, Skt. *vyavahāra-naya*), the soul (ādā, referring to the jīva) exerts agency over (*kattā*, Skt. *kartā*) the material world of karma, etc. (*puggalakammādīṇaṃ, pudgala-karma+ādī*). But (du) from a more precise perspective (*ṇiccayado*, Skt. *niścaya-naya*), a more pure perspective (*suddhaṇayā*, Skt. *śuddha-naya*) the soul (*ādā*) is removed from karma (*cedaṇakammāṇādā*) exerting agency over (kattā, Skt. kartā) over purely psychological conditions (*suddhabhāvāṇaṃ*, Skt. *śuddha-bhāva*).

16. In his commentary, Brahmadeva notes that this is an assertion of the agency of the soul on the part of Jain philosophy in contrast to the lack of agency (*udāsīna*) of the soul posited by Sāṅkhya philosophy (Ghoshal 1989, 25–26). We might also note that here "psychology" also refers to karmic, material reality.

17. *DS* 9: *vavahārā suhadukkhaṃ puggalakammaphalaṃ pabhuñjedi | ādā ṇiccayaṇayado cedaṇabhāvaṃ kau ādassa* || From a worldly perspective (*vyavahāra-naya*), the soul (*ādā*, referring to *jīva*) experiences (*pabhuñjedi*, Skt. *upabhojana*) pleasure (*suha*, Skt. *sukha*) and suffering (*dukkaṃ*, Skt. *duḥkha*) which are the results of (phalaṃ) material karma (*puggalakammaphalaṃ*). From a more precise perspective (*ṇiccayaṇayado*, Skt. *niścaya-naya*) the soul only (*kau ādassa*) experiences psychological conditions (*bhāvaṃ*) that are separate (cedaṇa, Skt. cedana) [from material karma].

18. *ĀS* 1.7.147: *je ajjhatthaṃ jāṇai, se bahiyā jāṇai | je bahiyā jāṇai, se ajjhatthaṃ jāṇai* | One who (je) knows (*jāṇai*) the inner-self (*ajjhatthaṃ*, Skt. *antar-ātman*) knows (*se bahiyā*) the external world (*bahiyā*); one who (*je*) knows (*jāṇai*) the external world (*bahiyā*) knows (se *jāṇai*) the inner-self (*ajjhatthaṃ*).

19. The proposition of "essences" would be objectionable to Hillman.

20. *YŚ* 12.7: *ātma-dhiyā samupāttaḥ kāyādiḥ kīrtyate 'tra bahir-ātmā | kāyādeḥ samādhiṣṭhāyako bhavaty antar-ātmā tu* || It is said that (*kīryate*) [identity with] the body etc. (*kāya+ādīḥ*) is constructed (*sampāttaḥ*) by perceiving the self (*ātma-dhiyā*) as the external self (*bahir-ātmā*). And (*tu*) that which governs over (*samādhiṣṭhāyakā*) the body etc. (*kāyādeḥ*) is constructed as (*sampāttaḥ*) the internal self (*antar-ātmā*).

21. *YŚ* 12.8: *cidrūpānanda-mayo niḥśeṣopādhi-varjitaḥ śuddhaḥ | atyakṣo 'nanta-guṇaḥ paramātma kīrtitas taj-jñaiḥ* || The *paramātma* is mentioned (*kīrtitaḥ*) by those who know it (*taj-jñaiḥ*) as consisting of the form of consciousness and bliss (*cid-rūpa+ānanda-mayaḥ*), completely deprived of mistaken appearances (*niḥśeṣa+upādhi-varjitaḥ*), pure, beyond the purview of sensory perception (*atyakṣaḥ*), and with infinite qualities (ananta-guṇaḥ).

22. All from *satthaṃ*: this is how Yuvācārya Mahāprajña glosses the term *sattaṃ*, citing "the *Niryukti* (the earliest commentary) on the Āyāro" (Mahāprajña 1981, 18–19).

23. *Ācārāṅga Sūtra* 1.1.1.31: *ettha satthaṃ samāraṃbhamāṇassa icchete āraṃbhā apariṇṇātā bhavaṃti*|| Now (*ettha*) the [violent, *vihiṃsai*, from 1.1.1.27] one who desires (*icchaete*) to use (*samāraṃbhamāṇassa*) weapons or instruments that cause harm even when they are one's own internal conditions that can be used as weapons (from *satthaṃ*, Skt. *śastra*) [upon even the tiniest of elemental beings, from previous verses] becomes (*bhavaṃti*) one who lacks the wisdom of spiritual insight (*apariṇṇātā*, Skt. *aparijñātā*).

24. *Ācārāṅga Sūtra* 1.1.1.32: *ettha satthaṃ asamāraṃbhamāṇassa icchete āraṃbhā pariṇṇātā bhavaṃ*ti || On the other hand (*ettha*) one who desires (*icchete*) not to use (*asamāraṃbhamāṇassa*) weapons or other such instruments that cause harm such as one's own internal conditions (*satthaṃ*) [upon even the tiniest of elemental beings] develops (*bhavaṃ*ti) wisdom and spiritual insight (*pariṇṇātā*, Skt. *parijñātā*).

25. *Ācārāṅga Sūtra* 1.1.1.33: *taṃ pariṇṇāya mehāvī neva sayaṃ pudhavi—satthaṃ samāraṃbhejjā, nevaṇṇehiṃ puḍhavi—satthaṃ samāraṃbhāvejjā, nevaṇṇe puḍhavi—satthaṃ samāraṃbhaṃte samaṇujāṇejjā* || Having attained such insight (*taṃ pariṇṇāya*), a wise person should never allow for any instrument of harm, internally or externally (*sattaṃ*) against [even the tiniest] beings in the earth (*mehāvī neva sayaṃ pudhavi—satthaṃ samāraṃbhejjā, nevaṇṇehiṃ puḍhavi—*), neither should they cause others to do so (*satthaṃ samāraṃbhāvejjā, nevaṇṇe puḍhavi*), nor should they approve of the engagement of anything, internally or externally that causes harm (*satthaṃ samāraṃbhaṃte samaṇujāṇejjā*).

26. *ĀS* 1.2.23: *taṃ se ahiyāe, taṃ se abohīe* | That (*taṃ*) [participation in violence] is as harmful to those (*se*) [who engage in violence to living beings]. That (*taṃ*) [participation in violence] deprives one of spiritual wisdom (*se abohīe*).

27. *TAS* 6.14: *kaśāyodayāt tīvra-pariṇāmaś cāritra-mohasya* || The intense [karmic] consequences (*tīvra-pariṇāmaḥ*) [that occur] because of the arising of (*udayāt*) of materialistic desire (*kaṣāya*), [causes] one to behave in a way that is deluded (*cāritra-mohasya*).

28. *Jain Yoga Philosophy: Pragmatism as a Method for Interfaith Peacebuilding*, publication forthcoming.

References

Ācārāṅga-sūtra. 1981. Edited and Translated by Yuvācārya Mahāprajña. Today & Tomorrow's Printers and Publishers.

Bohanec, Cogen. 2022. "A Dialogical Encounter Between Christian Ecotheological Ethics and Gauḍīya Vaiṣṇava Theology." In *Religion and Sustainability: Interreligious Resources, Interdisciplinary Responses; Intersection of Sustainability Studies and Religion, Theology, Philosophy*, edited by Rita Sherma and Purushottama Bilimoria. Springer.

Dundas, Paul. 2002. "The Limits of a Jain Environmental Ethic." In *Jainism and Ecology*, edited by Christopher Key Chapple. Harvard University Press.

Ghoshal, S. C., ed. 1989. *Dravya-saṃgraha of Nemichandra Siddhānta-Chakravarttī*. Varanasi: Bharatiya Jnanpith.

Hillman, James. 1995. "A Psyche the Size of the Earth." In *Ecopsychology: Restoring the Earth, Healing the Mind*, edited by Theodore Roszak, Mary E. Gomes, and Allen D. Kanner. Sierra Club Books.

Kalpa-sūtra. 1999. Translated by Kastur Chand Lalwani. Motilal Banarsidass.

Kanner, Allen D., and Mary E. Gomes. 1995. "The All-Consuming Self." In Roszak, Gomes, and Kanner, eds., *Ecopsychology*.

Nelson, Lance E. 1998. *Purifying the Earthly Body of God: Religion and Ecology in Hindu India*. State University of New York Press.

Roszak, Theodore. 1995. "Where Psyche Meets Gaia." In Roszak, Gomes, and Kanner, eds., *Ecopsychology*.

Tucker, Mary Evelyn. 2006. "Religion and Ecology: Survey of the Field." In *The Oxford Handbook of Religion and Ecology*, edited by Roger S. Gottlieb, 398–418. Oxford University Press.

Umāsvāti/Umāsvāmī. 2011. *Tattvārtha-sūtra: That Which Is*. Translated by Nathmal Tatia. Yale University Press.

Uttarādhyayana-sūtra. 2011. Edited by Shrut Acharya Pravartak Shri Amar Muni and Srichand Surana Saras, translated by Surendra Bothara. Padma Prakashan.

Wiley, Kristi L. 2004. *The A to Z of Jainism*. Scarecrow Press.

Yogaśāstra of Hemacandra. 2002. Translated by Olle Quarnström. Department of Sanskrit and Indian Studies, Harvard University.

Part V

Interfaith Engagement

13

Engaged Virtues

Cultivating Friendliness, Joy, Compassion, and Equanimity in Jain Thought

ALBA RODRÍGUEZ JUAN

The cultivation (*bhāvanā*) of friendliness (*maitrī*), joy (*pramoda*), compassion (*kāruṇya*), and equanimity (*mādhyasthya*) occupies a significant place within Jain religiosity. According to Umāsvāti in the *Tattvārthasūtra* (*TS*), friendliness is to be practiced toward all living beings; joy toward the virtuous; compassion toward the afflicted; and equanimity toward the unvirtuous.[1] Later Jain authors redefined and explained these practices in different ways, sometimes referring to them as "the four *bhāvanā*s." As part of Jain praxis, these four *bhāvanā*s or cultivations seem to have been used by Jains to lead a life of minimal harm.

While much has been written in academic scholarship regarding the ways in which Jains are engaging with topics such as the global ecological crisis, animal exploitation, or food consumption, the current study of the four *bhāvanā*s refocuses our attention on our everyday social interactions with members of our own species with whom, it seems, interactions are becoming more difficult in today's social and political climate. The *bhāvanā*s indeed offer guidance regarding how we should conduct ourselves when exposed to different situations in everyday life, providing a spiritual framework within which to interpret challenging social engagements.

The four *bhāvanās* or cultivations have similar counterparts in other South Asian religious traditions with which Jains have been intellectually engaged since very early times. For instance, they correspond to the four *brahmavihāras* outlined in many Buddhist scholastic treatises, rendered in Pali as *mettā, karuṇā, muditā,* and *upekkhā*. Detailed descriptions can be found, for example, in the second book of the *Abhidhamma Piṭaka,* dating from the early centuries BCE.[2] There are also references in the *Saṃyuttanikāya* and the *Saṃyuktāgama* suggesting that these practices were cultivated by those who were not Buddhists (Bronkhorst 1993, 68). In the Mahāyāna lore in particular, the *brahmavihāras* came to be considered a preliminary practice to inspire the Bodhisattva path. Mahāyāna Buddhist texts often recognize three scopes in Buddhist practice: (1) the low scope, where the practitioner basically aims for a higher rebirth; (2) the middle scope, which includes practices such as contemplating on the faults of *saṃsāra*; and (3) the highest scope, which includes further practices for the development of *bodhicitta*.[3] The *brahmavihāras* are included in the early stages of the highest scope, indicating their foundational role in the progression toward advanced states in Buddhist meditation practice.

There also references to the four *bhāvanās* in brahmanical literature. The cultivation of friendliness, joy, compassion, and equanimity appears in some Upaniṣads. Sometimes, these terms are listed in the same order,[4] and other times they occur in isolation, though with similar meanings.[5] Patañjali also included the four *bhāvanās* in his well-known *Yogasūtra* as part of a set of ethical observances intended to purify and clarify the mind.[6]

However, scholarship on these four cultivations in the Jain context is very limited. This chapter attends to this gap by paying attention to how the *bhāvanās* were defined in four Jain Śvetāmbara texts. I explore various interpretations of these practices by prominent Jain philosophers such as Umāsvāti, Haribhadra, and Hemacandra, followed by a more significant consideration of their culmination in the work of Yaśovijaya, who elaborated upon the *bhāvanās* thoroughly. I will show how the *bhāvanās* developed in engagement with Buddhist and brahmanical intellectual environments, and share a common notion of ethical good across traditions. They are deeply rooted in a process of ascetic detachment and pursuit of the self that nevertheless considers ethical engagement with, and commitment to, one's social world.

The Many Meanings of *Bhāvanā*

The word *bhāvanā* is polyvalent, having been used in the Jain tradition in a number of ways. The most common English translations of the Sanskrit word *bhāvanā* are "cultivation," "contemplation," "reflection," and "meditation." The term *bhāvanā* comes from the Sanskrit root *bhū-*, meaning "to be" or "to become." Monier Monier-Williams suggests that the stem *bhāvanā* can be taken to have a causitive sense of the root *bhū*, as "causing to be" (1899, 755). In addition to the fourfold model that I focus upon in this chapter, *bhāvanā* is also a designation used by Śvetāmbaras for twelve themes of reflection that are often called *anuprekṣās* by Digambaras (Wiley 2004, 56). Some late Jain authors have used the words *bhāvanā* and *anuprekṣā* interchangeably.[7] Furthermore, the term *bhāvanā* can also refer to a list of twenty-five observances or supporting practices that reinforce the mendicant vows (*mahāvrata*). There are five observances for each of the five mendicant vows, listed in *TS* 7.3–7.8 (Dg.) and 7.3 (Śv.).[8] While both Śvetāmbaras and Digambaras might have used the term *bhāvanā* in these ways, only Digambara authors of medieval texts on lay conduct (*śrāvakācāra*) used it to refer to yet another, different set of sixteen mental attitudes or observances to be followed by lay Jains in order to advance on their respective religious paths (Joshi 1981, 8; Dundas 2002, 158). These are identical with the list of sixteen virtues in the *TS* (Dg. 6.24; Śv. 6.23) that lead to the binding of the variety of karma that causes rebirth as a Tīrthaṅkara (Wiley 2004, 56–57).

Consistent with these meanings, in the context of contemporary Jain meditation, *bhāvanā* can refer, in general, to practices for the purification of the soul. For example, Ācārya Mahāprajña, the well-known Śvetāmbara Terāpanthī leader, included *bhāvanā* in his eightfold model of Jain meditation or *prekṣā-dhyāna*, designed for both Jain mendicants and laity. Upon my question on what *bhāvanā* means in this model, Samani Pratibha Pragya, a Jain scholar and longtime teacher of *prekṣā-dhyāna*, explained that it means "preparing your mind for meditation." That is to say, *bhāvanā* is to be practiced before meditation, in preparation for it.[9]

Furthermore, *bhāvanā* can also refer to a kind of religious intention similar to devotion (*bhakti*). John Cort defines it as an "intentionally generated meditational sentiment" (Cort 2001, 206). The same word is also used to refer to some Jain devotional songs, hymns, or singing sessions.[10] Although there are more ways in which Jains have used the word *bhāvanā* throughout history, these are some of the most common. For the purposes of this chapter, I draw our attention to some examples from Jain texts that discuss a set of four *bhāvanās*.

The Four *Bhāvanā*s in the *Tattvārthasūtra*

In the *Tattvārthasūtra* (*TS*), practices comprising what are more widely referred to as "the four *bhāvanās*" are included in chapter 7, which discusses the five vows of nonviolence (*ahiṃsā*), truthfulness (*satya*), non-stealing (*asteya*), proper sexual conduct (*brahmacharya*), and non-attachment (*aparigraha*). The *bhāvanās* are presented as practices for strengthening both the vows of the Jain mendicants (*mahāvrata*s) and the vows of Jain householders (*aṇuvrata*s) and are complementary to other religious observances. Umāsvāti writes that the *bhāvanā*s are:

> Friendliness (*maitrī*) for all living beings,
> joy (*pramoda*) at the sight of the virtuous,
> compassion (*kāruṇya*) for the afflicted,
> and equanimity (*mādhyasthya*) towards the ineducable.[11]

Early commentators provided different interpretations of this verse. For example, Kawasaki has pointed out that, in the Digambara tradition, Pūjyapāda defines *maitrī* in his *Sarvārthasiddhi* as "the wish for non-arising of the sufferings of others,"[12] a definition adopted by his successors Akalaṅka, Vidyānandin, Bhāskaranandi, and Śrutasāgara. For instance, Akalaṅka, in his *Tattvārthavārtika* defines compassion (*anukampā*)[13] as "*maitrī* toward all living beings"[14] therefore considering compassion (*anukampā*) and friendliness (*maitrī*) as roughly synonymous (Kawasaki 2022, 120).[15]

Following the verses on the *bhāvanā*s, we find in the *TS* brief definitions of the five great vows (*mahāvrata*s) and the five lesser vows or limited vows of restraint (*aṇuvrata*s) (Dg. 7.8–7.14; Śv. 7.13–7.19). Then, seven supplementary practices for the householders are listed (Dg. 7.16; Śv. 7.21), followed by the practice of fasting to death (Dg. 7.17; Śv. 7.22). After these, transgressions of the vows are explained (Dg. 7.18–7.32; Śv. 7.23–7.37); and ultimately, we find the benefits and worth of charitable acts (Dg. 7.33–34; Śv. 7.38–7.39). The location of the four *bhāvanā*s in the *TS* suggests that they are included in a broad Jain ethical and soteriological framework that gives priority to the vows, aiming to minimize harm (*hiṃsā*). The commentator on the *TS* Saṅghavī Sukhlāl has highlighted the close relationship between the *bhāvanā*s, the vows, reflections on the nature of suffering (what he calls *duḥkha-bhāvanā*), and other complementary practices included in chapter 7 of the *TS* (Sukhlalji 1974, 308).

As we can gather from their location in the *TS*, the four *bhāvanā*s require an inward focus, which nevertheless first requires an outward process of discernment. Indeed, one must begin by determining the category into which each person with whom one interacts belongs: Are they happy, suffering, virtuous, or non-virtuous? Only after doing so, can one cultivate the appropriate *bhāvanā* for that person and situation (Chapple 2010, 101–112). Because the *bhāvanā*s require this kind of engagement with one's social environment, they differ from other Jain meditative or contemplative practices that have a marked inward focus, such as, for example, the practice of *kāyotsarga* ("abandonment of the body").

The Four *Bhāvanā*s in Later Jain Textual Sources

Jain texts written between 700 CE and 1300 CE are marked by tremendous innovations in Jain philosophical thought. During this period, Jain authors interested in yoga reconstructed Jain yoga through comparative studies with other yoga systems and in engagement with their surrounding intellectual and religious environments (Jain 2016; Chapple 2003). They adopted the framework of the Three Jewels of correct knowledge (*samyag-jñāna*), correct worldview (*samyag-darśana*), and correct conduct (*samyak-cāritra*), and discussed the Jain vows as applying to the three levels of mind (*manas*), speech (*vāc*), and body (*kāya*). Although they still abided by Jain karma doctrine, they did not only use the word "yoga" to refer to action that causes the influx of karma as understood in the *TS* and earlier Jain canonical sources; instead, they often used it to refer to Jain religious practices in a broad sense, with the main goal of producing auspicious karma (*puṇya*) and eliminating negative karma (*pāpa*).

In what follows, I will consider the *bhāvanā*s in these four Jain texts: the *Yogabindu*, the *Yogadṛṣṭisamuccaya*, the *Yogaśāstra*, and the *Dvātriṃśaddvātriṃśikā*. While exact dates cannot be determined for these texts, they are presented here in a relative chronological order. The four texts were written by Śvetāmbara authors who appear to be building upon one another's work but are also simultaneously engaging with thought found in other non-Jain traditions of their respective times. There are other texts that also mention the four *bhāvanā*s, such as the *Jñānārṇava* by the Digambara mendicant Śubhacandra (1000 CE), which describes them as essential supports for meditation, particularly *dharma-dhyāna*.[16] Furthermore, non-scholarly Jain writings and media material on the topic abound, particularly regarding friendliness and compassion. Therefore, clearly much remains to be done to provide a more precise genealogy of these *bhāvanā*s, especially if we intend to know how they are practiced in contemporary times.

The Four *Bhāvanā*s in the *Yogabindu*

The *Yogabindu* (*YB*) is a text attributed to Haribhadra[17] and probably written in the mid-to-late first millennium of the Common Era. It discusses yoga practices found in various religious traditions, such as worship, ethical training, discernment skills, and meditation. The starting point in the text is that suffering is inevitable in the human condition and that it can only be overcome by spiritual practice that diminishes the effects of past karma. Haribhadra presents a fivefold yoga consisting of (1) introspection or self-reflection (*adhyātma*); (2) ethical cultivation (*bhāvanā*);[18] (3) meditation (*dhyāna*); (4) equanimity (*samatā*); and (5) the quelling of *vṛttis* (*vṛtti-saṃkṣaya*).[19]

The beginning of the last section of the *YB* offers a recapitulation of four modalities of yoga explained in earlier parts of the text: mantra recitation (*YB* 381–387), self-assessment (*YB* 388–396), deity-worship (*YB* 397–399), and deliverance from sin (*YB* 400–401). To these, Haribhadra adds the four *bhāvanā*s (*YB* 402):

> One should develop friendliness (*maitrī*) toward those who possess goodness, sympathetic joy (*pramoda*) for those who have superior qualities, compassion (*kāruṇya*) for those afflicted with pain, and equanimity (*mādhyasthya*) toward those who are without knowledge.[20]

Taken together, these practices are believed to assist in destroying negative karmas (*vṛtti-kṣaya*), the final phase of the *Yogabindu*'s fivefold yoga (Chapple, forthcoming, 36).

In the *YB*, Haribhadra engages extensively with non-Jain thinkers, and discusses extant practices prevalent in his time. In his detailed analysis of several central works by Haribhadra, Anil Mundra explains how the Jain philosopher engages with doctrinal diversity in various ways. He shows that Haribhadra is interested in both commonality and difference, in integrating and negotiating the two. In fact, one of Haribhadra's main concerns in his whole corpus is to negotiate both agreement and disagreement (Mundra 2022). In the example of the four *bhāvanā*s in the *YB*, Haribhadra seems to embrace commonality and agreement more than difference. He draws freely on the thought of other religious traditions, portraying the *bhāvanā*s as a shared practice that aims to perfect the ascetic self, a self that remains embodied and engaged with the social world.

The *Bhāvanā*s in the *Yogadṛṣṭisamuccaya*

The *Yogadṛṣṭisamuccaya* (*YDS*) was likely written by Haribhadra[21] around the end of the first millennium CE. Consisting of 228 verses, it discusses how to maintain moral conduct in religious life. The author demonstrates a particular interest in various yogic traditions (Chapple 2003). Like the *YB*, *JĀ*, and *TS*, the *YDS* is based on the Jain view that sees karma as the cause of suffering. Yoga, in its different modalities, is presented as a means to overcome it. Among other practices, we find a verse with somewhat conceptually similar ideas to the four *bhāvanās*:

> Boundless compassion (*dāya*) toward the afflicted, non-malevolence (*adveṣa*) toward those with noble qualities and fitness for service (*sevana*), in all circumstances, without exception.[22]

Here, the Sanskrit word *dāya* is used for compassion.[23] Non-malevolence (*adveṣa*) is advised toward the virtuous instead of joy (*pramoda*). Friendliness (*maitrī*) is not mentioned directly. Instead, service (*sevana*) is prescribed, and equanimity does not appear. What is particularly noteworthy here is that, whereas compassion (*dāya*) and non-malevolence (*adveṣa*) may be primarily enacted as internal dispositions, service clearly entails a strong dimension of social engagement. This verse is included in the second section of the text, which deals with preliminary yoga practices that Haribhadra refers to as "friendly" (*mitrā*). Other preliminary practices of this stage are writing, worship, giving, listening, speaking, teaching, study, reflection, and meditation (*YDS* 28).

Like in the *YB*, Haribhadra here also includes the *bhāvanās* as part of a broader self-purificatory goal that has resemblance in other traditions. For example, we find in the *YDS* a reconstruction of Jain yoga that directly engages with Patañjali and draws parallels with other yoga systems, such as the Vedānta yoga of Bhagavaddatta, the Buddhist yoga of Bhāskara, and the tantric goddess systems prevalent at Haribhadra's time (Chapple 2003, 97). While some of the verses of the *YDS* seem to dispute non-Jain ideas—such as the central Buddhist teachings of non-self, or the tantric premise that desire can be transformed by its enactment—other verses such as the aforementioned on compassion and service, the premise that there is suffering in life, and the final goal of liberation have a more ecumenical tone. This points to shared ethical concerns held by South Asian intellectuals who were most probably engaging with one another.

The Four *Bhāvanās* in the *Yogaśāstra*

The *Yogaśāstra* (*YŚ*) is a twelfth-century Sanskrit text written by Hemacandra (1088–1173) and is often considered the most comprehensive text for lay Śvetāmbara Jains. It includes a wide variety of practices under the label of "yoga," such as which food to eat, which form of giving (*dāna*) is appropriate, physical practices to cleanse the body, etc. The four *bhāvanās* are included too but they are not called *bhāvanās* per se. Having described the Three Jewels in detail, Hemacandra moves to discuss the Four Passions (anger, pride, delusion, and greed), the significance of controlling the senses to achieve purity of mind and high levels of mental equanimity or tranquility (*sāmya* or *samāyika*), and the Twelve Contemplations.[24] Then, he defines the four *bhāvanās* as follows:

> In order to reconnect [the broken] virtuous meditation, [an unenlightened mendicant] should practice friendliness (*maitrī*), appreciation (*pramoda*), compassion (*kāruṇya*), and tolerance (*mādhyasthya*). These [four] are [like] elixirs of life for him.
>
> May no one commit evil. May no one suffer. May the entire world be liberated.
>
> Such a sentiment is called friendliness (*maitrī*).
>
> Appreciation (*pramoda*) is predilection for the virtuous of those whose defects have been removed and who sees reality as it is.
>
> The will to remove the conditions of those who are in a miserable condition, tormented, excessively terrified, and begging for their life, is called compassion (*kāruṇya*).
>
> That which remains unconditionally neutral towards cruel acts, towards those who blaspheme against the Jinas (*devatā*) and the teachers (*guru*), [and] towards those who praise themselves, that is called tolerance (*mādhyasthya*).
>
> When a man of great intellect meditates on the self by means of these [four practices], even if the continuity of pure meditation is broken, it is reconnected.[25]

This exposition of the four *bhāvanās* is followed by a section on yogic postures. While Hemacandra offers little elaboration on the four *bhāvanā*s themselves, their placement in the text suggests that they serve to prepare both the mind and the body for meditation. Hemacandra wrote the *YŚ* (as well as other texts) for a Śaiva Caulukya king named Kumārapāla (r. 1143–c. 1172) to show the king how to live as a lay Jain (Dundas 2002, 135). Nonetheless, the text still contains influences from the Trika Śaiva and the Nāth traditions (Qvarnström 2002; 2003). There is also evidence of Hemacandra having taught the predecessor king Siddharāja the importance of paying attention and respect to different philosophical systems (Tawney 1901, 105–106). Gary A. Tubb, drawing on a point made by Cort, notes that the primary aim of this attitude was to attract the king's attention to the Jains in a court otherwise dominated by the Śaiva tradition (Tubb 1998, 61). While inner, religious conviction should not be disregarded as influential, it was likely more crucial for the king to prioritize preserving the Jain community's place within society. In any case, Hemacandra's decision to include the four *bhāvanā*s alongside other Jain teachings in his long treatise indicates an engagement of Jain practices with the tantric and Śaiva religious sensibilities of his time. Hemacandra's definitions of the four *bhāvanā*s closely resemble those of previous authors; however, the next author examined here introduces important nuances. We now turn to Yaśovijaya, often regarded as the last great Jain intellectual of the early modern period.

The Four *Bhāvanā*s in the *Dvātriṃśaddvātriṃśikā*

The *Dvātriṃśaddvātriṃśikā* (*DD*)—*Thirty-Two (Chapters) with Thirty-Two (Verses)*—is a Sanskrit text with an auto-commentary composed by the Tapā Gaccha monk Yaśovijaya (1624–1688). Yaśovijaya wrote in several Indian languages on a wide range of topics. While navigating a different sociohistorical and religious landscape, his thought remained deeply influenced by earlier Jain philosophers, particularly Haribhadra. Yaśovijaya reinterpreted many of Haribhadra's ideas, particularly on yoga. In fact, the *DD* is a long compendium on Jain mendicant conduct that includes various chapters on yoga. The four *bhāvanā*s are discussed in chapter 18—"The Divisions of Yoga" (*yoga-bheda*)—which starts in the following manner: "It is mentioned by the skilled in the yoga path that yoga has five main parts: self-reflection, ethical cultivation, meditation, equanimity, and the quelling of *vṛttis*."[26]

This is a direct reference to verse number 31 in the *Yogabindu* (*YB*).[27] Indeed, in this chapter, Yaśovijaya discusses the fivefold yoga of the *YB* reinterpreting some ideas and adding nuances. It is noteworthy that the *bhāvanās* are discussed at the beginning of chapter 18. In verses 2–6, Yaśovijaya gives definitions of each *bhāvanā* and differentiates four subtypes of each. I have not found this fourfold subdivision in other sources, so it seems to be an innovation. He says:

> Appropriately following the teachings [in the Jain *āgamas*] on the observance of the Jain vows [for lay people and mendicants], those who know about the self, understand it as a reflection on the *tattvas* [and are] endowed with feelings (*bhāva*) such as friendliness, etc.[28]

> Friendliness (*maitrī*) is considered to be a kindly mental disposition. [It is to be practiced] gradually towards four kinds of subjects: one's teachers, one's fellow monks, one's students, and everyone.[29]

> Compassion (*karuṇā*) is the desire to remove suffering. [It arises in four different manners]: from ignorance, from seeing the suffering [of others]; from the higher wish to overcome the sufferings of *saṃsāra*; [and] from one's one nature (*svabhāva*). [This last form is towards everyone], towards those who are happy and those who are not.[30]

In his auto-commentary, Yaśovijaya explains further these four kinds of compassion. The first type, he says, arises from ignorance and is characterized, for example, by the desire to give something that is not wholesome to someone who is unsuitable.[31] The second kind of compassion, according to him, would for example arise when seeing someone who is suffering, such as a very poor person, and giving them food, clothing, bedding, a seat, and other worldly things.[32] The third kind of compassion is the desire to overcome worldly suffering, even among happy beings who have a strong desire for liberation.[33] The last type of compassion arises from one's own nature (*svabhāva*) and is directed toward all beings when one understands that all beings suffer to some extent, even those who are usually happy.[34] After the discussion on compassion, joy and equanimity are defined:

> Joy (*muditā*) brings contentment.
> [It arises in four different circumstances]:
> towards unwholesome worldly pleasures;
> towards that with true cause [like eating healthy food];
> towards wholesome beings still bounded [to *saṃsāra*];
> and towards the happiness of all living beings.[35]

> Due to compassion, considering future consequences,
> from non-attachment, and from reflecting on reality,
> one practices equanimity (*upekṣa*) towards the unwholesome,
> the untimely, the pleasant, and the worthless.
> [Ultimately], towards everyone.[36]

Once the four qualities have been cultivated, Yaśovijaya explains that the practitioner reaches higher levels of introspection and other positive results:

> One should abandon envy for the happy, indifference for the suffering, enmity for the virtuous, [and] attraction and aversion towards the unrighteous.
> Having obtained these qualities, one should abide in oneself (*adhyātma*).[37] From this, there is destruction of sin, strength, good conduct, and eternal knowledge.
> This is indeed the nectar derived from direct experience.[38]

Interestingly, an alternative definition of *bhāvanā* comes next, composed of five main parts:

> The continuous and discerning practice [of *adhyātma*] is called *bhāvanā*. Its result is ceasing from impure practice and progressing towards a pure state.[39] This (*bhāvanā*) is considered fivefold, including: knowledge, faith, conduct, asceticism, and non-attachment. It is the cause of firm conditions.[40]

Following this alternative definition of *bhāvanā*, Yaśovijaya explains that meditation occurs when consciousness is continuously held, and not hindered by eight kinds of obstacles:

> In active consciousness (*upayoga*),[41] different thoughts might arise. Meditation (*dhyāna*) is when there is no interruption [of active consciousness]. It partakes in a pure and singular awareness, along with a subtle enjoyment.[42]

> Progress in meditation occurs when abandoning the eight faults of mind, one by one: exhaustion, agitation, confusion, over-exertion, distractibility, clinging, enjoying what is not supposed to be enjoyed, and interrupting [religious practices].[43]

The rest of the chapter discusses the positive fruits of meditation, the interconnection between meditation and a proper understanding of reality, the three restraints (*gupti*), and the five observances (*samiti*). Some of these practices are further discussed in later chapters.

Altogether, Yaśovijaya's explanations of the four *bhāvanā*s and the place where they are discussed within the text suggest that the category of *bhāvanā* requires more than just focusing one's time and energy on mediation. It also requires adjusting one's attitude toward others in this world, specifying how one ought to cultivate an appropriately ascetic perspective within the overarching notion of *vairāgya*. This would be important both for lay Jains and for mendicants who are still invested in the welfare of the Jain community, as most were.[44] Furthermore, according to Yaśovijaya's alternative definition of *bhāvanā* as knowledge, faith, conduct, asceticism, and non-attachment, the term also refers to a practice of purification intended to prepare one for advanced meditation practices.

In addition to the *DD*, in the opening chapter of the *Adhyātmopaniṣatprakaraṇa*, another of Yaśovijaya's texts, he outlines two distinct perspectives on the self. From an etymological standpoint, the self is conceived as the agent responsible for various actions. In contrast, in the context of everyday language, it is identified with the mind, endowed with virtuous qualities like friendliness (1.2–4) (Ganeri 2008, 6). In the *Dharmaparīkṣā*, Yaśovijaya argues that "moral qualities such as compassion evinced by those belonging to non-Jain paths can be viewed positively, in the same way as qualities in general, whether worldly or transcendent, can also be readily approved of" (Dundas 2002, 164).

Finally, it is noteworthy that Yaśovijaya engages with Buddhist terminology. In the *DD*, he writes the words *maitrī*, *muditā* (instead of *pramoda*), *karuṇā* (instead of *kāruṇya*), and *upekṣa* (instead of *mādhyasthya*). Many occurrences of Buddhist ideas in Yaśovijaya's corpus are quotations or paraphrases of earlier Sanskrit authors who had engaged with Buddhists when the Buddhist tradition was still philosophically dominant. This is arguably the case for many textual traditions where Buddhists remained influential as interlocutors long after Buddhism had disappeared from India, with their ideas continuing to shape and inspire subsequent intellectual developments. It is particularly visible and concrete in the case of Jain literature.[45]

Conclusion

In the Jain texts explored in this chapter, the four *bhāvanā*s primarily function to eliminate karma, prepare the practitioner for meditation, and enable the attainment of advanced meditative states. Compassion and equanimity have received the most attention in existing scholarship. Equanimity[46] lies at the basis of Jain meditative practices and the entire religious life.[47] Compassion is considered one of the four main signs of *samyag-darśana* or *samyaktva*. Jaini explains that this moment of insight "fills the individual with an unselfish desire to help other souls towards *mokṣa*" (1979, 150). It is also seen as a form of karma that ultimately needs to be removed. But given the fact that, for Jains, liberation is not possible in this era of the cycle of time in this world, the Jain *bhāvanā* of compassion remains part of the modus operandi in daily life that aims to ensure a better rebirth while also having positive consequences on well-being in this very life.

Along with compassion and equanimity, the Jain philosophers presented in this chapter consider friendliness and joy for others to be common human capacities that are crucial to advance in the religious path. All of these four *bhāvanā*s are dependent on the situation one is engaging with: One should be able to deploy the appropriate quality according to the situation by continuously cultivating all four by inner means. In this way, the *bhāvanā*s seem to be states reflective of a well-cultivated, self-possessed person.

The textual placement of the discussion on *bhāvanā* explored in this chapter suggests that this category entails more than simply dedicating time and effort to silent and static meditation. It also involves a transformation of one's attitude toward other living beings, articulating how an ascetic disposition should be cultivated within the broader framework of *vairāgya*. Jain intellectuals often celebrate and even praise positive virtues of character. This emphasis would have been significant for both lay Jains and mendicants, many of whom remained engaged with the well-being of the Jain community. Although we cannot know for certain how the Jains used their texts in the past, and it is also unclear how Jain texts influenced religious practices on the ground, this preliminary exploration also shows that central figures in Jain intellectual history were engaging with shared forms of religious praxis in their respective sociohistorical contexts. The four *bhāvanā*s are shared across traditions as part of a shared vocabulary of what constitutes a well-cultivated, self-reflective person. In this sense, they could be considered pan-Indic. Given the internally transformative, ascetic nature of the *bhāvanā*s for one pursuing *adhyātma* (and eventually *mokṣa*), it can be argued that the orientation of these four qualities or attitudes toward others is deeply rooted in ascetic detachment and pursuit of the higher self. The history of Jain ethics draws out general principles from ascetic vows, and this explains well the shift toward thinking of ascetic self-cultivation with the goal of rescuing the self from *saṃsāra* as a platform for ethical engagement with (and improvement of) the world.[48]

The four Jain *bhāvanā*s suggest that ethical worldly engagement constitutes a dimension of the religious path. The cultivation of friendliness, joy for others, compassion, and equanimity is presented as an ideal that seeks to reconcile what may initially appear contradictory: The ascetic committed to the path of liberation (*mokṣa-marga*) is both constrained by *saṃsāra* and striving to transcend it, yet remains actively engaged with the world. This ideology of the *mokṣa-marga* coexists with a sustained emphasis on everyday ethical practice, refinement, and commitment to the welfare of others.

Notes

1. *TS* 7.6 (Dg.), *TS* 7.11 (Śv.): *maitrī-pramoda-kāruṇya-mādhyasthyāni ca sattva-guṇādhika-kliśyamānāvineyeṣu* |

2. See, for example, Thiṭṭila 1969, 357–375.

3. See, for example, Sonam 1997, 27–55.

4. *Varāhopaniṣad*, I.13.

5. *Maitrī*: *Mahopaniṣad*, V.71, VI.30; *Karuṇā*: *Nāradaparivrājakopaniṣad*, IV.2; *Mudita: Akṣyupaniṣad*, II.35; *Maitrī Upaniṣad*, III.16; and *Upekṣā: Bhāvanopaniṣad*, V.2; *Sarasvatīrahasyopaniṣad*, V.63 (Bohanec 2012).

6. *PYS* 1.33. *maitrī-karuṇā-muditā-upekṣāṇāṃ sukha-duḥkha-puṇya-apuṇya-viṣayāṇāṃ bhāvanātaś citta prasādanam* |

7. The literature on the twelve *anuprekṣās* is extensive. For a thorough historical perspective, see Hooper 2020.

8. The abbreviation "Dg." refers to Digambara, and "Śv." refers to Śvetāmbara.

9. Mahāprajña's eightfold model of *prekṣā-dhyāna* includes (1) bodily relaxation with self-awareness (*kāyotsarga*); (2) inner journey (*antaryātrā*); (3) perception of breath (*śvāsa-prekṣā*); (4) perception of the body (*śarīra-prekṣā*); (5) perception of psychic centers (*caitanya-kendra-prekṣā*); (6) perception of psychic colors (*leśyā-dhyāna*); (7) meditation or contemplation (*anuprekṣā*); and (8) autosuggestion (*bhāvanā*). Pratibha Pragya clarified that this eightfold model is not a sequence because all these elements are to be cultivated together. Personal communication, March 5, 2024. For more details, see Pratibha Pragya 2020, 195–196.

10. See examples in Kelting 2001, 93–94, 165, 178–180; 2009, 132, 224; 2020b, 720; Kelting and Cort 2020, 813.

11. 7.6 (Dg.) and 7.11 (Śv.): *maitrī-pramoda-kāruṇya-mādhyasthyāni ca sattva-guṇādhika-kliśyamānāvineyeṣu* | Translations are mine unless otherwise stated, with reference to Tatia 1994.

12. *SS* 683: *pareṣam duḥkhānutpatty-abhilāṣo maitrī* |

13. Note that Akalaṅka is using the Sanskrit word *anukampā* for compassion instead of *kāruṇya* as found in the *TS*.

14. *TV* 1.2: *sarva-prāṇiṣu maitrī anukampā* |

15. For more details on compassion in Jainism, see, for example, Wiley 2006; Kawasaki 2022.

16. *JĀ* 27.4: *catasro bhāvanā dhanyāḥ purāṇa-puruṣāśritā* | *maitry-ādayaś ciraṃ cite dhyeyā dharmasya siddhaye* ||

17. Although Haribhadra has often been treated as a single author, there may have been more than one figure with this name. The author of the *Yogabindu* is sometimes referred as Haribhadra Virahāṅka (Williams 1965, 4; Chapple 2016, 125), and the author of the *Yogadṛṣṭisamuccaya* as Haribhadra Yākinī-putra (Williams 1965, 7; Chapple 2003, 2).

18. Note the broader use of the word *bhāvanā* here, referring to ethical cultivation that includes the Jain vows and other practices, including the four cultivations (*bhāvanās*) that are the focus of this chapter.

19. *YB* 31: *adhyātmaṃ bhāvanā dhyānaṃ samatā vṛtti-saṃkṣayaḥ* | *mokṣeṇa yojanād yoga eṣa śreṣṭho yathottaram* ||

20. *YB* 402: *maitrī-pramoda-kāruṇya-mādhyasthya-paricintanam* | *sattva-guṇadhika-kliśya-mānāprajñāpy-agocaram* || The English translation is by Chapple (forthcoming), and I have also consulted K. K. Dixit (1967).

21. See footnote 17.

22. *YDS* 32: *duḥkhiteṣu dayā'tyantam adveṣo guṇavatsu ca aucityāt sevanaṃ caiva sarvatraivāviśeṣataḥ* | The English translation is by Chapple 2003, 110.

23. From tracing the terms for "compassion" in early Buddhism and Jainism, we find that *karuṇā* is employed almost exclusively as a technical term in the context of the *brahmavihāras*; while *anukampā*, and sometimes *dāya*, are used in other contexts. Vesna Wallace, personal communication, Nov. 8, 2021.

24. The twelve contemplations consist of reflecting on (1) the impermanence of all things (*anitya*), (2) the lack of refuge in external forces or self-reliance (*aśaraṇa*), (3) the cycle of transmigration (*saṃsāra*), (4) the aloneness of every soul (*ekatva*), (5) the separation of body and soul (*anyatva*), (6) the impurity of the body (*aśuci*), (7) the influx of karmas (*aśrava*), (8) the stoppage of karmas (*saṃvara*), (9) the wearing away of karmas (*nirjarā*), (10) the true religion (*dharma*), (11) the nature of the universe (*loka*), and (12) the means of acquiring right cognition (*bodhi*). Hemacandra exposes them in this order.

25. Translation by Qvarnström 2002, 97–98. Note Qvarnström's use of the words "appreciation" and "tolerance" for *pramoda* and *mādhyasthya*, respectively. I have decided to retain these word choices here to show the complexities of the translation process.

26. *DD* 18.1: *adhyātmaṃ bhāvanā dhyānaṃ samatā vṛtti-saṃkṣayaḥ* | *yogaḥ pañca-vidhaḥ prokto yoga-mārga-viśāradaiḥ* || English translations of the *DD* are my own, done with the help of Christopher Key Chapple, Anil Mundra, and McComas Taylor.

27. *YB* 31: *adhyātmaṃ bhāvanā dhyānaṃ samatā vṛtti-saṃkṣayaḥ* | *mokṣeṇa yojanād yoga eṣa śreṣṭho yathottaram* ||

28. *DD* 18. 2: *aucityād vṛtta-yuktasya vacanāt tattva-cintanam | maitry-ādi-bhāva-saṃyuktam adhyātmaṃ tadvido viduḥ ||*

29. *DD* 18. 3: *sukha-cintā matā maitrī sā krameṇa caturvidhā | upakāri-svakīya-svapratipannākhilāśrayā ||*

30. *DD* 18. 4: *karuṇā duḥkha-hānecchā mohād duḥkhita-darśanāt | saṃvegāc ca svabhāvāc ca prītimat-svapareṣu ca ||*

31. *DD* 18. 4 com. line 1: *sā ca mohād ajñānād ekā | yathā glānayā citāpathya-vastu-pradānābhilāṣa-lakṣaṇā |*

32. *DD* 18. 4 com. line 2: *anyā ca duḥkhitasya dīnāder darśanāt tasya loka-prasiddhā-hāra-vastra-śayanāsanādi pradānena |*

33. *DD* 18. 4 com. lines 2–3: *saṃvegān mokṣābhilāṣāc ca sukhiteṣv api sattveṣu prītimatsu sāṃsārika-duḥkha-paritrāṇecchā chadma-sthānāṃ aparā |*

34. *DD* 18. 4 com. lines 3–4: *aparā punar apareṣu ca prītimattā-saṃbandha-vikaleṣu sarveṣv eva svabhāvāc ca pravartamānā kevalinām iva bhagavatāṃ mahā-munīnāṃ sarvānugraha-parāyaṇānām ity evaṃ caturvidhā |*

35. *DD* 18. 5: *āpāta-ramye saddhetāvanubandha-yute pare | santuṣṭir muditā nāma sarveṣāṃ prāṇināṃ sukhe ||*

36. *DD* 18. 6: *karuṇāto 'nubandhāc ca nirvedāt tattva-cintanāt | upekṣā hy ahite 'kāle sukhe 'sāre ca sarvataḥ ||*

37. *DD* 18. 7: *sukhīrṣyāṃ duḥkhitopekṣāṃ puṇya-dveṣam adharmiṣu | rāga-dveṣau tyajan netā labdhvādhyātmaṃ samāśrayet ||*

38. *DD* 18.8: *ataḥ pāpakṣayaḥ sattvaṃ śīlaṃ jñānaṃ ca śāśvatam | tathānubhava-saṃsiddham amṛtaṃ hy ada eva nu ||*

39. *DD* 18.9: *abhyāso vṛddhimān asya bhāvanā buddhi-saṃgataḥ | nivṛttir aśubhābhyāsād bhāva-vṛddhiś ca tat-phalam ||*

40. *DD* 18.10: *jñāna-darśana-cāritra-tapo-vairāgya-bhedataḥ | iṣyate pañcadhā ceyaṃ dṛḍha-saṃskāra-kāraṇam ||*

41. *Upayoga* is a technical term in Jainism that refers to the application of the capacity of consciousness. It includes two main cognitive capacities: (1) *darśana*, an initial perception that provides general information about an object; and (2) *jñāna* or knowing, which provides a more in-depth understanding of the object.

42. *DD* 18.11: *upayoge vijātīya-pratyayāvyavadhāna-bhāk | śubhaika-pratyayo dhyānaṃ sūkṣmābhoga-samanvitam ||*

43. *DD* 18. 12: *khedodvega-bhramotthāna-kṣepāsaṃgānyam-udrujām | tyāgād aṣṭa-pṛthak-citta-doṣāṇām anubandhy adaḥ ||*

44. Steven M. Vose, personal communication, May 21, 2024.

45. Anil Mundra, personal communication, April 20, 2024.

46. *Sāmāyika* or *samatva-yoga* are technical terms often used in Jain sources to refer to equanimity. For more details, see, for example, Jain 2016; Kelting 2020a, 531–542; Hooper 2020, 543–563; Jaini 1979, 190 and 221.

47. Dundas says: "Strictly speaking, the entire ascetic life is regarded as an act of *sāmāyika* so that its ritual performance is in fact merely a temporary actualization of it" (2002, 170).

48. I am very grateful to all the scholars who read drafts of this chapter and offered me feedback: Christopher Jain Miller, Cogen Bohanec, Anil Mundra, Ana Bajželj, Christopher Key Chapple, Steven Vose, and John Cort.

References

Bohanec, Cogen. *The Brahmavihāra: A Hindu and Buddhist Sample of Pandharmic Virtues.* Unpublished seminar paper, Graduate Theological Union, Fall 2012.

Bronkhorst, Johannes. 1993. *The Two Traditions of Meditation in Ancient India.* 2nd ed. Motilal Banarsidass.

Chapple, Christopher Key. 2003. *Reconciling Yogas: Haribhadra's Collection of Views on Yoga.* State University of New York Press.

———. 2010. "Brahmā Vihāra, Emptiness, and Ethics." In *Freeing the Body, Freeing the Mind: Writings on the Connections Between Yoga and Buddhism,* edited by Michael Stone. Shambhala.

———. 2016. "The Jaina Yogas of Haribhadra Virahāṇka's Yogabindu." In *Yoga in Jainism,* edited by Christopher Key Chapple. Routledge.

———. Forthcoming. *The Yogabindu: A Raindrop of Singular Yoga in an Ocean of Dispute.* Publisher to be determined.

Cort, John E. 2001. *Jains in the World: Religious Values and Ideology in India.* Oxford University Press.

Dixit, K. K. 1967. *The Yogabindu of Ācārya Haribhadrasūri.* Lalbhai Dalpatbhai Bharatiya Sanskriti Vidyamandira.

Dundas, Paul. 2002. *The Jains.* Routledge.

Ganeri, Jonardon. 2008. "Worlds in Conflict the Cosmopolitan Vision of Yaśovijaya Gaṇi." *International Journal of Jaina Studies* (Online) 4 (1): 1–11.

Hooper, Giles Ross. 2020. "A Study of the 'Twelve Reflections' (*dvādaśa bhāvanāḥ*) Depicted by the Eleventh-Century Jain Digambara Scholar Ācārya Śubhacandra in his 'Ocean of Knowledge' (*Jñānārṇava*) and an Analysis of his Contribution to the Development of Jain Meditation Practice." Doctoral dissertation, University of Sydney.

Jain, Sagarmal. 2016. "The Historical Development of the Jaina Yoga System and the Impacts of Other Yoga Systems on Jaina Yoga." In Chapple, ed., *Yoga in Jainism.*

Jaini, Padmanabh S. 1979. *The Jaina Path of Purification*. Motilal Banarsidass.

Joshi, Lal Mani. 1981. *Facets of Jain Religiousness in Comparative Light*. L. D. Institute of Indology.

Kawasaki, Yutaka. 2022. "A Note on the Concept of Compassion in Early Jainism." In *Nagabharana: Recent Trends in Jainism Studies*. BlueRose Publishers.

Kelting, M. Whitney. 2001. *Singing to the Jinas: Jain Laywomen, Maṇḍaḷ Singing, and the Negotiations of Jain Devotion*. Oxford University Press.

———. 2009. *Heroic Wives Rituals, Stories and the Virtues of Jain Wifehood*. Oxford University Press.

———. 2020a. "*Tapas* and Asceticism." In *Brill's Encyclopedia of Jainism*, edited by Khut A. Jacobsen, John E. Cort, Paul Dundas, and Kristi L. Wiley. Brill.

———. 2020b. "The Process of Pilgrimage." In Jacobsen et al., eds., *Brill's Encyclopedia of Jainism*.

Kelting, M. Whitney., and Cort, John E. 2020. "Śvetāmbara Jain Devotional Literature in Gujarati." In Jacobsen et al., eds., *Brill's Encyclopedia of Jainism*.

Monier-Williams, Monier. 1899. *A Sanskrit-English Dictionary: Etymologically and Philologically Arranged with Special Reference to Cognate Indo-European Languages*. Clarendon Press.

Mundra, Anil. 2022. "No Identity Without Diversity: Haribhadrasūri's Anekāntavāda as a Jain Response to Doctrinal Difference." Doctoral dissertation, University of Chicago.

Pratibha Pragya, Samani. 2020. "Yoga and Meditation in the Jain Tradition." In *Routledge Handbook of Yoga and Meditation Studies*, edited by Suzanne Newcombe and Karen O'Brien-Kop. Routledge.

Qvarnström, Olle, trans. 2002. *The Yogaśāstra of Hemacandra: A Twelfth Century Handbook on Jainism*. Harvard University Press.

———. 2003. "Losing One's Mind and Becoming Enlightened: Some Remarks on the Concept of Yoga in Śvetāmbara Jainism and Its Relation to the Nātha Siddha Tradition." In *Yoga: The Indian Tradition*, edited by Ian Whicher and David Carpenter. Routledge Curzon.

Saṅghavī, Sukhlāl. 1974. *Commentary on Tattvarth Sutra of Vacaka Umasvati*. Translated by K. K. Dixit. L. D. Institute of Indology.

Sonam, Rinchen. 1997. *Atisha's Lamp for the Path to Enlightenment: An Oral Teaching by Geshe Sonam Rinchen*. Translated and edited by Ruth Sonam. Snow Lion Publications.

Tatia, Nathmal, trans. 1994. *Tattvārtha Sūtra. That Which Is*. Motilal Banarsidas.

Tawney, Charles Henry. 1901. *The Prabandhacintamani Composed by Merutunga Acarya*. Asiatic Society of Bengal.

Thiṭṭila, Ashin, trans. 1969. "Analysis of the Illimitables." In *The Book of Analysis (Vibhaṅga): The Second Book of the Abhidhamma Piṭaka*. Pali Text Society.

Tubb, Gary A. 1998. "Hemacandra and Sanskrit Poetics." In *Open Boundaries: Jain Communities and Cultures in Indian History*, edited by John E. Cort. State University of New York Press.

Yaśovijaya Gaṇi. 1909. *Dvātriṃśaddvātriṃśikā*. Srī Jaina Dharma Prasāraka Sabhā.

Wiley, Kristi. 2004. *Historical Dictionary of Jainism*. Scarecrow Press.

———. 2006. "Ahiṃsā and Compassion in Jainism." In *Studies in Jaina History and Culture: Disputes and Dialogues*, edited by Peter Flügel. Routledge.

Williams, Robert. 1963. *Jaina Yoga: A Survey of the Mediaeval Śrāvakācāras*. Motilal Banarsidass.

14

Engaging Difference

Approaches to Religious Pluralism in Haribhadra's *Yogabindu*

CHRISTOPHER KEY CHAPPLE

One of the persistent difficulties in world cultures entails dealing with issues of difference, disagreement, and discord. Each word employed to describe this phenomenon stems from an ancient Indo-European prefix rendered as *duḥ* in Sanskrit and variant forms of *dis* or *dif* in English. Cultures define themselves through mandates and taboos. To enter into a sense of belonging, one conforms. By rebelling, one runs the risk of being shunned. To be *dif*ferent makes one an outsider. To be disagreeable sets one at odds with others. To be *dis*cordant aligns oneself with singing out of tune.

Without the many, we would live in a monochromatic world. Thomas Berry, citing Thomas Aquinas, proffers the perspective that variegation is essential for the fullness of life (Berry, 1968, 5). As species become extinct, never again can their consciousness enrich and form the awareness of others.

India in the sixth century bustled with all forms of religious difference. The rich tapestry of difference prompted at least three ways to engage with the religious other: celebration, antagonism, and hegemonic inclusion. Buddhists, Jains, Vaiṣṇavas, and Śaivas maintained distinct literary- and institution-building endeavors. The Buddhists, whether followers of the Theravāda or Mahāyāna, agreed on three core teachings (suffering, impermanence, no-self) and three pillars of the faith (Buddha, Dharma, Saṅgha). The Jains sought freedom from karmic affliction through strict adherence to the vows of nonviolence, adherence to truth, honesty, celibacy (or fidelity in marriage for married Jains), and minimization of possessions. The Vaiṣṇavas chanted mantras and studied texts such as the *Bhagavad Gītā* within the *Mahābhārata*, the *Rāmāyaṇa*, and the burgeoning Purāṇas. Śaivas took up practices of meditation and told and enacted stories in different Purāṇas. Buddhist stupas and Jain, Śaiva, and Vaiṣṇava mandirs sprouted throughout the landscape.

On the one hand, the flourishing of multiple religious cultures during the Gupta and post-Gupta period seems to have signaled a period of peaceful coexistence. On the other hand, texts and narratives indicate that each group competed in a vibrant identity marketplace. Philosophical and worship practices delineated stark differences. The Buddhists proclaimed that no self could be found. The Jains claimed that the self is eternal and the world is real. Some readers of the *Bhagavad Gītā* asserted that the self is eternal and the world is merely an illusion. Vaiṣṇava veneration of Kṛṣṇa, Rāma, and other avatāras concretized into a fixed theology and belief. Śaiva theology brought an interweaving of cosmos with body. Temples and monasteries offered surety in their structures and in their teachings. All were interwoven in the context of social structures that delineated and enforced difference through endogamy, with brahmins marrying within brahmin families to perpetuate the learning of Vedic rituals and the laws as mandated in the Dharmaśāstras; *kṣatriya*s marrying *kṣatriya*s and serving as landlords, kings, and queens; *vaiśya*s marrying *vaiśya*s and cementing power within the marketplace; and the majority *śūdra* worker classes creating and maintaining subcommunities. Reciprocity and inequality marked the social system, which persists even today despite a constitutional counter-mandate effected at the time following India's independence from colonial rule.

During this seeming golden age, a biographical tradition emerged suggesting that coexistence was not always peaceful. Several stories have been told about Haribhadra, an arrogant brahmin who undergoes a personal and religious conversion.[1] These stories can refer to either the sixth-century Haribhadra Virahāṅka or the eighth-century Haribhadra Yākinī Putra. They warn about the hunger for knowledge, the dangers of learning philosophical arguments for the purpose of subverting them, and the perils of holding firm views. The stories also offer a rationale for formulating a thought system that makes space for recognizing the validity of views held by others without surrendering one's own view.

Haribhadra, so the story goes, was born into a brahmin family. He memorized the Vedas, including the Upaniṣads. He mastered the theory behind ritual, the law manuals, the medicinal texts, and, above all else, the philosophical texts. Hence, he knew all six traditional *darśanas*: Vedānta, Sāṃkhya, Yoga, Nyāya, Vaiśeṣika, Mīmāṃsā. He became an expert in theology, psychology, spiritual practice, physical descriptions of the world, and ritual. He was awarded a special gold sacred thread, no doubt with great pomp and circumstance. The texts describe his physicality and personality: portly and proud.

At one point he announced that he had learned and mastered all things and dared anyone to challenge him with new knowledge, reminiscent of Bhaddā Kuṇḍalakesā, the early Buddhist nun who moved from town to town, placing a branch in the town square, inviting others to best her in debate (Kema 1982, 23–27). A Jain nun who went by the name Yākinī caught the ear of Haribhadra. She was reciting a Prakrit Jain verse unknown to him, and he sought to learn from her and her teacher. This presumably brought him to understand the basic principles as articulated in the fifth century by the Jain scholar Umāsvāti, who composed a masterwork of philosophy, the *Tattvārthasūtra*. Its ten chapters encapsulate and directly communicate the core teachings of Jainism.[2] Like Patañjali's *Yoga Sūtra,* it can be easily memorized. Its lyrical, enticing use of language lends itself to street preaching, one premise cascading dramatically into the next. It starts with three jewels that point the path to freedom (*mokṣa mārga*): Laudatory Outlook (*samyag-darśana*), Laudatory Knowledge (*samyag-jñāna*), and Laudatory Comportment (*samyag-cāritra*). It outlines the cosmos and the imbrication of human-induced karma. It describes human physicality and the call to take up an ethical life. Its commentaries delineate a fourteen-fold ladder of spiritual ascent (*guṇasthāna*) leading to perfect freedom and omniscience. Haribhadra heard the nun Yākinī in public performance reciting and declaiming the Jain teachings. He paused, listened, queried, and converted, learning even more details from her teacher. Haribhadra renounced the early tradition that shaped him and embraced Jain faith and practice.

The Buddhists were also actively teaching, operating a major university in Nālandā. Most likely both Haribhadras lived in western India, perhaps in Chittor, Rajasthan (Shukla 1989). Nālandā was hundreds of miles to the east. Although he had mastered the Vedic and Jain traditions, he yearned to learn the arguments made by the Buddhists that continued to recruit persons to the Saṅgha.

Haribhadra's two nephews agreed to help him in his quest for Buddhist knowledge.[3] The two young men, Haṃsa and Paramahaṃsa, traveled for weeks before they arrived. They presented themselves as aspiring novices and asked for admission to the course of study at Nālandā University. Dutifully, the two young men attended all the lectures, took notes, and participated fully in the rigorous daily monastic regimen. However, their countenance drew suspicion. Rather than nodding their heads in assent as the teachings of Nāgārjuna systematically disassembled any notion of abiding essence in self or other in favor of the no-self-essence teaching (*niḥsvabhāva*), their eyes darted between each other, obviously unconvinced by the arguments. They were hauled into the courtyard, where one of the wardens overseeing the orthodoxy of the students drew an image of the Jina Mahāvīra with chalk and ordered the students to stamp on it. From a Buddhist perspective, Mahāvīra taught the heresy of self, in direct opposition to Buddhist doctrine. The boys looked at each other and sprinted, running through the gates of the monastic university, which you can still visit today. The Buddhist police caught up with one of the boys and beat him to death. The other dashed down a lane, donned a disguise, and shouted to the police: "He went that way!" Through this deception his life was spared. He made his way back to Haribhadra and, over the course of several hours, explained Buddhist philosophy, painstakingly conveying every nuance and example. At the end of his discourse, he became overwhelmed with grief at the death of his brother and died.

Haribhadra grieved deeply for the deaths of both nephews. He set out on a course of philosophical revenge. He challenged any and all Buddhists to come forth and debate the nature of the self.

Is the self real? Does it suffer? Does it undertake the philosophical quest? Does it resolve to overcome past karma? Does it meditate? Does it experience bliss? Does consciousness persist? Does energy persist? Using everyday examples and sophisticated argumentation, he won the argument again and again, convincing 1,400 Buddhists of their fallacy in regard to no-self. The stakes were high. Each and every defeated Buddhist entered a vat of boiling oil and died as set forth in the rules of engagement.

When this last debate ended, remorse overcame Haribhadra. How could he possibly expiate the sins accrued by these repeated acts of violence? How could 1,400 deaths legitimate the death of his two nephews? From the depths of despair, he arrived at a solution. His voracious and rapacious pursuit of knowledge caused a hardening of the heart. This hardening of the heart obscured right view, right knowledge, right action. For him, as a scholar, the only appropriate response would be to correct the impulse to be right at all costs. Under strict instructions from his teacher Jinabhaṭa, he devoted his life not to teaching correct knowledge in absolute categories but to inviting others to learn multiple perspectives, see them as valid within their own context, and seek out some thread of common intent across traditions. Hence, according to the *Prabandhakośa* of Rājaśekharasūri, 1,400 texts came to be attributed to Haribhadra, one for each life lost.

Engaging Religious Difference: Haribhadra's *Yogabindu*

The *Yogabindu*, the earliest text attributed to Haribhadra that employs this approach, was most likely composed in the sixth century. K. K. Dixit published an English translation of the *Yogabindu* in 1968 and the *Yogadṛṣṭisamuccaya* in 1970. Although Dixit does not take a firm position on the different dates that can be attributed to the Haribhadras, I posit that the *Yogabindu* can be dated from the sixth century for several reasons. First, it ardently engages with Buddhism. Haribhadra directly quotes Dharmakīrti, a Buddhist logician whose dates have been given as 550 to 610 (Balcerowicz 2016, 437–483). Second, although the text carefully critiques both Sāṃkhya and Vedānta, it does not utilize a key term associated at a later time with Śaṅkarācārya: *māyā*. Third, it does not engage traditions of *tantra* or goddess worship.

This brings us to the method and content of the *Yogabindu*. Although it ostensibly was composed to expiate for the sin of harsh judgmentalism, it approaches the topic obliquely. The rhetorical strategy employed by Haribhadra begins with a positive assertion—all traditions, regardless of their philosophical particularity, share one concern in common: the purification and extirpation of karma. Haribhadra goes on to describe in detail special religious practices held in common across traditions such as prayer and ritual. At the very end of the text, arguments are presented against the unchanging self of Vedānta, the non-doing self of Sāṃkhya, and the absence of self in Buddhism. He cleaves to the importance of the self in both the transactional and transcendent realm. Hence, Haribhadra remains a Jain, and though asserting commonality across religious traditions throughout the bulk of the text, he concludes by asserting their differences.

The following section cites five examples of practices held in common: Yoga, *pūjā*, *japa*, past life remembrance, and the importance of dreams. In a few places, Haribhadra provides a summary that highlights his arguments against key Buddhist teachings, indicating differences with Jainism. The chapter ends with an examination of his juxtapositional strategy for engaging with philosophical difference, pointing to a philosophical variety of "engaged Jainism" that seeks a way to cultivate tolerance and acceptance.

Yoga in the *Yogabindu*

In order to make space to engage with other religious traditions, the *Yogabindu* opens with a six-verse discourse on the commonly held doctrine of karma.[4] Haribhadra's rhetorical appeal is clear: People, no matter which religious tradition they belong to, desire freedom from the fetters of karma. Yoga, universally conceived, is the process and practice to achieve this goal:

> 1. Having bowed to the celebrated, auspicious,
> eternally liberated Lord of Yogīs,
> I will proclaim the *Yogabindu*,

which I put forth to demonstrate truth.
2. Each impartial, knowledgeable person
who is established in the way of authenticity
knows the harmonious nature of truth
among all Yoga texts.
3. Because the purpose of Yoga is liberation,
there can be no splintering.
Since there is no difference in the final goal
there is no true difference between types of Yoga.
4. Due to its goal of liberation,
Yoga is followed with effort by the intelligent ones.
This pure, true system, beneficial to one's being,
should be sought with great longing.
5. To the extent that a system results in
in joining one to one's true nature,
such a Yoga connects one with
the most eminent of intentions.
6. Due to the linking (*saṃyoga*) of the self with the other
(karma), one remains trapped in *saṃsāra.*
Through disconnection (*viyoga*) from that (karma),
One is indeed liberated . . .

In verse 6, Haribhadra clearly aligns himself with the mechanics of Yoga as described in Patañjali's *Yoga Sūtra,* employing the technical term *saṃyoga* (*YS* II:17, 23, 25), which refers to linking with a mistaken identity due to karma in contrast with disconnecting from that karma through a process known in Jain tradition as *viyoga.* Buddhists might not agree with his appeal to the notion of self (*ātman*) but would not argue with the premise that karmas must be set aside. Thus while engaging religious difference, Haribhadra maintains space for finding common ground.

Pūjā in the *Yogabindu*

Haribhadra gives a robust description of the importance of honoring one's parents, elders, and teachers. Like with the description of karma, this discourse, while giving specific instructions, can be applied universally, regardless of caste or creed. In fact, this sequence concludes with a strong appeal that all traditions must be respected and that one must avoid negative judgments:

> 110. *Pūjā* is to be practiced to honor
> the knowledge of those who see connections
> and to acknowledge the service provided by
> wise gurus and gods.
> 111. The list of those to be honored
> is long and detailed, including women and men,
> mothers and fathers, teachers of the arts,
> the elderly, and teachers of dharma.
> 112. These vaunted people are to be acknowledged
> three times each day through bowing (*namakriya*)
> or at least thinking about them.
> 113. This Yoga entails standing when they enter,
> not taking a seat before they do,
> not flaunting their names in public,
> and not listening to any off-color talk (about them).
> 114. And, within one's power,
> always offer them the best of clothing
> and sublime actions and undertakings.
> 115. Renouncing undesirable things,
> turn to things desired.
> These are to be known with refinement.
> It is said they must not conflict with dharma.
> 116. After dispatching the bodies of the dead in the
> highest manner, do not sit on their furniture.
> Offer their wealth to a place of pilgrimage.
> Memorialize them with a blessed portrait.
> 117. In a spirit of purity and faith,
> one should know how to do *pūjā* for the gods
> with flowers (*puṣpa*), food offerings (*bali*),
> garments (*vastra*), songs (*stotra*), and turmeric.
> 118. Householders should honor
> all the great souls and gods
> with a will and inclination
> that does not discriminate against any of them.
> 119. All gods merit honoring,
> not just one preferred god.

> Those (who worship all gods) have controlled their senses
> and have overcome their fears and difficulties.

We can see that *pūjā* for Haribhadra acknowledges religious difference, but simultaneously advocates for the worship of all deemed worthy, whether they are a god or a human.

Japa in the *Yogabindu*

The first instance of commonality in religious practice previously mentioned clearly engaged with vocabulary used in Patañjali's *Yoga Sūtra* as seen in the terms *yoga* and *saṃyoga*. The second instance cited, *pūjā*, does not appear in the *Yoga Sūtra*, though it does play an important role in the *bhakti* yoga of the *Bhagavad Gītā*. The third topic in the *Yogabindu* returns us to the descriptions of yoga practice delineated by Patañjali, the process of mantra recitation. Though Patañjali specifies that the syllable to be intoned is the *praṇava*, associated with the ideation of Īśvara, the teacher of all teachers (*YS* I: 23–29), explained in the commentaries as the syllable *Oṃ*. Haribhadra's verses concern themselves not with any specific deity or syllable but with the process to be undertaken regardless of one's religious tradition:

> 381. *Japa* is said to be the initial practice
> to attain spirituality (*adhyātma*).
> From the essence of this limb arises divine grace (*devatā anugraha*). Hence this is a way of cultivating insight (*abhidhīyate*).
> 382. The object of *japa* is noble recitation.
> It is said to be a hymn to the gods (*devatā-stava*).
> It is seen that through this sins dissolve (*pāpa-hāra*).
> Poisons are thus removed (*viṣa-apaharaṇa*).
> 383. It is advised for it (*japa*) to be performed
> either in front of a deity (*devatā-apurata*)
> or in a place where the water is pure
> or in a beautiful grove of trees.
> 384. Counting the joints of the fingers
> or telling the mala beads like giving life to a son,
> one witnesses (breath) stability at the tip of the nose.

By oneself, one finds inner peace (*praśānta antarātmanā*).
385. [*Japa* requires] focusing the mind
on the qualities of the desired deity,
as well as its meaning and associations.
If one is distracted, then one should stop.
386. When one gets over improper behavior,
then one can, through the breath, resume.
It purifies desires.
In this way, a person, by stopping, is not stopping.
387. In *japa* the measure of time is celebrated.
From this, in not doing (*akaraṇe*),
one acquires the dispositional/emotional behaviors
(*bhāva-vṛtti*) that characterize awakening (*vidur-buddhā*).
388. This is praised by the noble sages.
Purity (arises) from effort at holding (to this practice).
From this, dharma always arises,
both at the time of doing it and following its
performance.

Just as the overcoming of karma and practice of veneration can be seen across traditions, the same can be said about the recitation of sacred syllables through *japa*, which may be performed to any deity according to the instructions Haribhadra provides.

The Remembrance of Past Lives (*punar janma smṛti*) in the *Yogabindu*

The mechanics of reincarnation are very mysterious.[5] Nonetheless, the philosophies of Buddhism, Jainism, and Sāṃkhya-Yoga utterly depend on this premise. Afflictions and obstacles have been identified variously across traditions: the Buddhist and yogic *kleśa*s, the Jaina *kaṣāya*s, the Vedantic *upādhi*s. They dwell and fester in subconscious memories known as *saṃskāra*s or *vāsanā*s. They govern present and future behavior. All beings carry the subtle influences of past actions into their present life as they take birth. They also bring self-power, as evidenced by acts of will. If business remains unresolved in one life, it carries over into another life. The difficulties inherent in past karmas can only be extirpated through sustained *tapas* (austerity) and meditation. As part of the process, one might begin to unravel the stories or at least the feelings that carry over from one life to the next.

The following passage from the *Yogabindu* would pertain to all persons seeking self-understanding, regardless of their religious differences. A bit like the gentle approach taken to the recitation of mantra where one might become distracted yet is urged to resume the practice, this segment suggests that the recollection of past lives will by nature be hazy and tentative. Furthermore, it requires a great deal of preparation and intense desire. Even then, such recollections may or may not arise.

> 57. Through *brahmacarya* (celibacy), through *tapas,*
> though reflection on sacred literature,
> through special wisdom mantras,
> through service at places of pilgrimage,
> 58. Through the correct honoring of one's parents,
> through offering medicine to the sick,
> and through the cleansing of deity images and the like,
> one can remember past lives.
> 59. This is not the case for all those who arrive here from the other world,
> as the hold-over (memories of past births) are very thin.
> 60. This is not for everyone due to connecting with deluded grasping.
> The specifics of experience may not be recalled by all people.
> 61. There is a similarity (of past life experiences) to the impulse of a baby being drawn to the breast[6]
> or the remembrance of a recurring dream.
> 62. Hence, just as one fails to remember specific actions in dreams,
> so, also, holding (memories of prior) birth can be elusive even for the accomplished ones with subtle intellect.
> 63. The great souls hear about this and they see it.
> Therefore, their testimony regarding the self and other matters has certainty.
> 64. Indeed, from success in this knowledge,
> one holds fast to yoga.

> Hence, whoever has this ascertainment
> is no longer influenced by karmas (*anya*).[7]

This last statement indicates the importance that past life remembrance can hold: If one remembers and understands and ascertains the past life story, then the sway of karma falls away. The Buddha remembered and spoke 550 stories regarding his past lives, recorded by his disciples. In each he demonstrated both self-understanding and an understanding of the lives of those around him in this life, who played roles in the past life recollections. Jain literature abounds with tales wherein protagonists and antagonists meet life after life, sometimes as humans, often as animals. The *Yogavāsiṣṭha* includes a charming tale, the story of Puṇya and Pavana, wherein seeing and remembering the immensity of one's past lives and the past lives of others can assuage grief. These verses from Haribhadra, which engage with the broader assertion found across Indic traditions that past lives can be remembered, acknowledge the difficulty of retrieving such memories, while at the same time signaling their restorative power.

The Importance of Dreams (*Svapna*) in the Yoga *Bindu*

Dreams play an important role in a number of Indic religious traditions and texts. The *Māṇḍūkya Upaniṣad* delineates four levels of consciousness: awake, dreaming, deep sleep, and the ineffable fourth state. As part of a cascade describing auspicious activities, *Yoga Sūtra* I:28 proclaims that sleep can generate meditative states (*svapna-nidrā-jñānālambanaṃ vā*). The Sevenfold Yoga of the *Yogavāsiṣṭha* includes a stage wherein the world itself is seen as if it were a dream, cultivating a state of dispassionate remove. This would not accord with the Jain insistence on the reality of things. Nonetheless, Haribhadra engages extant religious traditions concerned with the world of dreaming, highlighting what he considers as the important supporting role dreams play in the cultivation of the spiritual life:

> 43. From even a little bit of faith
> generated by the external practices of Yoga,
> beautiful dreams arise such as visions of one's chosen deity.

> 44. The yogīs, established in good action,
> mainly see thrilling gods, gurus, brahmins, and sadhus
> in their dreams,
> driving away all lower states.
> 45. The process of driving away these (lesser states)
> establishes the efficacy (of yoga).
> Because they cut away time and circumstance
> they are not to be faulted.
> From the yoga of sleep and mantra,
> the dream of truth (*satya svapna*) is made real.
> The knowing person, in a state of harmony,
> thus attains goodly success.

The linkage here of dream (*svapna*) and truth (*satya*) points to an aspiration that seeks to convert the desire, wish, or dream of freedom into a reality.

We have examined five theologically neutral practices or techniques that can be found across traditions: yoga, devotional practice, mantra recitation, recollection of past lives, and divination via dreams. While engaging with religious differences of his time, Haribhadra sees implied commonality in the five shared practices. Haribhadra thereby holds forth both an olive branch and a debating stick. From the perspective of philosophical views, he devotes a significant part of the text to pointing out differences between Jainism, Buddhism, Sāṃkhya, and Vedānta, particularly on the topics of human agency and individual identity. We will take up his arguments against the Buddhist teaching on no-self and then conclude with examples of how the *Yogabindu* reconciles differences through a process of friendly juxtaposition.

Argument Against the Buddhist Philosophy of No-Self, No-Essence

During the time of Haribhadra, the Mādhyamika school of Nāgārjuna was in full bloom, which Haribhadra quotes directly. The Mahāyāna position asserts a four-cornered negation of positivity, negativity, neutrality, and the idea of transcendence, claiming that no essence can be found in self or others. Simply put, the Mahāyāna enlightenment experience removes all attachments. As a result, this state of elevated equanimity sees even the idea of *nirvāṇa* itself as an illusion, proclaiming it to be inseparable from *saṃsāra*. Haribhadra carefully rebuts this Buddhist position, engaging it with his own Jain stance in the following verses in the *Yogabindu*:

> 75. Each person arises due to the constructs of his or her (karmic) essence.
> Only through a subtle intellect can knowledge (of the constructs) be discerned.

Haribhadra here asserts the reality of karmic residue and the necessity of its removal through the various practices listed previously.

> 76. An event (*kāryam*) does not happen randomly.
> An event always occurs through the union
> of the embodied soul with its being (*sattva*).

The next two verses emphasize the power of karma that manifests as events, or things to be done, using the future participial form of the common root *kṛ*.

> 77. Each state (*bhāva*) is distinct (*citra*).
> Its future order (*ṛta*) arises from its past.
> There can be no other cause.
> Thus, let this (the operations of karma) be accepted.

Hence, Haribhadra disputes the Buddhist notion that no essence (*niḥsvabhāva*) can be found in things or in persons. In direct opposition, he claims the opposite to be true. He asserts the Jain position that the soul or self is in a real relationship with karma. One's karmic being (*bhāva*) determines the experience of the soul.

> 78. It might be asked if this assent
> to the teaching of self-essence (*svabhāva*) is in error.
> How could there not be a teaching about the "other"
> (karma) in relationship to one's state?

Furthermore, Haribhadra proclaims the reality of time as an essential truth. The operations of karma throughout past, present, and future must be maintained as factual.

> 79. The great souls (*mahātmas*) agree that
> teachings regarding time and other topics are agreeable.
> One who always rejects this view is out of touch.[8]
> 80. Due to karmic bondage,
> the soul undergoes transformations (*pariṇāma*).
> It experiences suffering (*duḥkha*) in (real) time.
> How can all this future order (*ṛta*) arise
> other than from self-essence (*svabhāva*)?

These verses directly contradict Buddhist teachings that presumably were taught to Haribhadra by his nephew as indicated in the previous story.

The Bodhisattva and the Jain Saint

As he engages the Buddhist tradition, Haribhadra shows common intent between the Buddhist Bodhisattva and the person who treads the Jain path to freedom, the *mokṣa mārga.* Rather than lingering on the differences between Buddhism and Jainism, Haribhadra gives praise to the Buddhist Bodhisattva ideal and shows once again a common intent. He aligns the Buddhist awakening (*bodhi*) with the fourth Jain level of spiritual ascent, correct view (*samyak-dṛṣṭi*).

> 271. The Bodhisattvas descend into the body, indeed,
> from on high.
> Although joined (to the world) here in body,
> their consciousness does not descend.[9]
> 272. These two (Bodhisattvas and Saṃyagdṛṣṭīs) are the
> same in all ways.
> They have a taste for higher purpose. They are visionary.
> They tread the path.
> They are of noble disposition. They have lovely qualities.

> 273. Correct vision and awakening arise from the same source (*pradhāna*).
> It is clear that the Jain saint[10] is of the same being as the Bodhisattva.
> 274. Whether a person desires to be joined in the space of awakening (the Bodhisattva)
> or making pilgrimage (the Jain saint's journey to the Siddha Loka),
> it is known that excellence can be found
> in both the Bodhisattva and the Jain saint.

Rather than castigating the Buddhist for holding an incorrect view, Haribhadra sees parallelisms of intent and action between the practitioner of Buddhism who takes a vow to help others and the Jain saint who through his or her own commitment to karmic purification brings great benefit through adherence to vows.

Juxtapositionalism: Engaging Five Philosophies of Freedom

As a rhetorical method, Haribhadra urges reconciliation rather than dispute in several sections of the *Yogabindu*. He lays out terms that indicate the goal of Hinduism, Buddhism, and Jainism, respectively.

> 302. Liberated, Buddha, Arhant:
> these are all terms that possess the meaning of (attaining) lordship (*aiśvarya*).
> That lord would be known as independent (from karma).

He criticizes any attempt to speculate about or rationalize the process of freeing oneself from bondage, preferring experience over analysis. Haribhadra warns against falling into conflictual sectarianism:

> 303. Trying to cut all this conceptually is an endless endeavor at cleansing,
> trying to sort the threads of one tradition from another.
> I think this is without purpose.

> 304. From obsessing on what distinguishes (one from another) one would be engaging in sectarianism.
> Mainly, this (would foster) conflict, a state akin to cutting up fruits.
> 305. Ignorance, affliction, karma and so forth:
> these are the cause of worldly existence.
> They are indeed known as the occurrence of the root of karma.
> 306. The cutting that arises from opposing one with another
> (puts) the various positions (*upādhis*) at odds.
> Visionary persons call this irrational and without purpose.
> 307. Hence, mainly instability would result
> from pointing to and cutting up things.
> The result, presumably, would be (mere) analogies and speculation.

Whether Hindu, Buddhist, or Jain, Haribhadra considers the yoga path to be common to all. The rigors of keeping vows or abiding by strict dietary observances help undo the self-inflicted harmful patterns of karma. In the doing, one approaches freedom:

> 66. It is said that those who know the yoga path,
> whose stains have been shaken off by the rigor of their *tapas*,
> that those elevated ones who are established and possessed of yoga,
> are the same whether in darkness or in light.
> 67. The opinionated, decisive ones who speak arguments and counterarguments
> do not arrive at the place of ultimate truth.
> Rather, they tread a path like an ant carrying a sesame seed.

Echoing remarks made at the beginning of the text, he reiterates the ubiquity of karma and specifically delineates the usage for each tradition.

With rhetorical grandeur Haribhadra juxtaposes, but does not prioritize or develop a hierarchy, when describing the goal of five different philosophies of freedom:

> 422. "Cloud of Dharma," "Undying Self,"
> "The Uprising of Powerful Auspicious Being,"
> "The Bliss of Pure Being," "The Highest":
> these names are all used to describe the purpose of yoga.

Cloud of Dharma (*dharma-megha*) is the tenth and final accomplishment of the Bodhisattva in Mahāyāna Buddhism and also the culminating description of freedom in the *Yoga Sūtra,* after which all fettering karmas cease. Undying self (*amṛta-ātmā*) carries allusions of both the state of the soul in the Jain Siddha Loka and overtures from the Upaniṣads and the second chapter of the *Bhagavad Gītā*. The Uprising of Powerful Auspicious Being (*bhava-śakra-śiva-udaya*) contains allusions to Śaivism in the words chosen, while not contradicting the Jain description of freedom. The Bliss of Pure Being (*sattva-ānanda*) echoes passages from the Upaniṣads and the emphasis in Sāṃkhya and Yoga on the cultivation of lightness of being (*sattva*). The Highest (*para*) encapsulates the intent and goal of the spiritual journey: to reach the summit.

Regardless of tradition, the process requires a steady process of purification. Haribhadra uses the graphic metaphor of a burned frog. It cannot rise from its ashes. Likewise, great sages burn the seeds of past karmas and thereby attain the auspicious state.

> 423. Logic states that a frog reduced to ashes (does not return).
> So it is with the seeds of behavior of the great sage.
> Having burned (the seeds) and having left behind connection (with karma),
> the sage attains the auspicious state.

Freedom arises with the abandonment of karma, regardless of one's religious tradition.

Conclusion

This chapter began with a gripping tale of jealousy, intrigue, murder, revenge, remorse, and reformation. The *Yogabindu* uses a gentle tone to praise the common intent of all religions: the purification of the human person. Rather than asserting Jain superiority, Haribhadra engages a common idea shared by most philosophers of India: the reality of karma and the efficacy of yoga. He cites select examples of practices held in common, including *pūjā, japa,* past life remembrance, and the importance of dreams. Nonetheless, he also uses the *Yogabindu* as an opportunity to elucidate difference, delineating arguments against Buddhism and other non-Jain thinkers. However, he also criticizes the entire process of analytical debate, using the metaphor of an ant treading a path with a sesame seed, perhaps weaving from side to side and looking silly in the process. Hence, he sets forth a process of juxtaposition, not unlike the method used by Huston Smith in his groundbreaking 1958 work *The World's Religions* (Smith 1991). Rather than emphasizing critique, this method lets each tradition stand on its own. Without eliding differences through hegemony or trying to subsume traditions into an all-inclusive monism, Haribhadra simply lets stand the goal proclaimed by each: Cloud of Dharma, Undying Self, Auspicious Pure Blissful Being, and simply, the Highest.

> "What's in a name? A rose by any other name would smell as sweet." (Shakespeare, *Romeo and Juliet,* Act II, Scene II)

Notes

1. Phyllis Granoff points out that the stories of Haribhadra's two nephews summarized and amplified below are told in various forms citing more than five sources. They appear two hundred years after a similar story discusses the escapades of Akalaṅka and Niṣkalaṅka at a Buddhist monastery. See Granoff 1989 and Dundas 2020.

2. A new translation was sponsored in 1994 by Charles, then Prince and now King of England. See Tatia 1994.

3. The sources for these stories are the *Prabhāvakacarita* of Prabhācandra (1277 CE) and the *Prabandhakośa* of Rājaśekharasūri (1349 CE), which, as noted above, seem to be modeled after the earlier *Kathākośa* (1077 CE).

4. All translations are by the author with acknowledgment given to the help of Alba Rodríguez Juan, Anil Mundra, Robert Zabel, and others.

5. See the online open access journal *Religions: Perspectives on Reincarnation: Hindu, Christian, and Scientific*, https://www.mdpi.com/journal/religions/special_issues/reincarnation.

6. This perhaps indirectly correlates with the documented ability of very young children to remember past lives as documented by Ian Stevenson of the University of Virginia. See Stevenson 1997.

7. The word *anya*, "other," carries multivalent meanings, including karma, reliance on an external deity, belief in a faulty worldview, and so forth.

8. Haribhadra Virahāṅka argues here that the operations of karma through moments of time must be affirmed.

9. Haribhadra is making a series of fascinating arguments. First, the praise of the Bodhisattva helps account for the praise given to the Samyakdṛṣṭi/Bhinnagrantha for reentering the world. The metaphor of descent keeps returning. Though not using the word *avatāra* directly, it seems abundantly implied. Second, although the body of the Bodhisattva descends (*patina*), the consciousness of the Bodhisattva does not descend, but rather remains elevated due to the lofty nature of the Bodhisattva vow, to do service for others.

10. Haribhadra uses the term Hanta, short for Arhat, to refer to the Jain saint.

References

Balcerowicz, Piotr. 2016. "On the Relative Chronology of Dharmakīrti and Samantabhadra." *Journal of Indian Philosophy* 44:437–483.

Berry, Thomas. 1968. *Five Oriental Philosophies*. Magi Books.

Dixit, K. K., trans. 1968. *The Yogabindu of Ācārya Haribhadrasūri*. Lalbhai Dalpatbhai Bharatiya Sanskriti Vidyamandir.

———. 1970. *The Yogadṛṣṭisamuccaya and Yogaviṃśika of Ācārya Haribhadrasūri*. Lalbhai Dalpatbhai Bharatiya Sanskriti Vidyamandir.

Dundas, Paul. 2020. "Haribhadra." *Brill's Encyclopedia of Jainism Online*. Brill. https://referenceworks.brill.com/display/db/bejo.

Granoff, Phyllis. 1989. "Jain Lives of Haribhadra: An Inquiry into the Sources and Logic of the Legends." *Journal of Indian Philosophy* 17 (2): 105–128.

Kema, Sister, trans. 1982. "Bhadda Kundalakesa: The Former Jain Ascetic." In *Buddhist Women at the Time of the Buddha: The Wheel*, by Hellmuth Hecker, no. 292–293. Buddhist Publication Society.

Shukla, R. S. 1989. *India as Known to Haribhadra Suri*. Kusumanjali Prakasan.

Smith, Huston. 1991. *The World's Religions: Our Great Wisdom Traditions.* HarperCollins. Originally published as *The Religions of Man,* 1958.
Stevenson, Ian. 1997. *Where Reincarnation and Biology Intersect.* Praeger.
Tatia, Nathmal, trans. 1994. *That Which Is: Tattvārthasūtra.* HarperCollins.

15

Fortuitous Jain Engagements with Nondualities

Jain Yoga in the *Yogapradīpa* and *Yogasāra*

CORINNA MAY LHOIR

This chapter focuses on the origins and philosophical heritage of the Jain medieval text *Yogapradīpa* (*YP*), serving as a part of a larger research project aimed at producing an annotated translation of the *Yogapradīpa* as well as a survey of Jain Yoga texts from the second millennium CE. It also introduces ideas of the *Yogasāra* (*YS*), a text presumably originating in the same milieu.[1]

With 141 verses, *Yogapradīpa* serves as a treatise emphasizing the perception of the soul within the body through meditation to achieve liberation. *Yogapradīpa*'s approach to yoga and meditation centers on *dhyāna* as a key aspect of its eightfold yoga path, mirroring Patañjali's Classical Yoga. My research investigates the philosophical foundations within the Jain tradition that influenced *Yogapradīpa*'s unique approach and adaptation of its eightfold path as well as the ways in which the text's author is engaging philosophical streams found in texts on early *haṭhayoga*[2] from other Hindu traditions.

This chapter's exploration raises research questions about Jain engagements with other philosophical systems in society. It seeks to understand how Jain adaptations to a world of diverse philosophical systems were influenced and how Jains added their distinctive Jain touch to it. By exploring these complexities, we will gain insights into how Jains navigated diverse philosophical systems while maintaining a commitment to their own foundational philosophical positions, as well as Jains' distinct impact on the second-millennium CE South Asian philosophical milieu. I will discuss the use of the term *laya* (dissolution) and the origins of ideas of defining *dhyāna* (meditation) in *haṭhayoga* and Jain Yoga texts as a case study to explicitly illustrate how Jain texts engage with broader *haṭhayoga* discourses and practices oriented toward nonduality, illustrating the unique ways in which Jains integrate these elements while steadfastly upholding their distinct soteriological commitments.

The adaptations of Jainism to the yoga milieu of pan-dharmic traditions demonstrate the social engagement inherent in textual engagement. Understanding these survival mechanisms is crucial for both scholarly and practical purposes, contributing to our knowledge of the interactions between different religious and philosophical traditions and shedding light on the dynamics of religious coexistence.

Beginnings of Yogic Thought

Liberation from the endless cycle of death and rebirth (*saṃsāra*) is the highest goal in most Indian religious traditions. The practice of yoga is one, although not the only, way to achieve this goal. From its ancient beginnings, a variety of yoga traditions developed primarily among heterodox, non-brahmanical ascetics and practitioners of the so-called *śramaṇa* movements, a group of independent ascetics and wandering monks representing the precursors of what would become Buddhism and Jainism (Bronkhorst 2007, 13–42). Recent research by Philipp Maas shows that the *Pātañjalayogaśāstra* (second to fourth century CE, according to Maas), a key summation of the yoga practices found in the *śramaṇa* culture, was sourced not only from brahmanical but also from the resulting Buddhist and Jain thought of Patañjali's milieu (Maas 2020). Yoga thereby transcended religious barriers even as its techniques gradually became a distinct feature of almost all of India's religious traditions.

There is unfortunately still only limited awareness among scholars of the significant impact that Jainism had not only on conventional Indian philosophical thinking but also on the evolution and development of yoga. In addition to its significance as a śramaṇic religion for the early roots of yoga, Jainism, over the centuries, like the other Indian religious traditions, has had a long history of interaction, exchange, and entanglement with other surrounding spiritual practices and beliefs. In time, Jains adopted, contributed, and exchanged various elements from yoga systems and techniques from neighboring traditions.

Beginnings of Yogic Thought in Jainism

Jainism, like other Indian spiritual traditions, places great importance on the practice of yoga and meditation (*dhyāna*) as a path toward spiritual enlightenment and liberation (Jain 2016, 14). According to lecture 28 of the *Uttarādhyayanasūtra*, an authoritative canonical root text (*mūla*) of the Śvetāmbara branch of Jainism, which is believed to carry the words of the ford-maker Mahāvīra himself,[3] one can gain understanding of one's true self through right knowledge (*samyag-jñāna*), develop faith through right vision or attitude (*samyag-darśana*), and gain the necessary requisite control of oneself through right conduct (*samyak-cāritra*) (Jain 2016, 14; Jacobi 1968, 152–157).

This triadic foundation is pivotal in Jainism's conceptualization of yoga as a disciplined path of self-purification and liberation. However, the purification of the self can only be achieved through the practice of penance (*tapas*), viewed as having two components: pure meditation (*śukla-dhyāna*) and non-attachment toward the body and worldly belongings (*kāyotsarga*) (Jain 2016, 14–16).

Early Jain texts, such as the *Sūtrakṛtāṅgasūtra*, articulate yoga as an exercise in restraint and self-control, prefiguring later elaborations in Jain literature. Samani Pratibha Pragya, in her examination of yogic terms in ancient Jain texts, highlights the continuity and evolution of these ideas, demonstrating how early Jain conceptions of yoga seamlessly transition into the structured frameworks seen in later works (Pratibha Pragya 2021, 171–188). This evolution underscores how Jainism has historically contextualized yoga not merely as physical or meditative practices but as a holistic discipline embodying the Three Jewels.

The integration of the Three Jewels into Jain Yoga serves as a strategic anchor, enabling Jain authors to assimilate and reinterpret external yogic influences, such as those from Patañjali's system, within their own doctrinal framework. This strategy is evident in Jain texts, where the synthesis of Jain values with broader yogic practices illustrates a dynamic engagement with the wider Indian philosophical milieu: In the eighth century CE, the Jain author Haribhadra revolutionized Jain Yoga by integrating aspects of Patañjali's eightfold system into his *Yogadṛṣṭisamuccaya*, while also redefining yoga to mean any practice that unites the self with liberation, as outlined in his twenty-verse Prakrit text, *Yogaviṃśikā* (Dixit 1970, 113).

In the twelfth century CE, Jain philosopher Hemacandra, in his extensive work *Yogaśāstra*, paralleled Umāsvāti's path to liberation from the *Tattvārthasūtra* by defining yoga through the Three Jewels: right faith, knowledge, and conduct. While initially focusing on these in the *Yogaśāstra*'s first chapters, he later incorporates Patañjali's eightfold yoga, including postures and breath control techniques, which in Jainism, unlike in Classical Yoga, serve as health aids and meditation supports rather than as liberating practices. Hemacandra also explores aspects of meditation, and, in classifying *dhyāna* as twofold only, significantly altered Jain meditation classifications for the first time. Influenced by the cultural context under Śaiva King Kumārapāla, he integrated tantric and mantra practices, reflecting Jainism's adaptive nature in assimilating external elements while maintaining its doctrinal commitments (Jambūvijaya 1977, 1981, 1986; Qvarnström 2012, 7–13).

Such integration is also reflected in the *Yogapradīpa*, which, as we will see, while drawing upon external yogic models, retains a distinct commitment to Jain soteriology, showcasing the adaptability and resilience of the Jain philosophical tradition. In verse 113, yoga is characterized by (*ātmaka*) the Three Jewels of knowledge, vision, and conduct (*jñāna-darśana-cāritra-rūpa-ratna-traya*) and proclaimed as the means (*upāya*) for attaining the state of liberation (*muktipada*) (*YP* 113),[4] thereby underscoring Pratibha Pragya's conclusion: "Thus, throughout the medieval period, Jain yogic tradition assimilated many common elements from contemporaneous traditions and

'Jainised' them into suitable forms, perhaps foreshadowing developments in the modern period" (Pratibha Pragya 2021, 181).

Mapping the Environment of the *Yogapradīpa*: Language and Jain Identity in Gujarat

The *Yogapradīpa* traces its origins to the region of present-day Gujarat, with the oldest manuscripts I have identified housed in the Hemacandra Jñān Mandir, a Jain library in Patan (presumably fourteenth century). Significant collections in Ahmedabad's manuscript libraries, such as the L. D. Institute of Indology and the Acharya Shri Kailasasagarsuri Gyanmandir, along with a sixteenth-century manuscript at the B. L. Institute of Indology in Delhi, feature translations into Old Gujarati. This practice of rendering the text into Old Gujarati contributed significantly to the broadening of its reach, making the profound teachings of the *Yogapradīpa* accessible to a wider demographic that may not have been well-versed in Sanskrit. The existence of these vernacular translations and commentaries is a testament to the rich and adaptive heritage of the text, reflecting a dynamic interplay between scholarly rigor and cultural engagement with the text's broader place and time period.

The Jain community's strategic use of language, as evidenced by their transition from Prakrit to Sanskrit and eventually to regional languages like Old Gujarati, reflects a deeper philosophical and cultural agility (Dundas 2020, 739–755).[5] This linguistic adaptability has not only allowed Jains to maintain their unique religious identity but also facilitated their engagement with broader philosophical and cultural milieus. The Jain tradition's multilingual approach, thus, is more than a mere survival mechanism; it is a dynamic process of cultural engagement and adaptation, which has cultivated a rich intellectual tradition.

The strategic use of Sanskrit in Jain texts such as the *Yogapradīpa* and *Yogasāra* is emblematic of the Jain community's skill in engaging diverse philosophical and religious landscapes. By composing these texts in Sanskrit, a language with pan-dharmic resonance, Jains not only facilitated a dialogue with adherents of other traditions but also reaffirmed their unique doctrinal stance. This linguistic choice underlines the dual purpose of these texts: to serve as a bridge of understanding to followers of different religious paths, and to articulate the distinctiveness of Jain philosophy.

Origins and Significance of the *Yogapradīpa* and the *Yogasāra*

The *New Catalogus Catalogorum* of the University of Madras (2011, vol. 22, 80–81) reveals four different works entitled *Yogapradīpa*. One of these, identified as a Jain work, has eight manuscripts in various catalogs. In the Descriptive Catalogue of the Amer Shastra Bhandar, a large archive of Jain literature in Jaipur, Rajasthan, the text is described in more detail: The author is unknown, the script is Devanāgarī, the number of folios is seven, the theme is *yogaśāstra* (manual of Yoga), and the text is complete with 141 verses (Birch and Hargreaves 2017). A critical edition of the text exists, compiled by Amṛtlāl Kālidās Kośī in 1960, based on a total of four manuscripts and two earlier editions (from 1911 and 1922), together with a translation into Gujarati (Kośī 1960). The fact that there are multiple editions of this text and that it has been considered noteworthy by various Jain scholars of the twentieth century testifies to its importance for a Jain audience, despite it having remained under the radar of global yoga scholarship until now.

John Cort has pointed out that the misidentification of the author in the case of one manuscript from Patan as Śubhacandra is also of interest, as at least one copyist puts this text in the orbit of the *Jñānārṇava* ("Ocean of Wisdom of Meditation"), an important Jain text on meditation from the eleventh century (John Cort, email to author, Oct. 24, 2023). Interestingly enough, one chapter of the *Jñānārṇava* is also called by another name, the *Yogapradīpādhikāra*.

The author of the other text I describe in this chapter, the *Yogasāra*, also remains unidentified. While I discovered a reference to a palm-leaf manuscript of this text, purportedly housed in Patan, the actual manuscript could not be located there. If this manuscript indeed existed, it would suggest that the *Yogasāra* predates the fourteenth century, aligning its age with that of the thirteenth-century *Dattātreyayogaśāstra*.

Some of the multi-text manuscripts (MTMs; i.e., manuscripts that contain more than one text) I found during my research in

Gujarat contained copies of the *Yogasāra* as well as of the *Yogapradīpa*. Consultations with Jain *munis* in Patan suggested a common heritage or even a common author of these two texts, although I must, for the time being, defer providing evidence to support this assertion.

Elements of Early Haṭhayogic Practice

Samādhi in Classical and in Early Haṭhayoga

In Classical Yoga, particularly in the context of the *Pātañjalayogaśāstra* from the fourth century CE, we encounter the concept of *samādhi* as a twofold experience, with each part of it representing a unique facet of meditative absorption.

The first, *saṃprajñāta samādhi*, is a state accompanied by mental states or cognition, suggesting a level of awareness or understanding within the meditative experience. This state is marked by a deliberate and sustained contemplation on an object, concept, or image. The practitioner's consciousness, rather than dissolving into the void of the no-mind, maintains a laser-like focus, facilitating a profound understanding and absorption into the nature of the object of meditation (Mallinson and Singleton 2017, 333–334).

The second, *asaṃprajñāta samādhi*, is a noncognitive state where the fluctuations of the mind are completely suppressed. It is akin to reaching a profound silence within the mind, where all chatter, all movement of thought, and mental stirrings are extinguished. This is the quintessential state of "no-mind," a level of contemplation so deep that the practitioner emerges beyond the normal confines of conscious thought into a realm of pure being, unencumbered by the typical mental noise that characterizes human consciousness.

The conception of *samādhi* in early *haṭhayoga*, which began to emerge around the eleventh century (Mallinson and Singleton 2017, 333–334), shifts entirely from a cognitive to a more somatic experience and is described as being more of a "death-like" state (Cestola 2024, 7; Birch 2020a, 227ff.). This implies a profound level of detachment and disengagement from the physical senses and external consciousness. *Haṭhayoga* systems focus on physical engagement and highlight the body's crucial role in yoga practice, aiming to achieve *samādhi* through methods distinct from those in Classical Yoga. Physical methods[6] are affirmed and utilized to achieve a state of deep, transformative tranquility, the prerequisite for the highest goal: "On the whole, *samādhi* is the necessary and sufficient cause for liberation in Hatha- and Rājayoga texts" (Birch 2020a, 200).

Building upon this understanding of *samādhi* in Classical Yoga and its evolution in *haṭhayoga*, it is essential to recognize the diverse methodologies and interpretations that have emerged over the first centuries. The *Haṭhapradīpikā* (*HP*), a fifteenth-century compendium, draws from a multitude of earlier texts[7] to present a layered and multifaceted view of *samādhi*, not just offering a single pathway but rather illustrating a confluence of techniques and definitions that reflect the wisdom and practices of numerous lineages in verses 3 and 4 of chapter 4: "*rājayoga, samādhi, unmanī, manonmanī, amaraugha, advaita, nirālamba, nirañjana, amanaska, laya, tattva, śūnyāśūnya, para pada, jīvanmukti, sahaja* and *turya* are synonyms" (*HP* 4.29 and 4.30).[8]

The terms mentioned in this verse include *rājayoga* (king of yoga), *samādhi* (absorption), *unmanī* (the condition beyond the mind), *manonmanī* (the condition of the mind without the mind), *amaraugha* (a stream [*ogha*] of immortals [*amara*]), *advaita* (non-dual state), *nirālamba* (unsupported, self-supported), *nirañjana* (spotless, pure), *amanaska* (no-mind state), *laya* (dissolution), *tattva* (the true or real state), *śūnyāśūnya* (void and non-void state), *para-pada* (highest state), *jīvanmukti* (liberation-in-life), *sahajā* (condition of innate bliss), and *turya* (the "fourth condition" of the soul, highest condition of consciousness), which are to be considered as different expressions or names that denote the same ultimate state. The use of *ekavācaka* (with *eka* meaning "one," and *vācaka*, which can be translated as "expressing," "signifying," or "denoting"), therefore, conveys the idea that despite the linguistic diversity and the seemingly different concepts these terms represent, they all signify one truth or reality in the realm of spiritual experience. This state is not monolithic, but a culmination of various spiritual experiences, accessible through a spectrum of practices from the physical to the auditory, such as, for example, the tuning into the subtle resonance of (*anāhata*) *nāda*, as referred to in verse 49 of the fourth chapter of the *Haṭhapradīpikā*, used to achieve *laya*: "When the mind dissolves into that which is the most subtle object of perception in the unstruck sound, that is the supreme state of Viṣṇu. The tone of that sound is that of the unstruck sound. The object of perception is inside the sound [and] the mind is inside the object of perception. When the mind dissolves [in it] (*layaṃ yāti*), that is the supreme state of Viṣṇu" (*HP* 4.49).[9]

The term *laya* is pivotal in understanding the concept of *samādhi*, particularly in the context of its role in the dissolution of the mind in early *haṭhayoga* texts. *Laya*, often translated as "absorption" or "dissolution," denotes a state where the usual functions of the mind are transcended, culminating in a profound state of *samādhi*. In this state, the individual consciousness merges or dissolves into a higher or universal consciousness, indicating a cessation of the ordinary mental activities and fluctuations, and "the Yogis hear a centrally aroused sound and lose themselves in that sound; and thus, reduction of life activity or absence of ordinary consciousness in Laya Yoga is absorption of mind in Nāda of which the content is the great unknown symbolized by internally aroused sound. It is a state of Higher Consciousness" (Digambaraji 2016, 142). In most medieval yoga texts, the unstruck sound, *anāhata-nāda*, is noted as a main focus for meditation (Birch 2013, 269).

Trans-Sectarianism in Haṭhayogic Texts

Mallinson has pointed out that despite the Śaiva "appropriation" of *haṭhayoga* techniques, Svātmārāma's *Haṭhapradīpikā* lacks detailed philosophical teachings and explicit Śaiva sect-markers, suggesting a move toward a more universal yoga approach, albeit subtly indicated through its *maṅgala* verses and invocations. This trend mirrors a broader historical shift where yoga practices began transcending sectarian confines to appeal to a wider audience, aiming for a pan-Indian identity that could serve as an alternative to mainstream religious expressions (Mallinson 2014, 229).

This phenomenon of trans-sectarian yoga is visible in verses 41 and 42 of the thirteenth-century *Dattātreyayogaśāstra* (*DYS*) (Mallinson and Singleton 2017, xx), one of the texts the *Haṭhapradīpikā* extensively borrowed from: "Whether a Brahmin, an ascetic, a Buddhist, a Jain, a Skull-Bearer or a materialist, the wise man who is endowed with faith and constantly devoted to the practice of [*haṭha*] yoga will attain complete success" (*DYS* 41 and 42)[10] (trans. by Mallinson 2014, 230).

The diversity within the *Haṭhapradīpikā* echoes the broader yogic philosophy that while the destination of *samādhi* remains constant—a state of profound peace and unity—the routes by which one may arrive there are as varied as the practitioners themselves. Mallinson outlines how the *Haṭhapradīpikā* assimilates various non-dual yogic systems to achieve *samādhi,* reflecting *haṭhayoga*'s integration of Vedāntic nonduality and metaphysical concepts, particularly in the context of *samādhi,* during a transitional period from the Śaiva to the Vedāntic dominant paradigm, aligning with yoga's goal as a unificatory, liberating experience. Citing the work of Bouy (1994), Mallinson writes, "The texts of the early haṭhayogic corpus quickly floated free of any sectarian moorings and became common property, allowing them to be used not only to compile the *Haṭhapradīpikā,* but, in the 17th century, to create a corpus of yoga Upaniṣads" (2014, 238). In light of this, Mallinson concludes, "*Haṭhayoga* is a practical soteriology independent of metaphysical speculation" (2014, 237).

In the following part of the chapter, I aim to demonstrate how the *Yogapradīpa* and *Yogasāra* exemplify Jain engagements with their broader religious landscape by showing their creative adaptation of the *haṭhayoga* corpus and of Sanskrit traditions. Despite drawing from a framework of non-dual practices and concepts such as *laya* and *nāda,* the authors maintained a unique, pluralistic perspective that aligns with Jain ontological and metaphysical principles. The following analysis illuminates how Jains maintained their pluralistic ontological commitments while simultaneously adopting influential practices from their religious milieu that were more frequently used to achieve non-dual soteriological outcomes.

The Yoga of the *Yogapradīpa* and the *Yogasāra*

The *Yogapradīpa* and the *Yogasāra* presumably predate[11] the *Haṭhapradīpikā* by one or two centuries. Neither text focuses on physical practices, but on meditation as the means of liberation. Birch has shown that the *Yogapradīpa* manifests distinctive Jain elements in its exposition of meditative and soteriological practices. The text underscores the centrality of the Jain paradigm of the Three Jewels—knowledge (*jñāna*), faith (*darśana*), and conduct (*cāritra*)—as the essential pathway toward liberation. Furthermore, it articulates the *aṣṭakarma*, explicating the eightfold nature of karmic matter, and integrates veneration for Pārśvaprabhu, acknowledging the twenty-third Tīrthaṅkara Pārśvanātha's place within its spiritual framework. Birch also illustrates: "The salient theme of the *Yogapradīpa* is to see the Self (*ātman*) in the body by means of meditation" (Birch and Hargreaves 2017).

The unique Jain quality of this *ātman* is best witnessed in verse 14 of the *Yogapradīpa*: "The own *ātman* is to be meditated upon by the wise men as having the appearance of a pure crystal, adorned with the qualities of the all-knower [the *jina*] and connected with the aspects of the highest self" (*YP* 14).[12] While interpreting concepts such as *ātman* within a Jain framework, the *Yogapradīpa* and Yogasāra add special perspectives to the trans-sectarianism of early *haṭhayogic* texts.

Trans-Sectarianism

The *Yogasāra* presents the same fascinating perspective on the transcendent and trans-sectarian nature of spiritual truth as the *Dattātreyayogaśāstra* (and the later *haṭhayoga* corpus at large). Given that both texts are approximately contemporaneous, this parallelism underscores a broader, era-specific exploration of spirituality that transcends individual sectarian boundaries as clearly expressed in the *Yogasāra*: "Whether Buddha or Viṣṇu, or whether Brahma or Īśvara, let him be called Jina or the supreme conqueror, indeed, there is no difference in meaning. 'Only my god is god. Yours isn't.' To say this is just a manifestation of small-mindedness, which appears to the ignorant" (*YS* 36–37).[13]

These verses in the first chapter of the *Yogasāra* articulate the notion that whether one venerates Buddha, Viṣṇu, Brahma, Īśvara, or Jina, the essence of the divine remains constant and undifferentiated. This wisdom asserts that the diversity of divine representation is merely a play of names and forms, not altering the underlying reality. The text critiques the divisive tendencies that arise from possessiveness over one's chosen deity, attributing such sentiments to ignorance and jealousy, which are portrayed as distortions of truth propagated by those who lack true understanding.

Similarly, the *Yogapradīpa* echoes this sentiment in verse 32: "This untainted [Lord] alone is perceived as Brahmā by Brahmins, Viṣṇu by mendicants in yellow robes and it is seen as Rudra by ascetics. Having been made Buddha by the Buddhists, this eternal [Lord] is the Lord of the Jinas praised by the Jains and it is called Śiva by the Kaulas" (*YP* 32)[14] (trans. by Birch and Hargreaves 2017). This illustrates that the divine is perceived differently by various groups: Brahmā by the Brahmins, Viṣṇu by those in yellow garments, and Rudra by ascetics. These verses from *Yogapradīpa* and *Yogasāra* indeed place all deities and the Jina on an equal footing, reflecting the ecumenical stance similarly observed in early haṭhayogic texts, and which was also familiar to prior first millennium Jain authors of yoga texts such as Haribhadra (see Chapple in this volume). Such an approach does not dilute Jain ontology, soteriology, or distinct elements but rather embraces a more inclusive, universal perspective on spiritual practice. By acknowledging the validity of various paths toward the ultimate goal of liberation, the *Yogapradīpa* and *Yogasāra* align with the broader yogic tradition of recognizing multiple avenues to spiritual realization, while, as we will see, still preserving a Jain core through specific practices and philosophical underpinnings.

Dissolution (*laya*) in the *Yogasāra*

The *Yogasāra* gives the following definitions for *laya* in the third chapter: "This is the natural bliss (*sahajānanda*), that very state is considered self-enjoyment. That which is the making of mindlessness (*unmanīkaraṇaṃ*), is the absorption (*laya*) in the essence of tranquility for the sage" (*YS* 15/99).[15] Later in the same chapter, the author states, "Just as a traveler scorched by the sun finds relief upon reaching a good tree, in the same way, a yogi who has undergone penance (*tapas*) and is on the path of liberation attains the supreme dissolution (*paraṃ layam*)" (*YS* 30/114).[16]

By integrating concepts from *haṭhayoga* traditions such as the incorporation of specific no-mind terminology (*laya*) common in haṭhayogic texts of the same era, the *Yogasāra* demonstrates a willingness to engage with and adapt ideas that resonate with the core principles of Jain thought. The utilization of these terms in the *Yogasāra* further indicates a nuanced understanding of meditative states and processes, aligning with the Jain emphasis on internal spiritual experience and the progression toward liberation. This underscores Jainism's capacity to maintain doctrinal integrity while fostering dialogue with a spectrum of yogic philosophies and practices.

Laya and the Unstruck Sound (*anāhata-nāda*) in the *Yogapradīpa*: The Bell and the Uninterrupted Flow of Oil

Verse 116 of the *Yogapradīpa* stands out as particularly intriguing, as it offers a concept of *dhyāna* characterized by the analogy of an uninterrupted flow of oil or the resonant, prolonged sound of a bell, a metaphor that echoes and can be traced back to similar depictions found in other traditional sources: "Uninterrupted like the flow of oil, like the long sound of a bell, he who knows this as the dissolution (*laya*) of the sound of *oṃ*, he is a yogi" (*YP* 116).[17] This imagery is not unique to the *Yogapradīpa* but has roots presumably in the classical exegesis of the *Bhagavadgītā* by Śaṅkara, as given in his commentary on *Bhagavadgītā* (*BhG*) 13.24: "Meditation (*dhyāna*) is a continuous and unbroken thought (*avicchinnapratyaya*), like a stream of oil (*tailadhārāvat*)" (*BhG* 13:24).[18] The later *Yogayājñavalkya* (*YY*), traceable to its earliest manuscript from the tenth century CE, presents an even more strikingly similar verse to the one we find in the *Yogapradīpa*: "Like an uninterrupted continuous flow of oil, like the long sound of a bell, he who knows this as the most prominent (*agra*) sound of *oṃ* (*pranava*), not produced by the voice (*avāgjaṃ*), he is a knower/ he who knows the Veda (*vedavit*)" (*YY* 117 and 118).[19]

Noteworthy in this intertextual dialogue is the *Yogapradīpa*'s deliberate substitution of *veda* with *yoga*, and the subsequent shift from *vedavit* ("one who knows the Veda") to *yogavit* ("one who knows yoga"), emphasizing the Jain orientation toward a soteriology not anchored in Vedic authority but in the direct experiential knowledge of the soul. The wordplay of *veda sa vedavit* loses its double entendre and is pragmatically adapted to *yas taṃ vetti, sa yogavit,* reinforcing the Jain doctrinal emphasis on individual, personal spiritual experience as the path to liberation.

This nuanced substitution underscores the Jain text's departure from Vedic primacy, as also discussed by Ellen Gough in an unpublished article.[20] Through her analysis of *Dhyānvicār*, a study by Śvetāmbara Tapāgaccha Ācārya Kalāpūrṇasūri, it is evident that the *Yogapradīpa* is recognized for aligning the *anāhata-nāda*, or the unstruck sound, with the soul's direct experience. Gough states that in "including 'yoga' instead of 'Veda,' the *Yogapradīpa* rejects the primacy of the Vedas and promotes Jain soteriology" (2021, 10). Gough observes that verse 116 of the *Yogapradīpa* also echoes verse 18 of the *Dhyānabindu Upaniṣad* (*DU*), a text belonging to a corpus of yoga Upaniṣads that have been chronologically situated in the seventeenth century (Mallinson 2014, 238):[21] "He who understands that the true essence of *oṃ* lies in its silence truly comprehends the Veda, likened to an unbroken flow of oil or the continuous toll of a bell" (*DU* 18)[22] (Gough 2021, 10).

Prior to discussing the concept of *anāhata-nāda*, the *Yogapradīpa* clearly defines yoga within the Jain framework of liberation, identifying it with the foundational principles of right perception, knowledge, and conduct. Consequently, the text integrates the meditative focus on the dissolution of *nāda* as a critical element within the Jain schema of spiritual liberation. This analysis, as meticulously presented by Gough, underscores the ability of the Jain text's author to reinterpret and integrate *nāda* within the Jain tradition's soteriological framework (2021, 10).

Conclusion

This brief exploration of the *Yogapradīpa* and the *Yogasāra* reveals the nuanced ways in which Jain authors of meditation and yoga have engaged with broader yogic traditions, reflecting Jainism's adaptability and its simultaneous commitment to its doctrinal distinctiveness. This simultaneous synthesis and distinctiveness of ideas not only positions Jain Yoga within the larger religious landscape of India but also underscores its contributions to the diversity of thought in second-millennium yoga traditions. The texts analyzed here exemplify Jain thinkers' capacity to integrate external influences while maintaining the Jain tradition's own soteriological goals.

Instead of presenting a singular, absolute path to spiritual realization, the *Yogapradīpa* acknowledges the diversity of spiritual experiences and the individuality of the meditative journey, aligning with the Jain ethos of embracing multiple truths and perspectives (*anekāntavāda*). And yet, both the *Yogapradīpa* and the *Yogasāra* maintained a distinctive commitment to Jain soteriology: The Jain texts under examination adopt haṭhayogic practices and concepts aimed at nonduality but repurpose them toward distinct Jain soteriological objectives grounded in a pluralistic ontology. Therefore, while texts such as the *Haṭhapradīpikā* may represent a "fortuitous union of non-dualities" aimed at a universal experience of *samādhi* (Mallinson 2014), Jain texts utilize *haṭhayoga*'s practices aimed at nonduality to underscore the *duality* between the soul (*jīva*) and non-soul (*ajīva*). Indeed, while discussing *laya*, *anāhata-nāda*, and *samādhi*, the *Yogapradīpa* may parallel classical (*haṭha*-) yoga descriptions in its portrayal of the transcendental state achieved through meditation, but it also infuses this discussion with a uniquely Jain perspective, which respects the complexity and plurality of spiritual experiences and the individuality of the soul (*jīva*).

Notes

1. All translations are my own unless otherwise noted.

2. James Mallinson defines *haṭhayoga* as follows: "*Haṭhayoga* is a Sanskrit term used in Indian texts from approximately the twelfth century onwards to denote a type of yoga in which physical practices predominate. Between the fourteenth and eighteenth centuries *haṭhayoga* was gradually assimilated into several mainstream Indian religious traditions" (Mallinson 2021, 2526). While Jain Yoga texts from this time period appear to lack overt characteristics of *haṭhayoga*'s physical practices, my research reveals subtle yet significant exchanges of ideas and methodologies discernible within the textual evidence.

3. Concerning the dating of the *Uttarādhyayanasūtra* and the *Sūtrakṛtāṅgasūtra*, Jacobi vaguely concludes that the texts "were collected in course of time, probably in the first centuries before our era, and that additions or alterations may have been made in the canonical works till their time of the first edition under Devardhiganin (980 A.V. = 454 A.D.)" (Jacobi 1968, xl), while Samani Pratibha Pragya follows the traditional dating "fourth century BCE" for the *Sūtrakṛtāṅgasūtra* (Pratibha Pragya 2021, 171).

4. *jñānadarśanacāritrarūparatnatrayātmakaḥ | yogo muktipadaprāptāv upāyaḥ parikīrtitaḥ ||* (Kośī 1960, 57).

5. In his article, Dundas describes how Jain communities from the early centuries CE strategically used vernacular Prakrits like Ardhamagadhi to establish a distinct identity from the Sanskrit-centric brahmanical culture. Over time, as Prakrit languages became standardized yet less understood by the masses, Jains, responding to changing linguistic landscapes, embraced Sanskrit. This shift was particularly evident from the twelfth to the seventeenth centuries, as Jains adapted Sanskrit for various literary forms, tailoring its grammar to suit their unique narrative and doctrinal expressions. Starting in the second millennium CE and predominantly in the medieval period, there was a notable shift back to vernacular languages, particularly Old Gujarati, which served not only to make Jain texts more accessible to broader audiences but also to maintain a resonant cultural and doctrinal connection within the region.

6. Mallinson summarizes these physical methods as follows: ". . . are used to make the breath enter the central channel and to raise *bindu*, semen, up to its source in the head and keep it there" (Mallinson 2014, 226).

7. Jason Birch has pointed out the importance of the *Hathapradīpikā*: "Svātmārāma incorporated a larger repertoire of techniques than earlier works and synthesized diverse teachings of various yoga traditions into a cohesive system, which he called *Haṭhayoga*" (Birch 2020b, 455).

8. *rājayogaḥ samādhiś ca unmanī ca manonmanī | amaraugho'pi cādvaitaṃ nirālambaṃ nirañjanam || amanasko layas tattvaṃ śūnyāśūnyaṃ paraṃ padam | jīvanmuktiś ca sahajaṃ turyaṃ cety ekavācakāḥ || ekavācakāḥ* (Hanneder and Mallinson, 2024, trans. by Hanneder and Mallinson 2024).

9. *anāhatadhvaner antar jñeyaṃ yat sūkṣmasūkṣmakam | manas tatra layaṃ yāti tad viṣṇoḥ paramaṃ padam ||* (Hanneder and Mallinson 2024, trans. by Hanneder and Mallinson 2024).

10. *brāhmaṇaḥ śramaṇo vāpi bauddho vāpy ārhato 'thavā | kāpāliko vā cārvākaḥ śraddhayā sahitaḥ sudhīḥ || yogābhyāsarato nityaṃ sarvasiddhim avāpnuyāt | kriyāyuktasya siddhiḥ syād akriyasya kathaṃ bhavet ||*

11. This is the conclusion of the current author based on the age of the manuscripts that the author was able to retrieve.

12. *śuddhasphaṭikasaṃkāśaḥ sarvajñaguṇabhūṣitaḥ | paramātmākalāyukto dhyeyaḥ svātmā manīṣibhiḥ ||* (Kośī 1960, 8).

13. *buddho vā yadi vā viṣṇur yad vā brahmāthaveśvaraḥ | ucyatāṃ sa jinendro vā nārthabhedas tathāpi hi | mamaiva devo devaḥ syāt tava naiveti kevalam | matsarasphūrjitaṃ sarvam ajñānānāṃ vijṛmbhitam |* (Bhadrankarvijay 1967, 28).

14. *brāhmaṇair lakṣyate brahmā viṣṇuḥ pītāmbarais tathā | rudras tapasvibhir dṛṣṭa eṣa eva nirañjanaḥ |* (Kośī 1960, 18).

15. *sahajānandatā seyaṃ saivātmārāmatā matā | unmanīkaraṇaṃ tad yad muneḥ śamarase layaḥ* | (Bhadrankarvijay 1967, 28).

16. *sadvṛkṣaṃ prāpya nirvāti ravitapto yathā'dhvagaḥ | mokṣādhvasthas tapas taptas tathā yogī paraṃ layam* | (Bhadrankarvijay 1967, 28).

17. *tailadhārām ivācchinnam dīrghaghāṇṭāninādavat | layaṃ praṇavanādasya yas taṃ vetti, sa yogavit* | (Kośī 1960, 18).

18. *tailadhārāvat saṃtato'vicchinnapratyayo dhyānam* (Vasudeva 2016, 23).

19. *tailadhārāvad acchinnaṃ dīrghaghāṇṭāninādavat | avāgjaṃ praṇavasyāgraṃ yas taṃ veda sa vedavit* (Vasudeva 2016, 10).

20. Ellen Gough, "The Jain Yogapradīpa and the Depiction of Silence," unpublished article, sent to the author on Nov. 11, 2023.

21. There is another work that contains two verses that bear great similarity to verse 116 of the *Yogapradīpa*: The *Yogacūḍāmaṇi Upaniṣad*, the "Crown Jewel of Yoga," also part of the corpus of yoga Upaniṣads originating in the early eighteenth century. Notably, it replicates the opening line, *tailadhārām ivācchinnaṃ dīrghaghāṇṭāninādavat*, and concludes with a parallel phrase, *yas tam veda sa vedavit*, akin to that in the *Yogayājñavalkya*. This textual resemblance might suggest that the *Yogacūḍāmaṇi Upaniṣad* similarly draws from the earlier source, illustrating the prevalent sharing of philosophical concepts not only within but also across different spiritual traditions.

22. *tailadhārām ivācchinnaṃ dīrghaghaṇṭāninādavat | avācyaṃ praṇavasyāgraṃ yas taṃ veda sa vedavit* | (trans. by Gough 2021, 10).

References

Bhadrankarvijay, and Amrutlal Kalidas Doshi, eds. 1967. *Yogasāra*. Jaina Sāhitya Vikāsa Maṇḍala.

Birch, Jason. 2013. *The Amanaska: King of All Yogas: A Critical Edition and Annotated Translation with a Monographic Introduction*. DPhil diss., University of Oxford.

———. 2020a. "The Quest for Liberation-in-Life." In *Hindu Practice*, edited by Gavin Flood. Oxford University Press.

———. 2020b. "Haṭhayoga's Floruit on the Eve of Colonialism." In *Śaivism and the Tantric Traditions: Essays in Honour of Alexis G. J. S. Sanderson*, edited by Dominic Godall, Shaman Hatley, Harunaga Isaacson, and Raman Srilata. Brill.

Birch, Jason, and Jacqueline Hargreaves. 2017. "The Yogapradīpa: A Premodern Jain 'Light on Yoga.'" *The Luminescent*, March 7. https://www.theluminescent.org/2017/03/the-yogapradipa-premodern-jain-light-on.html.

Bouy, Christian. 1994. *Les Nātha-yogin et les Upaniṣads: Étude d'histoire de la littérature hindoue*. Collège de France, Institut de civilisation indienne.

Bronkhorst, Johannes. 2007. *Greater Magadha: Studies in the Culture of Early India*. Brill.

Cestola, Rocco. 2024. "Fading into Death Through Pātañjalayoga: On the Apparent Dead-Like State of the Yoga Practitioner Absorbed into Contentless Samādhi." In *Journal of Yoga Studies [Online]* 5 (May 2).

Digambaraji, Swami, ed. 2016. *Hathapradīpīkā of Svātmārāma*. 3rd ed. Kaivalyadhama, S. M. Y. M. Samiti.

Dixit, K. K. 1970. *The Yogadṛṣṭisamuccaya and Yogaviṃ śika of Ācārya Haribhadrasūri*. Lalbhai Dalpatbhai Bharatiya Sanskriti Vidyamandira.

Dundas, Paul. 2020. "Jainism and Language Usage." In *Brill's Encyclopedia of Jainism*, edited by John E. Cort, Paul Dundas, Knuth A. Jacobsen, and Kristi L. Wiley. Koninklijke Brill N. V.

Gough, Ellen. 2021. "The Jain Yogapradīpa and the Depiction of Silence." Unpublished article.

Hanneder, Jürgen, and James Mallinson. 2024. *Light on Hatha Yoga: A Critical Edition and Translation of the Haṭhapradīpikā, the Most Important Premodern Text on Physical Yoga.* Project founded by Arts and Humanities Research Council (AHRC) and the German Research Foundation Deutsche Forschungsgemeinschaft (DFG). http://hathapradipika.online/.

Jacobi, Hermann, trans. 1968. *Jaina Sutras, Part II: The Uttarâdhyayana Sûtra; The Sûtrakritâṅga Sûtra*. Dover edition. Dover.

Jain, Sagarmal. 2016. "The Historical Development of the Jaina Yoga System and the Impacts of Other Yoga Systems on Jaina Yoga. A Comparative and Critical Study." In *Yoga in Jainism*, edited by Christopher Key Chapple. Routledge.

Jambūvijaya, Muni, ed. 1977, 1981, 1986. *Yogaśāstra and Svopajñavṛtti*. Vols. 1–3. Jaina Sāhitya Vikāsa Maṇḍala.

Kośī, Amṛtlāl Kālidās, ed. 1960. *The Yogapradīpa*. Jaina Sāhitya Vikāsa Maṇḍala.

Maas, Philipp André. 2020. "Pātañjalayogaśāstra." In *Brill's Encyclopedia of Hinduism Online*, edited by Knut A. Jacobsen, Helene Basu, Angelika Malinar, and Vasudha Narayanan. http://dx.doi.org/10.1163/2212-5019_BEH_COM_1010071178.

Mallinson, James. 2014. "Haṭhayoga's Philosophy: A Fortuitous Union of Non-Dualities." *Journal of Indian Philosophy* 42, no. 1 (March): 225–247.

———. 2021. "Yoga: Haṭha." In *The Encyclopedia of Philosophy of Religion*, edited by Stewart Goetz and Charles Taliaferro. Wiley-Blackwell.

Mallinson, James, and Mark Singleton. 2017. *Roots of Yoga*. Penguin.

Pratibha Pragya, Samani. 2021. "Yoga and Meditation in the Jain tradition." In *Routledge Handbook of Yoga and Meditation Studies*, edited by Suzanne Newcombe and Karen O'Brien-Kop. Routledge.

Qvarnström, Olle. 2012. *A Handbook on the Three Jewels of Jainism: The Yogaśāstra of Hemacandra*. Revised and expanded edition. Hindi Granth Karyalay.

Vasudeva, Somadeva. 2016. "The Yogayājñavalkya." HYP Workshop, presentation handout. All Souls College, Sept. 16, 2016. http://hyp.soas.ac.uk/all-souls-2017-somadeva-vasudeva/.

16

The Anuvrat Movement

A Case of Socially Engaged Jainism

SHIVANI BOTHRA

Scholars have recently begun to show interest in the Anuvrat Movement in the growing body of Western scholarship on Jainism (cf. Qvarnström and Birch 2012; Bothra 2013; Jain 2016; Kothari 2016; Reading 2019; 2020). The movement is sometimes referred to casually in the context of sectarian branches. At other times, it is regarded in a general way as another Śvetāmbara Terāpantha innovation or outreach program. Therefore, there remains a need for a more comprehensive exploration of the movement and its implications across various facets of human experience—political, economic, socio-ethical, and environmental. Adopting the constructive-reproductive model of engaged Jain studies (see Miller's introduction to this volume), this chapter contributes to this objective by offering a concise historical overview of the movement, outlining eleven *aṇuvrata* vows associated with it and analyzing how these vows can be engaged to address contemporary global crises.

Understanding Jainism's Role in Social Change

Traditionally, *ahiṃsā* is a quintessential Jain ethical principle of inaction for the purification of the soul (cf. Bronkhorst 2007). Keeping this principle as a central focus, the late Acharya Tulsi's (1914–1997) Anuvrat Movement reconceived traditional Jain vows oriented around *ahiṃsā,* formulating eleven vows for Jains, as a practical form of active engagement in spirituality and ethical living. These vows could also serve as resolutions for non-Jains. In this chapter, I argue that while the Anuvrat Movement (henceforth referred to as AM) did not explicitly manifest as a politically or socially active movement, it encompasses elements that resonate with what we might refer to as a form of socially engaged Jainism. I will show how Tulsi tackled the task of rebuilding post-independence India and will examine whether his AM can address contemporary global issues, such as social inequality, political corruption, economic instability, environmental degradation, and sustainability. With this background, the chapter poses two fundamental questions: (1) How can a mass movement, rooted in a complex system of vows, bring about social change? (2) What distinguishes the AM from conventional perceptions of Jainism? The chapter shows AM as a nonsectarian, ethical movement that applies traditional principles in the framework of what we might refer to as engaged Jainism today. It further shows how the movement emerged as a distinctive phenomenon when Jainism was often perceived solely in terms of liberation or extreme asceticism. The institutionalization of the AM serves as a prime example of contemporary socially engaged Jainism and forms the central focus of this chapter.[1]

A key aspect distinguishing the Jain tradition from the diverse Indian traditions is its dedicated approach to both ascetic and lay practices. The ascetic path, which is encompassed by the *mahāvrata*s (higher vows), is distinct from the lay path that includes the *aṇuvrata* (lesser vows). The ascetic path comprises a relatively small number of monks and nuns. Despite the small numbers compared to the lay community, their impact on the tradition remains substantial. This significant influence and their visible presence have led scholars to characterize Jainism as a religion primarily centered on asceticism. Another factor feeding such a notion is the large number of canonical texts enumerating the conduct of monks and nuns compared to the later texts that expand on lay practices.

Nevertheless, since the 1990s, scholars have increasingly realized that the Jain tradition is complex and dynamic, not reducible to asceticism (cf. Cort 2001). Moreover, Acharya Tulsi's various social and spiritual initiatives compel us to revisit such notions in a new light. He argues for the social significance of Jain principles, particularly *ahiṃsā* (nonviolence), as the highest value with a universal appeal. He demonstrates the social dimension of *ahiṃsā* through the AM. Initially focused on middle-class and affluent Terāpanthī Jains, the movement gradually embraced individuals from all backgrounds to advocate a peaceful and just global society.[2] Let us explore how Tulsi addresses ethical, social, economic, and political concerns by developing a nonsectarian movement.

Origin of the Anuvrat Movement

This section sets the stage for discussing AM within the context of engaged Jainism. It proposes the need for a movement that transcends religious boundaries. It briefly introduces the founder's vision of applying Jain principles to address societal issues and economic instability. But first, let us begin with the fundamental questions: What is AM, who is the founder, and why did it emerge?

The AM is a nonreligious movement that was initiated by a sectarian monk leader, Acharya Tulsi, in a small town in Rajasthan in 1949. Unlike traditional religious movements, it does not impose any specific belief system or religious practices on its followers. The movement also does not interfere with an individual's belief system or ritualistic practices. Instead, it respects freedom to worship in one's chosen manner, be it in temples, mosques, churches, or other places of worship. The movement primarily focuses on developing character through ethical engagement in one's personal and commercial/work life. In that sense, the AM favors *samyak-cāritra* (right conduct), although without disparaging *samyak-jñāna* (right knowledge) or *samyak-darśana* (right vision), which all together comprise the threefold Jaina path to liberation. In fact, *aṇuvrata* seeks to bridge the gap between knowledge and conduct to build a healthy society (Vibha 2012).

The term *aṇuvrata* comprises two words: *aṇu*, meaning "small," and *vrata*, meaning "vow." Thus, the movement emphasizes the observance of smaller ethical commitments or resolutions in daily life rather than imposing rigid religious doctrines. Individuals without any discrimination of caste, color, creed, or region can be an Aṇuvratī (practitioner of the tradition). On May 15, 1950, at the first major gathering (*adhiveśana*) of Aṇuvratīs, founder Acharya Tulsi said, as reported in *The New York Times*, "If an atom (*aṇu*) has the demonic power to destroy the world, demonstrated in the unprecedented holocaust at Hiroshima and Nagasaki, I want to tell the world that we have its counterpart in *aṇuvrata*—atomic vow—which has the power to counter the threat of an atomic bomb" (Tulsi 1992, 137–138).

Acharya Tulsi was not known as an armchair philosopher but as a man of action with the sole concern of moral upliftment of humanity (Tulsi 1993, 1). As the ninth Śvetāmbara Terāpantha monk, Tulsi served as the leader of his community from 1936 to 1994, achieving a pan-Indian stature. He was a prolific poet and author of more than one hundred books, and he emerged as a distinguished twentieth-century religious leader. The tradition maintains a record of his 62,000 miles of walking, on foot, to spread AM, among other initiatives, and to inspire Indians toward ethical living. Qvarnström and Birch (2012) see this effort as part and parcel of the missionary nature of the movement.

In the mid-twentieth century, against the backdrop of global recovery from devastating world wars and colonization, India was also engaged in its own reconstruction process. In this post-independence era, the tragic demise of Mahatma Gandhi triggered outbreaks of violence that further compounded the challenges faced by the nascent nation. India grappled not only with the aftermath of colonialism but also with deep-seated issues of caste oppression, untouchability, sectarianism, communal tensions, and internal discord. This dark side of Indian society cast a pall over all aspects of life—social, religious, political, and economic—fueling widespread dissatisfaction with the emerging nation.

In response, many post-independence political and nonpolitical movements emerged, each aimed at addressing the prevailing challenges. Examples include the Bhoodan and Chipko Movements, which sought to tackle various environmental issues plaguing Indian society. Additionally, several social and religious reformers and leaders, such as Ram Manohar Lohia and Jayaprakash Narayan, stepped forward with action plans aimed at contributing to the enormous task of rebuilding India. Similarly, Acharya Tulsi became disillusioned with the prevailing human psyche characterized by selfishness, excessive competitiveness, over-consumerism, and the pursuit of profits through unethical means. These, along with the preceding conditions prevalent in post-independence India, served as the driving factor for the inception of the movement. Therefore, inspired by Gandhian thought and with the goal of rebuilding India, Acharya Tulsi expanded the scope of traditional vows beyond the religious realm, applying Jain values to address the pressing issues of the time. He believed that he could draw from his own tradition, which would raise individual moral consciousness, lead to societal purification, and ultimately prepare the ground for broader global changes.

In August 1948, on the anniversary of India's independence, Acharya Tulsi issued a public call urging Indians to embrace true freedom (*asalī āzādī apanāo*) as a means of awakening their consciousness. Through this slogan, he emphasized the importance of character development and self-determination. At this event, a young man asked, "Is it possible to lead a moral life in today's time?" This inquiry, coupled with the slogan, marked the inception of the AM, officially introduced in March 1949 from a small town in Rajasthan, India. In explaining Acharya Tulsi's vision of the AM, Sādhavī Kaṇakprabhā notes that neglecting ethical values undermines the effectiveness of infrastructural development and will not resolve problems. For any nation, infrastructural growth is crucial to enhance the economic status of the public. However, what is even more important is fostering ethical and moral values. Without advancing in the highest morality, material progress lacks meaningful significance (Kanakprabha 2005).

The above view suggests that Tulsi was not opposed to advancing or raising the economic standards of the Indian public. Rather, he aimed to complement the existing practices with a broader moral framework to elevate their character. This inclusive ethos is vividly depicted on the cover page of the book, which documents fifty years of Tulsi's journey with an emphasis on the movement. The book cover features Acharya Tulsi alongside two monks against the backdrop of a diverse gathering of the Indian public. At the center of attention is a wheel adorned with spokes bearing religious symbols representing Hinduism, Sikhism, Islam,

Christianity, and Jainism—prominent traditions in India. The book's cover and title, *Turning the Wheel of Dharma* (*Dharam Cakra Ke Pravartan*), exemplify the movement's commitment to engaging Jain principles and inclusivity (Mahāprajña 1997).

In the beginning, Acharya Tulsi encountered the difficult situation of naming the movement. The name was important to him, as it would define and defend the movement. He was aware that if he chose a term drawn directly from his own tradition, then the movement might appear sectarian and lose its wider appeal. Conversely, adopting a term like "nonviolent" could overlook the nuanced essence of small vows, which formed the core of the movement. Striving to bridge tradition with contemporary relevance, he envisioned *aṇuvrata* as a catalyst for societal wellness, emphasizing the cultivation of ethical values and individual transformation through self-discipline. His aim was not to sever ties with tradition but to reinterpret it in a way that resonated with the multireligious Indian society. *Aṇuvrata*, therefore, emerges not merely as a name but as a philosophy encapsulating the ideals of harmony, self-improvement, and collective betterment. Through embracing small vows, adherents embark on a journey of personal regeneration, contributing to the fabric of a more compassionate and virtuous society. Acharya Tulsi's vision transcends mere nomenclature, embodying a profound commitment to both tradition and progressive change.

Core Principles of the Anuvrat Movement

The Traditional Vow System

Whether we are speaking of the *mahāvrata* (great vows for renunciates) or the *aṇuvrata* (lesser vows for laity), the concept of vows constitutes a fundamental aspect of Jain practice—both in its spiritual dimensions and in its socially engaged forms. The *mahāvrata* are meant to be absolute and permanent, whereas the *aṇuvrata* are goals that laypersons strive to attain and could be undertaken for limited periods of time, depending on one's capacity, in order to bring one closer to the ideal way of life exemplified by the renunciates. The vows are constructed as follows: *ahiṃsā* (nonviolence), in which the renunciates vow not to destroy any life and the laity vow to take care whenever possible to minimize harming life; *satya* (truthfulness), in which the renunciates vow not to lie and the laity vow to take care and not to behave in a deceitful way or to spread gossip; *asteya* (non-stealing), in which the renunciates vow not to take what is not given and the laity vow not to covet or steal the possessions of others; *brahmacarya* (celibacy), in which the renunciates vow to abstain from sexual relationships, and the laity vow not to commit adultery and to be modest; and *aparigraha* (non/limited possession), in which the renunciates vow to renounce all interest in worldly things and the laity vow to limit their possessions to only what is essential whenever possible. The difference in the above scheme of vows lies in the intensity of practice. From this description, the laity's vows can be regarded as the Jain middle path. Acharya Tulsi used these five categories of vows as a foundation for his movement because they have been pervasive in many religious traditions in India.

Reinterpreting the Role of Religion

Clearly, the vows are meant to stress proper conduct. While the scholarship of William Robertson Smith carries many Eurocentric assumptions, he offers a helpful insight when he notes that "religion did not exist for saving of souls but for the preservation and welfare of society" (1927, 29). While he was referring to Judaism, Christianity, and Islam, Smith's insight concerning the importance of religion's behavioral function also applies to Tulsi's non-transcendental approach. Tulsi neither explicitly associated his movement with any religion nor rejected religion; instead, he reinterpreted religion according to contemporary needs. In a personal communication, one senior nun associated with the movement from its early stages authoritatively summed up Tulsi's behavioral approach to religion as follows:

> Acharya Tulsi unraveled three fundamental aspects of religion: First, religion is ritualistic and limited to a sacred space like a temple, church, synagogue, or monastery

> where people offer prayer or worship. Secondly, religion is ethical, which guides one to distinguish between right and wrong deeds. Thirdly, religion is spiritual, which leads a practitioner to raise his consciousness and lead a pure life. The AM does not interfere with any ritualistic practice. However, it only seeks to inspire people to adopt ethical values like restraining from telling lies, cheating people, violence, etc., to lead a spiritual life. (Rajimatī 2012)

Transitioning Vows to Resolutions

One major way the movement embodies the philosophy of vows is encapsulated in AM's slogan: "Self-restraint is life." The majority of monks and nuns I interacted with emphasized this slogan. Interestingly, one nun in her interview quoted Mahāprajña[3] and said "Self-restraint is life, and an unrestrained life is death. Vows develop self-control, and modern-day diseases are caused by an unrestrained lifestyle" (Kanakshri 2013).

The discussion thus far has established that the Tulsian movement is rooted in the lesser vows (*aṇuvrata*). However, it does not clarify how this traditional scheme differentiates from the Tulsian vow system. On further inquiry, a non-Jain responded: "There is a metaphysical difference between the two sets of vows. The prime objective of the *aṇuvrata* vows, as elucidated in *Śrāvakācāra*,[4] is the liberation of the soul (*mokṣa*), whereas the objective of the AM is the purification of the soul" (Bhargava 2012). He further explained that the traditional vows are tied to a belief system and require a higher degree of self-restraint as compared to Tulsi's version of *aṇuvrata* vows. The views convey that the AM has deviated from the traditional understanding of the Jain path and its goals for the laity. Thus, the Tulsian vows were a new approach to generating the spirit of self-restraint among the masses.

I turn now to the action-oriented eleven vows that form the kernel of the AM. In today's global society, some socially harmful customs and practices persist despite efforts to address them. I have therefore included some of the global implications of Tulsi's vows below. A comprehensive examination of the vows must encompass their potential impact and efficacy in tackling these multifaceted challenges (Tulsi 1993).[5]

Jainism in Action

The first vow states: *I will not intentionally kill any innocent creature. I will not commit suicide, and I will not commit feticide.* This vow clearly belongs to the category of *ahiṃsā*, exhibiting great reverence for all living beings. The traditional *ahiṃsā* vow entails five infractions: "The treatment of humans and animals in one's care and include holding beings in captivity, beating, mutilating or branding, loading excessive weight on the back or head and providing insufficient food or water" (Jaini 1979, 173). This vow, primarily focused on safeguarding animals, was particularly relevant in an agrarian-centric India where household practices relied heavily on agricultural activities. In the AM of the mid-twentieth century, Tulsi expanded on the *ahiṃsā* vow by specifically singling out the issues of suicide and abortion, as he was aware that they were topics of great public debate in modern Indian society, in addition to those related to animals.

This commitment to nonviolence, particularly in the context of AM, epitomizes engaged Jainism—a philosophy that transcends individual practice to address contemporary societal concerns. Tulsi's expansion of the *ahiṃsā* vow to encompass issues like suicide and abortion reflects a proactive engagement with pressing issues of modern Indian society. By incorporating these challenges into the vow, Tulsi not only acknowledges their significance but also advocates for compassionate responses grounded in Jain ethical principles. Moreover, the vow has important global implications, addressing issues of gender-based violence, including practices such as domestic violence, sexual assault, female genital mutilation, and forced marriage, which disproportionately affect women and girls worldwide.

The second vow, which states that *I will not attack anybody, support aggression, and endeavor to bring about world peace and disarmament,* is also a continuum in the commitment to nonviolence. Here, Tulsi is again acknowledging a widespread modern concern about combating the fears of terrorism and traumas of war inflicted upon humanity. Tulsi imagined that the Jain experiences with the action of taking vows could be beneficial to secular society when combined with a willingness to be consciously aware of how actions, whether actions of an individual or of a whole nation, affect other beings. Mahāprajña provides an analogy of a house where these small vows are like screens or covers, which protect the interior against the detriments of variable weather patterns. By undertaking a vow, an individual redirects his or her energy inward and attempts to fight the coercive power of hatred, jealousy, anger, and greed that reside within oneself. With children being recruited and forced to participate in armed conflicts that expose them to violence, trauma, and long-term psychological harm, this vow also has important global implications.

The third vow—*I will not participate in violent agitations or any destructive activities*—is once again rooted in the principle of nonviolence, addressing a pertinent social issue in India's diverse, post-independence society. Instances of violent protests, such as the burning of police vehicles or vandalism in educational institutions, underscore the prevalence of extreme emotional turmoil. However, these destructive acts often overlook the long-term consequences and the essential needs they jeopardize. Engaged Jainism prompts us to consider how undertaking such a vow can curtail individual participation in such detrimental activities. The vow is relevant for global issues such as the recruitment and transportation of individuals for forced labor or sexual exploitation, as well as organ trafficking.

While falling under the umbrella of *ahiṃsā*, the fourth vow—*I will believe in human unity. I will not discriminate based on caste, color, etc., and I will not treat anyone as an untouchable*—also encompasses elements of *satya* (truth), inviting profound reflection on a fundamental question concerning humanity. The notion of inherent disparities based on factors such as caste, creed, color, or sex, stemming from circumstances beyond individual control, challenges the very essence of human equality. The Tulsian AM, as an example of engaged Jainism, prompts us to confront such societal constructs and question the underlying theories that perpetuate these divisions within humanity. The entrenched caste system in India, delineated initially by birth or profession, has persisted across Indian society. However, the interpretation and implementation of this system have often exacerbated disparities rather than promoting social cohesion. By undertaking this vow, individuals commit to challenging and dismantling systems of discrimination and inequality. Engaged Jainism calls upon adherents to actively advocate for truth and equality, fostering a more inclusive and compassionate society grounded in the principles of nonviolence and truthfulness. In terms of its global implications, this vow touches upon issues such as persistent discrimination and prejudice based on race, ethnicity, religion, gender identity, sexual orientation, or socioeconomic status in various forms, which lead to and sustain inequalities and marginalization.

The fifth vow, which enjoins followers to *practice religious toleration* and *not rouse a sectarian frenzy*, is similar to the fourth vow and demonstrates Tulsi's commitment to modernizing Jain principles by addressing a specific challenge prevalent in pluralistic Indian society: interreligious violence and intra-religious conflicts. Despite evolving circumstances, issues of hatred and intolerance toward other sects and religions persist. Furthermore, Tulsi's emphasis on raising awareness of internal prejudices within his own community signifies his unwavering dedication to fostering inclusivity and harmony. Engaged Jainism encourages introspection and action, challenging adherents to confront and overcome sectarianism and minor disputes within Jainism itself. Through this vow, Acharya Tulsi's tireless efforts to resolve sectarianism within Jainism are underscored, reflecting the principles of engaged Jainism that advocate for proactive engagement with societal challenges and the promotion of unity and understanding. Globally, this vow provides a guideline to navigate contemporary societies that are increasingly marked by religious, cultural, and ethnic pluralism, diversity, complexity, and mixing.

Amalgamating principles of *ahiṃsā*, *satya* (truth), and *aparigraha* (limited possession), the sixth vow states: *I will observe rectitude in business and general behavior. I will not harm others to serve any ends, and I will not practice deceit.* This vow reflects AM's commitment to ethical conduct in all facets of life, including business practices. Rooted in the framework of engaged Jainism, it discourages individuals from resorting to unethical or immoral means to maximize profit. Within the business community, adherence to this vow entails refraining from engaging in activities such as trading stolen goods, using deceptive measures such as false weights or adulteration, evading taxes, and accepting bribes. My discussions with informants underscored the significance that Acharya Tulsi placed on righteousness in business dealings, emphasizing the importance of upholding moral integrity in economic transactions. By embodying this vow, individuals align themselves with the principles of engaged Jainism, actively promoting ethical behavior and social responsibility within the business sphere. Adherents are expected to create a more just and equitable society guided by the values of nonviolence, truthfulness, and non-possession. On a broader scope, this vow may serve to counter corruption in government, business, and society, which undermines democracy, economic development, and social justice, perpetuating inequality and injustice.

In the context of engaged Jainism, the seventh vow—*I will set limits to the practice of continence and acquisition*—delves deeper into the principle of *aparigraha* (limited possession) and extends to the realm of *brahmacarya* (celibacy) or controlling sexual behavior. Unlike the sixth vow, which primarily focuses on ethical conduct in business dealings, the seventh vow encompasses a broader scope, emphasizing the need to overcome internal emotions such as anger, ego, greed, and deceit.

Tulsi emphasized that these detrimental passions are often the root causes of violence and discord in society. By accepting the seventh vow, individuals commit not only to limiting external possessions but also to restraining negative emotions. While the complete eradication of these emotions may be challenging, the vow encourages individuals to exercise control over them, ensuring that they do not dictate one's actions. Through this vow, the founder strives to cultivate inner harmony and promote peaceful coexistence within society. By setting limits on passions and restraining negative emotions, individuals contribute to the creation of a more compassionate and equitable world guided by the principles of nonviolence and self-restraint.

Within the framework of engaged Jainism, the eighth vow enjoins AM followers *not to resort to unethical practices in elections,* highlighting ethical considerations that underscore the transformative potential of politics. Tulsi astutely acknowledged the pervasive corruption and instability prevalent in post-independence India, recognizing their detrimental impact on individuals' quality of life. His unwavering commitment to positive change, inspired by the principles of his vows, propelled him to engage in political spheres with the aim of fostering societal improvement.

It is noteworthy to witness a religious leader transition from advocating for work ethics to applying ethics in politics to cleanse the political environment. Through this transition, Tulsi exemplified the principles of engaged Jainism, demonstrating how ethical values can be applied to political change around issues ranging from marginalization and discrimination against groups such as Indigenous peoples, refugees, migrants, and people with disabilities. Often, marginalized groups are manipulated, even coerced, during elections.

With the ninth vow, AM members pledge *not to encourage socially evil customs*. Like the preceding vows, this vow aligns with *ahiṃsā*, despite not directly involving harm to sentient or non-sentient beings. Acharya Tulsi seeks to highlight the potential indirect harm caused by certain socially entrenched customs in societies. Practices such as purdah (the veiling of women and restrictions on their public presence), dowry (the payment of money to the groom's family upon marriage), and the stigmatization of widows, which can lead to gender-based violence and female feticide, are among those scrutinized by Tulsi. Hence, he introduced many reforms through his movement aimed at fostering a more equitable and progressive society. These initiatives included simplifying birth, death, and marriage ceremonies; promoting female literacy; and abolishing purdah. While acknowledging the role of tradition in shaping social identity, Tulsi urged his followers to examine customs critically, raise awareness of their potential harm, and remain open to reform when necessary. The application of this vow can be extended to practices such as child marriage, which, despite legal prohibitions in many countries, persists, depriving young girls of their rights, education, and prospects.

Reflecting Acharya Tulsi's commitment to ethical conduct, AM's tenth vow imposes an unequivocal prohibition on intoxication and addictions, banning the use of alcohol, hemp, heroin, tobacco, etc. Rooted in the principles of engaged Jainism, this vow is underpinned by the belief that intoxicants obscure the clarity of the mind and tarnish one's character. Tulsi recognized that intoxication increases the likelihood of engaging in undesirable or criminal behavior, such as suicide, rape, or mass violence. By instituting this vow, Tulsi sought to address the pervasive issues of alcohol abuse and intoxication prevalent in society. Engaged Jainism emphasizes the importance of self-restraint and moral integrity in navigating the complexities of contemporary life. Adherents are encouraged to cultivate a clear and disciplined mind by prohibiting intoxication, fostering personal well-being, and contributing to a safer and more harmonious society.

The final vow—*I will be alert to the problems of keeping the environment pollution-free; I will not cut down trees and not waste water*—categorized under *ahiṃsā*—transcends individual well-being to encompass the preservation of the environment. In this commitment, Acharya Tulsi draws inspiration from Mahāvīra's concept of interdependence, recognizing the intricate web of connections among all living beings. Mahāvīra's teachings underscore humanity's interconnectedness with the elements of earth, air, fire, water, and vegetation. Neglecting the well-being of the environment ultimately jeopardizes our own existence. Furthermore, this vow stands in stark contrast to the resource-intensive and consumerist lifestyle prevalent in modern society. By pledging not to engage in deforestation and advocating for the prudent use of water resources, adherents of the AM align themselves with broader environmental movements, such as the Chipko Movement, which champion forest conservation. The final vow reflects a holistic commitment to *ahiṃsā,* extending compassion not only to sentient beings but also to the natural world. Through this vow, individuals reaffirm their responsibility to protect and preserve the environment, recognizing it as integral to their own well-being and the well-being of future generations. Arguably, this vow best exemplifies the AM's social dimensions. Environmental degradation, such as deforestation, pollution, overfishing, and unsustainable resource extraction, threatens ecosystems and biodiversity throughout the world, as well as human civilization at large.

In concluding the discussion on Acharya Tulsi's modified vows, it would be instructive to draw from Michael Tobias, a scholar of Jainism and professor of ecology, whose insights on self-restraint resonate deeply with the AM. Tobias emphasizes, "We humans are equipped with a conscience; we can make intelligent and sensitive choices . . . Amid the tumultuous sea of nature, we are like an island of choice . . . We can self-destruct or carry on. But we will not live on as a species if we fail to co-exist harmoniously with all other creatures sharing this island" (2000, 8). Tobias's reflection aligns seamlessly with the movement's central theme of *ahiṃsā* and the personalized practice of the small vows. Each of the eleven vows outlined above underscores the importance of making thoughtful decisions for both personal spiritual growth and global sustainability.

Assessing the Contemporary Relevance of the Movement

Undoubtedly, the *aṇuvrata* list of modified vows, its tone, and its examples make it appear as an Indian movement for uplifting the ethical and moral lives of the inhabitants of that country. However, while Tulsi's vows offer a timeless framework for ethical living, their relevance hinges on their adaptation to the evolving challenges faced by global societies. It is imperative to consider the implications of these vows in addressing pressing issues such as socioeconomic inequality and environmental degradation on a global scale. Tulsi introduced a concept that anyone could adopt to nurture their personal growth—a garden of self-development cultivated through the seeds of simplified small vows. The spirituality inherent in Tulsi's theory should be understood accurately and empathetically when viewed through a broader perspective.

Was it easy for a sectarian monk leader to devise a program that could presumably be applied to individuals regardless of any race, region, caste, or religion? Did he manage to achieve the desired transformation in his community and the nation at large? What were some of the challenges and criticisms that Tulsi encountered in his efforts to transcend religious boundaries? The discussion on the AM would be incomplete without addressing these questions.

From the start, Tulsi clarified that the social movement was not about converting people to Jainism or the Terāpanth tradition. He kept his approach nonsectarian. The movement holds on to the term *aṇuvrata,* which is rooted in Jain tradition because it best represents self-control and resolutions. Tulsi's approach to going beyond the Jain tradition raised questions from his followers and from members of other religions in India. Once, at a large gathering, someone asked him, "Are you Hindu or Muslim?" Tulsi replied, "I'm neither Hindu nor Muslim. I don't follow Hindu customs, nor do I practice Islamic traditions. I am a born human, and I am trying to conquer my inner passions and awaken myself, so I consider myself a Jain" (Mahāprajña 1997, 295).

The Anuvrat Movement: Success, Challenges, and Criticism

The Anuvrat Movement garnered praise from both Jains and non-Jains, yet it faced significant criticism from within Tulsi's own tradition. Let us first examine the success of the movement. The AM gained momentum gradually and achieved phenomenal success during the lifetime of its founder, Acharya Tulsi. This is evident in the six-hundred-page special issue commemorating fifty years of the *Anuvrat* monthly magazine. Over one hundred writers from various religious and nonreligious backgrounds contributed to this issue. In addition to tracing the trajectories of the movement, articles highlight Tulsi's efforts to engage with political and religious leaders of the time, effectively popularizing the movement amid other prominent Gandhian-led movements. The movement's success reminds us again of Max Weber's theory of the positive association between the exemplary charismatic role of a leader and the popularity and longevity of social movements in India.[6]

Let us now examine the criticisms. Jains traditionally see *aṇuvrata* as something exclusively Jain and timeless. Therefore, using it as a tool for a mass social movement was unacceptable to orthodox Terāpanthīs. Additionally, Tulsi's unclear strategies further fueled criticism, leading learned Jains to oppose his movement on theological grounds. Two main objections were highlighted in a special issue of *Anuvrat* magazine: First, Jain teachers stressed the importance of having the right understanding (*samyaktva*) before accepting the vows, and second, they believed that Acharya Tulsi was attempting to convert non-Jains to Jainism or the Terāpanth tradition.

The first objection stemmed from the radical perspective of Terāpanth regarding worldly (*laukika*) and transcendental (*lokkottara*) *dharma*.[7] Critics saw Tulsi as a sectarian monk who was involving himself in worldly affairs through the social movement. Tulsi defended his position by pointing out that thousands of people, including many non-Jains, met him during his foot travels. He wondered what he could offer to them and thus drew upon the concept of vows (*vrata*) from Jain scriptures, presenting it as a self-imposed resolution for the general public to regenerate their ethical and moral lives. The second objection focused on concerns about Acharya Tulsi accepting non-Jains as Aṇuvratīs while they continued to follow a non-Jain diet. Tulsi encountered this criticism repeatedly during his campaign for the movement. In response, as recounted by several monks and nuns, he emphasized that the movement does not impose any restrictions on individuals' eating habits, cultural activities, or religious rituals. Its primary aim is simply to promote the regeneration of humanity by cultivating ethical and moral values.

Although Tulsi's AM may no longer effectively serve its original specific purpose of bringing about social change to combat certain negative influences of modernization in post-independence India, his general underlying belief that some of the core concepts in Jainism could be applied to create forms of action that could have a positive influence on the improvement of secular society is still very relevant.

The proverb "A ship is safe in a harbor, but that's not why ships are built" aptly describes Acharya Tulsi, who emerged as one of the most prominent monks in mid-twentieth-century India. Recognizing the importance of inclusivity, he emphasized that religious teachings alone were insufficient. He believed that action was equally vital. Drawing from Jain traditions, he saw the concept of vows as a powerful tool for effecting social change in secular society. Tulsi explored vows as a vehicle for individual character regeneration and incorporated several reformative concepts on issues ranging from orthodox social customs to environmentalism. His movement was guided by the motto "Self-restraint is life," a phrase that summed up his philosophy, and continues to remain relevant into the present

Notes

1. In addition to an analysis of Tulsi's speeches and works and Anuvrat's materials, I will include interviews that I conducted with the Śvetāmbara Terāpantha community in India between 2012 and 2013.

2. My respondents were both Terāpanthi Jains. Non-Jain interviewees included members of the Muslim, Christian, and Sikh communities.

3. Mahāprajña was a Jain monk who later became Tulsi's successor in 1995 as the tenth Acharya of the Jain Śvetāmbara Terāpantha tradition.

4. A category of texts composed especially for the laity by medieval Jain teachers. For an exposition of these texts, see Williams 1963.

5. All the vows are drawn from the list in Tulsi 1993.

6. Weber develops his theory of charisma in his *Economy and Society* (1978, 241–254).

7. For a thorough discussion of *laukika* and *lokottara*, see chaps. 1 and 4 in Kothari (2013).

References

Bhargava, D. 2012. Interview by S. Bothra.

Bothra, Shivani. 2013. "The Anuvrat Movement: Theory and Practice." Master's thesis, Florida International University, Miami.

Bronkhorst, Johannes. 2007. *Greater Magadha: Studies in the Culture of Early India*. Brill.

Cort, John. 2001. *Jains in the World: Religious Values and Ideology in India*. Oxford University Press.

Dundas, Paul. 1992. *The Jains*. Routledge.

Jain, Andrea R. 2016. "Jain Modern Yoga: The Case of Prekṣā Dhyāna." In *Yoga in Jainism*, edited by Christopher Key Chapple. Routledge.

Jaini, Padmanabh S. 1979. *The Jaina Path of Purification*. University of California Press.

Kanakshri, S. 2013. Interview by S. Bothra, January.

Kanakprabha, Sadhvipramukha. 2005. "Dark Age and the Light of Anuvrat." *Anuvrta* (November): 27–32.

Kothari, Smita. 2013. "Dāna and Dhyāna in Jaina Yoga: A Case Study of Prekṣādhyāna and the Terāpanth." PhD diss., University of Toronto, Toronto.

———. 2016. "Preksā Dhyāna in Jaina Yoga: An Archetypal Ritual for the Proper Ordering of the Soul." In Chapple, ed., *Yoga in Jainism*. Routledge.

Mahāprajña, Y. 1997. *Turning the Wheel of Dharma*. Amṛt Mahotsava Rāśtṛya Samiti.

Qvarnström, Olle, and Jason Birch. 2012. "Universalist and Missionary Jainism: Jain Yoga of the Terāpanthī Tradition." In *Yoga in Practice*, edited by David Gordon White. Princeton University Press.

Rajimatī, S. 2012, June. Fieldwork interview by Shivani Bothra.
Reading, Michael. 2019. "The Anuvrat Movement: A Case Study of Jain-inspired Ethical and Eco-Conscious Living." *Religions* 10:636.
———. 2020. "Acharya Sri Tulsi, Anuvrat, and Eco-Conscious Living." In *Beacons of Dharma: Spiritual Exemplars for the Modern Age*, edited by Christopher Patrick Miller, Michael Reading, and Jeffrey D. Long. Lexington Books.
Smith, William Robertson. 1927. *Lectures on the Religion of the Semites: The Fundamental Institutions*. 3rd ed. Macmillan.
Tobias, Michael. 2000. *Life Force: The World of Jainism*. Jain Publishing Company.
Tulsi, Acharya. 1992. *Nonviolence: Man and Society*. Edited by M. Sukhlal. Jain Visva Bharati.
———. 1993. *Anuvrat: Gati-Pragati*. Edited by R. P. Bhatnagar. Jain Vishva Bharati.
Vibha, Sadhvi Vishrut. 2012. *Acharya Tulsi, A Legend of Humanity*. Acharya Tulsi Janam Shatabdi Samaroha Samiti.
Weber, Max. 1978. *Economy and Society*. University of California Press.
Williams, R. 1963. *Jaina Yoga: A Survey of the Mediaeval Śrāvakācāras*. Motilal Banarsidass.

17

Engaged *Anekāntavāda*

The Potential of Jain Philosophy for Grounding Dialogue Across Worldviews (with a Focus on *Vijñāna Vedānta*)

JEFFERY D. LONG

Much of the excitement generated by the Jain *anekānta* doctrine and its accompanying doctrines of perspectives (*nayavāda*) and conditional predication (*syādvāda*) arises from a perception that these doctrines have a great potential to serve as a philosophical foundation for mutually respectful dialogue across worldviews. If, whatever our perspective, we are willing to see other worldviews not simply as false (inasmuch as they differ from our own views), but as expressing some truth to which we have not previously had access, then an encounter with the religious or the philosophical other becomes not a confrontation to be feared but an opportunity for learning and growth, to be anticipated as a great adventure. Such an approach to truth, it seems, is not only most amenable to the cultivation of further knowledge and growth on the part of all involved. It is also a necessity in a world in which worldview differences are all too frequently invoked as justifications for violence against those whose perspectives diverge from our own.

This approach requires, however, people with diverse worldviews to agree on the basic premise that reality is amenable to a variety of different, yet valid, perspectives (*naya*s). Even if their view is that reality is ultimately simple, perhaps being reducible to one ultimate category, such as matter or consciousness, an openness to the perspectives of others entails some sense that reality is, at least as presented to our common experience, complex (*anekānta*). Our views may differ regarding whether this complexity is intrinsic to the nature of existence, whether it is merely apparent—that is, a function of our ignorance of its deeper unity—or whether the truth is somewhere in between. But even if it serves merely as a pragmatic starting point, some concept of *anekāntavāda*, it would seem, is a fundamental presupposition of a respectful dialogue across worldviews that is willing to grant the validity of the perspectives of others.

This chapter will explore the question "Can one arrive at *anekāntavāda*, at least in this minimalistic sense, from diverse philosophical starting points?" In other words, and perhaps more pointedly, "Given its rootedness in a distinctively Jain worldview and distinctively Jain ontological premises, can a non-Jain affirm *anekāntavāda*?" This chapter will argue that the answer to this question is "Yes," and then proceed to give examples of how various worldviews might engage in *anekāntavāda*. In the spirit of the present volume, the purpose of this chapter is also, therefore, to *engage* the Jain concept of *anekāntavāda* with other philosophical systems to see what the outcome of such an intellectual undertaking can be.

The chapter will focus chiefly upon the current author's own worldview, that of the Vijñāna Vedānta tradition of Sri Ramakrishna and Swami Vivekananda, arguing that *anekāntavāda* is deeply compatible with this tradition's spiritually cosmopolitan vision. This exercise in Hindu-Jain comparative theology will explore ways in which engaging the Jain teaching of the non-one-sidedness of reality (*anekāntavāda*) and its logical corollaries (*nayavāda*, the doctrine of perspectives, and *syādvāda*, the doctrine of conditional predication) can both inform and be informed by the teaching of *dharmasamanvaya* (or harmony of religions) that is central to the Vijñāna Vedānta, or Integral Vedānta, taught by Sri Ramakrishna and Swami Vivekananda.

Anekāntavāda is of great interest to philosophers and theologians who seek to apply this concept to the diversity of worldviews, in the name of developing a pluralistic philosophy that is aimed at cultivating greater harmony among the adherents of the world's religions and philosophies. It is also of great interest to a growing number of Jains who have come to see this doctrine as being aimed precisely at this goal: the promotion of intellectual *ahiṃsā,* or nonviolence practiced at the level of conceptual discourse. The philosophical methodology expressed in the Jain teachings of *anekāntavāda, nayavāda,* and *syādvāda* is an especially rich resource for potential applications both to interfaith dialogue and to the dialogue between religion and science, both of which are pressing needs of our current global era, particularly as polarization across worldviews has increasingly emerged as an element that fuels violence among human beings. This chapter aims to explore the idea that the multifaceted Jain approach to truth could be adopted by non-Jains in the effort to bridge the gaps that currently exist among diverse religions and between religion and science (as well as between religious and secular thought more generally). The aim of this effort would not be to produce agreement in all areas, but to foster mutual respect based on a shared commitment to the idea that reality is vast and mysterious and thus conducive to being explained and understood in a wide variety of ways. Rather than seeing worldviews that diverge from one's own as simply false, the multifaceted understanding of truth that underlies the Jain approach invites us to seek out the kernel of truth that can be discerned in the many diverse views of our shared reality that the world's varied religions and philosophies express.

Emerging from a similar sensibility and set of values, a central teaching of Vijñāna Vedānta, the worldview propounded by the Hindu teacher Sri Ramakrishna and his pre-eminent disciple, Swami Vivekananda, is *dharmasamanvaya,* or the harmony of religions, which claims that many religions can lead to the goal of the realization of humanity's true, divine nature. The idea here is not that all religions teach essentially the same things (though they do contain important overlaps), nor that they are true in the same sense or to the same extent, but that their practice can issue in a shared realization.

Though they emerge from quite distinct conceptual matrices and involve differing views about the nature of reality, there is sufficient overlap between these Jain and Vedāntic doctrines both in their content and in the concerns to which they are directed to allow for productive engagement between them. The aim here is not to "compare" these views in the sense of showing one to be superior to the other, but to pursue comparative theology in the sense that has been developed in the work of Francis Clooney (2010), who defines comparative theology as a process of "deep learning across religious borders." How can *anekāntavāda* and *dharmasamanvaya* shed light upon one another? How can each be enhanced by the other? How can they jointly point the way forward in a pluralistic world? Can they jointly encourage peaceful coexistence and mutually respective dialogue and learning?

Anekāntavāda: An Overview

Before bringing *anekāntavāda* into conversation with other worldviews, it is first necessary to understand it from within the context of the tradition in which it has emerged. *Anekāntavāda*, the doctrine of the non-one-sidedness of reality, is a Jain view that may have emerged, in its earliest forms, from discourse about the nature of existence presented in the canonical *āgama* literature of the Śvetāmbara Jain community as reflecting the teaching of the Jain tradition's twenty-fourth and final Tīrthaṅkara of our current cosmic cycle, Mahāvīra.[1] According to Jain teaching, in attaining *kevala-jñāna*, a Jina (conqueror of the self) such as Mahāvīra becomes literally omniscient (*sarvajña*). Mahāvīra's teaching on the nature of existence is thus seen as authoritative and ultimate.

The worldview that Mahāvīra proclaimed is ontologically pluralistic. It affirms that reality is made up of an irreducible variety of substances (*dravya*s). These substances are six in number and consist of the soul of life force of each living being (*jīva*), nonliving matter (*pudgala*), a principle of motion (*dharma*), a principle of inertia (*adharma*), space (*ākāśa*), and time (*kāla*).

According to Mahāvīra's teaching, as presented in the *āgama*s, many of the great philosophical questions that perplex human beings can be answered in seemingly opposed ways, depending on the perspective from which one examines the topic in question. The rise of diverse worldviews can thus be seen as a consequence of adhering to the truth of just one point of view without taking other perspectives into account. Mahāvīra is asked by one of his followers, Jamāli, for example, whether the soul is eternal or non-eternal, and whether the cosmos itself has a beginning and an end or not. In response, Mahāvīra says:

> The world is, Jamāli, eternal. It did not cease to exist at any time. It was, it is, and it will be. It is constant, permanent, eternal, imperishable, indestructible, [and] always existent. The world is, Jamāli, non-eternal. For it becomes progressive (in time-cycle) after being regressive. And it becomes regressive after becoming progressive. The soul is, Jamāli, eternal. For it did not cease to exist at any time. The soul is, Jamāli, non-eternal. For it becomes animal after being a hellish creature, becomes a man after becoming an animal and it becomes a god after being a man. (*Bhagavatī Sūtra* 9:386, as cited in Matilal 1981, 19)

In other words, if by "world" one is referring to the totality of reality itself, then the world is, according to Mahāvīra, eternal. As in the Hindu and Buddhist traditions, the world is held in the Jain tradition to have no beginning or end. But if by "world" one is referring to the current state of cosmic existence—to "this world"—then it is impermanent. It had a beginning, and it will have an end, as one cycle among many. Similarly, if by soul (again, *jīva*, or living being), one is referring to the living being in its current state of embodiment, then this is temporary. Beings are born and they die. But if one is referring to the living essence of the being, to the *jīva* as understood in Jain thought, then the living being is, in this sense, eternal, having no beginning or end.

Over the course of more than two millennia of philosophical reflection by thinkers within the Jain community, this "both/and" approach to fundamental philosophical questions was developed into the doctrines of *anekāntavāda, nayavāda,* and *syādvāda* as these are known today. The non-one-sided or *anekāṇta* nature of reality can be deduced from the ontological pluralism of the early Jain literature. Reality cannot be reduced to one single factor. One must take into account all the *dravya*s or substances that go into making up a moment of experience. Some elements of experience are impermanent while others are eternal. Neither is reducible wholly to the other.

From this understanding of reality emerges *nayavāda*. If an entity or a moment of experience can be said to have many facets or aspects, given the irreducible plurality of being, then it follows that any given entity can be viewed from perspectives that correspond to these facets or aspects.

From this understanding of epistemology as perspectival emerges *syādvāda*, which teaches us that our claims about the nature of reality, being conditioned by our perspective, are therefore able to convey only a limited portion of the truth about any given topic. Our claims are true, not in an absolute or dogmatic sense, but *syāt*—that is, in Jain technical usage, from a certain point of view, or in a certain sense. *Anekāntavāda* is a doctrine about the nature of reality. *Nayavāda* is a doctrine about the limits of knowledge that arise from reality being non-one-sided. And *syādvāda* is a doctrine about the limits of language that arise from the limits of knowledge.

As John Cort has pointed out, Jain thinkers have traditionally utilized these doctrines as a way to demonstrate the limitations—the one-sided, or *ekānta* nature—of the perspectives of rival *darśanas*, or schools of thought. Buddhists, for example, are thus depicted as having a partially correct view, in affirming the impermanent nature of any given entity, but as having captured only a piece of the truth, inasmuch as their perspective fails to grasp that in an entity there is something that is permanent and eternal. Similarly, adherents of various brahmanical (what would now be called Hindu) schools of thought are similarly depicted as having a partially correct view when affirming the permanent, eternal nature of substances, but as having captured only a piece of the truth, inasmuch as their perspective fails to grasp that in any entity there is something that is of an impermanent and changing nature.

While it is true that, as thus deployed—as polemical tools—these doctrines do say something positive about the perspectives of others and do not reject them as wholly false, they are ultimately acting in the service of establishing the more holistic and comprehensive nature of the Jain perspective (Cort 2000). Many contemporary Jain thinkers adopting what Miller has identified as a constructive-reproductive model of engaged Jainism (see Miller in this volume), however, focus on the degree to which these doctrines can draw our attention to the ways non-Jain schools of thought convey genuine insight into the nature of reality. Rather than seeing *anekāntavāda* as a tool for establishing the superiority of a Jain perspective, they see it, rather, as a conceptual tool for extending the practice of *ahiṃsā*—of nonviolence in thought, word, and action—to the intellectual realm. One should not reject the views of others as wholly wrong. One should rather, according to this way of thinking, appreciate and affirm what one can agree with in those perspectives. The idea here is that this way of approaching difference will mitigate the human tendency toward exclusivity and fanaticism.

Indeed, it is not only in the contemporary period that Jain thinkers have deployed *anekāntavāda* and its related doctrines as a way of affirming what is positive in other traditions and worldviews. The ancient parable of the blind people and the elephant (see Bridges in this volume) is often cited by Jain thinkers as a way to illustrate the main premise of *anekāntavāda*: that differences across worldviews can be explained by recourse to the idea that a shared, complex reality underlies the perceptions upon which these worldviews are based. This parable can be summarized as follows:

> As a joke, a king sent seven blind men to feel an elephant and describe its nature. Each approached the elephant from a different direction, seized a different part, and, being blind, assumed that what he perceived was the whole elephant. One grasped the ear and declared, "Elephant is like a large fan." Another grasped a leg and declared, "Elephant is like a great pillar." Another found the trunk, and feeling it, proclaimed, "Elephant is like a snake." Another grasped the tail and declared, "Elephant is like a rope hanging from the sky," while another, grasping only the tuft of the tail, said, "Elephant is like a broom." A sixth encountered the side of the elephant and maintained, "Elephant is like a wall." The seventh insisted that the others were all wrong, for he had grasped the tusk. He proclaimed, "Elephant is not any of those; elephant is like a spear." Each being certain of the truth of his own experience, they began to fight.
>
> A person who could see chanced to come by and found them quarrelling. After listening to their individual perceptions from their different points of view, he gently

> explained that there was no need for fighting over the issue, for each was partially right. But to have complete knowledge of the nature of the elephant, he said, one would have to be able to be aware of and combine all the different aspects of the creature.[2]

If we can grant that, however it may have been deployed by specific Jain thinkers at various points in the history of the tradition, *anekāntavāda* has the capacity to be deployed in the more positive and affirming way that has been adopted by many Jain philosophers—from the premodern era, such as Haribhadrasūri (ca. eighth century CE) and Yaśovijaya (1624–1688), and from the contemporary era, such as the late Acharya Mahapragya (1920–2010)—the question remains of whether this approach to truth and its expression is available from within many different worldviews, or if its rootedness in Jain ontology renders it exclusive to the Jain tradition.

Arriving at *Anekāntavāda* from Many Starting Points

Quite famously, Mohandas K. Gandhi (1869–1948), an eclectically minded Vaiṣṇava Hindu, on at least one occasion described himself as an adherent of *anekāntavāda*. In an editorial in one of his newspapers, *Young India*, Gandhi responded to a reader who pointed out that Gandhi sometimes seemed to speak as an adherent of nondualism (Advaita Vedānta) and sometimes in a more dualist or pluralistic mode, typical of Vaiṣṇava traditions and the Abrahamic religions. He wrote as follows:

> I am an *advaitist* and yet I can support *Dvaitism* (dualism). The world is changing every moment, and is therefore unreal, it has no permanent existence. But though it is constantly changing, it has a something about it which persists and it is therefore to that extent real. I have therefore no objection to calling it real and unreal, and thus being called an *Anekantavadi* or a *Syadvadi*. But my *Syadvada* is not the *syadvada* of the learned, it is peculiarly my own. I cannot engage in a debate with them. It has

> been my experience that I am always true from my point of view, and am often wrong from the point of view of my honest critics. I know that we are both right from our respective points of view. And this knowledge saves me from attributing motives to my opponents or critics. The seven blind men who gave seven different descriptions of the elephant were all right from their respective points of view, and wrong from the point of view of one another, and right and wrong from the point of view of the man who knew the elephant. I very much like this doctrine of the manyness of reality. It is this doctrine that has taught me to judge a Musalman [Muslim] from his own standpoint and a Christian from his. Formerly I used to resent the ignorance of my opponents. Today I can love them because I am gifted with the eye to see myself as others see me *and vice versa*. I want to take the whole world in the embrace of my love. My *anekantavad* is the result of the twin doctrine of *Satya* and *Ahimsa*. (Gandhi 1981 [1926], 30)

For Gandhi, this doctrine was a pragmatic one, a matter of learning to view others with empathy. As his example illustrates, one can arrive at the idea of *anekāntavāda* from conceptual points of origin other than that of the Jain tradition. And as we shall see in more detail shortly, Ramakrishna (1836–1886), although he was not strongly influenced by Jain thought, arrived at a similar concept of the inherent diversity of phenomenal reality through his practices of many *sādhanas*, or spiritual disciplines, rooted in many traditions (Hindu, Christian, and Islamic).

Conceptually speaking, how might adherents of other worldviews find their way to affirming the basic premise of *anekāntavāda*: the at least apparent complexity of reality and the consequent rise of a diverse array of valid perspectives upon it? Ultimately, it is the adherents of the diverse worldviews themselves who would need to develop ways of arriving at *anekāntavāda* (or a functional equivalent thereof) from their respective points of view. But a few comments can be made by way of a preliminary sketch of how a sampling of worldviews might be shown to yield some version of *anekāntavāda*.

One of the most obviously different ontologies from that of *anekāntavāda* is that of the nondualistic (*advaita*), or absolute monistic tradition of Vedānta. In contrast with the ontological pluralism of the Jain tradition, the Advaita Vedānta tradition affirms the ultimate unity of being in the form of *nirguṇa* Brahman, an ultimate reality with no limiting qualities whatsoever, composed of pure being, consciousness, and bliss (*sat-cit-ānanda*). The complex reality presented to our common experience is explained by this tradition as, finally, delusory: an effect of ignorance and of projection onto a reality that is, in fact, not diverse at all, and utterly beyond the realm of time, space, and causation that defines our ordinary experience. The complex realm described by Jain ontology is, from this point of view, an effect of *māyā* ("illusion" or "delusion"), which is how Brahman appears to itself as a world made up of many beings.

An adherent of Advaita Vedānta, however, can affirm *anekāntavāda* as reflecting the nature of relative reality, of the infinite Brahman as it appears through the lens of *māyā*. To be sure, the idea of the realm of relative or conventional truth (*vyavahāra satya*) is often deployed by thinkers in this tradition as a way of describing what they ultimately reject as a false appearance: "Brahman is alone real, the world an illusion" (*brahma satyaṃ jagan-mithyā, Vivekacūḍāmaṇi*, 20a). Yet, from within this tradition, the realm of *māyā* is the realm from which the search for ultimate reality must begin. At minimum, a pragmatic truth can be granted to *anekāntavāda* from this perspective, and the foundation built for a respectful dialogue with other worldviews.

An adherent of Buddhism can similarly affirm *anekāntavāda* in terms of our relative perceptions of existence and the Buddha's skillful means. The Mahāyāna tradition, for example, famously sees, not unlike Advaita Vedānta, reality as perceivable either from a relative or absolute perspective. Like an adherent of Advaita Vedānta, an adherent of this tradition can see relative truths as being necessary on the path to ultimate awakening. The famous parable of the burning house, found in the *Lotus Sūtra* (parable 3), illustrates this very concept: that the Buddha can teach in many ways, including ways that might not be, literally speaking, true, in the awareness that different kinds of teaching are helpful to different people depending upon where they currently are upon the spiritual path.

An adherent of theistic religions such as the Vaiṣṇava traditions of Hinduism and the Abrahamic religions can see the *anekānta* nature of our shared, given reality as a reflection of the infinite and ultimately inconceivable power of the Supreme Being. The world, as either God's creation or self-manifestation, is a reflection of the manifold dimensions of the divine mind. Within this vast and mysterious cosmos, which exists through the act of divine grace, one must make assertions about truth with modesty, with the understanding that it is finally only God who knows all things. All of our statements about reality must, in that sense, be provisional. In the Roman Catholic tradition, St. Thomas Aquinas, for example, affirms that, apart from the statement that "God exists," all other predications made about the divine reality are, by necessity, analogical in nature. Even the idea that "God is good" is limiting, given that our human understanding of "good" is incapable of truly encompassing divine goodness.

Finally, a materialist can affirm *anekāntavāda* as an expression of the mysterious nature of reality as it continues to unfold to our knowledge. There is always that truth which lies beyond the horizon of our knowledge. All of our statements about it are thus, again, always provisional, awaiting the eventual correction that ensues from the ongoing progress of science. Theories are superseded by other theories as knowledge advances, and there is no reason to expect an end to this process.

If these reflections are valid, they suggest that interlocutors coming from worldviews as diverse as Advaita Vedānta, Buddhism, various monotheisms, and materialism could conceivably enter into a mutually respectful conversation, with the understanding that all attempts to model reality have limitations. This is essentially what the Jain tradition affirms with its affirmation of the irreducible complexity of existence.

Let us turn specifically now to the Vijñāna Vedānta tradition of Ramakrishna and Vivekananda and see the ways in which a conversation between this particular worldview and *anekāntavāda* might be productive toward a mutually respectful, pluralistic, and cosmopolitan approach to worldview diversity. What is at stake here is an opportunity for Jains and Hindus in particular to develop a useful tool for engaging in productive and respectful interreligious dialogue.

Dharmasamanvaya: An Overview

Much as contemporary Jain thinkers seek to affirm *anekāntavāda* as an expression of intellectual *ahiṃsā*, there are also contemporary Hindu thinkers who affirm the ideal of "harmony of religions" (*dharmasamanvaya*) as a remedy to sectarianism, bigotry, and fanaticism, the "unholy trinity" condemned by Swami Vivekananda in his famous welcome address at the 1893 Parliament of the World's Religions in Chicago: "Sectarianism, bigotry, and its horrible descendant, fanaticism, have long possessed this beautiful earth. They have filled the earth with violence, drenched it often and often with human blood, destroyed civilisation and sent whole nations to despair. Had it not been for these horrible demons, human society would be far more advanced than it is now" (Vivekananda 1979 [1893], 4). To be sure, Hindus have taken a wide range of stances through the millennia regarding those who are regarded as religious "others" (including adherents of other traditions that would be regarded today as Hindu, such as in debates, for example, between Vaiṣṇavas and Śaivas, or between Naiyāyikas and Mīmāṃsakas). Like Jain thinkers, adherents of various Vedic systems of thought and practice have also sought to advance the superiority of their own views at the expense of others.

At the same time, there has also been a subcurrent within many Hindu traditions of affirmation of the validity and effectiveness of many systems of thought and practice as paths to liberation and to the realization of ultimate truth. There is the famous, and oft-quoted, verse from the *Ṛg Veda* (*RV* 1.164.46): *ekaṃ sad-viprā bahudhā vadanti* "The Real is one. The wise speak of It in many ways."[3] There are the verses from the *Bhagavad Gītā* and *Śiva Mahimna Stotra* mentioned by Swami Vivekananda in the welcome address just cited: "Whosoever comes to Me, through whatsoever form, I reach him; all men are struggling through paths which in the end lead to me" (*BG* 4.11). And, "As the different streams having their sources in different places all mingle their water in the sea, so, O Lord, the different paths which men take through different tendencies, various though they appear, crooked or straight, all lead to Thee" (Vivekananda 1979 [1893], 4; *SMS* 7). There has also been the widespread practice across many traditions of India of celebrating the holidays of multiple traditions, sharing sacred spaces, and paying respects to the sacred figures and at the sacred sites of many different communities: what one might call a "popular pluralism," or spiritual cosmopolitanism, which expands even beyond the boundaries of the Dharma traditions to include Abrahamic traditions such as Christianity and Islam.

It is in this context that one needs to understand the phenomenon of Sri Ramakrishna. Living from 1836 to 1886, this Bengali sage is famously believed to have practiced the paths of many traditions to the point where, in each, he experienced the culminating state of *samādhi*, or absorption in the sacred ideal of the tradition in question. On this experiential basis, Sri Ramakrishna and followers of the tradition based on his teaching affirm that many paths can lead to the liberating state of God-realization: the direct experiential awareness of the divinity present within all beings.

Engaging *Anekāntavāda* with *Dharmasamanvaya*: How Jain Philosophy and Vijñāna Vedānta Can Inform One Another

Like many contemporary Jains, adherents of the tradition of Ramakrishna and Swami Vivekananda see their teaching as having the potential to promote greater harmony among the followers of the world's diverse religions and philosophies. How can these two approaches complement one another? What can each derive from the other? And what challenges remain for both as part of a solution to the wider problem of interreligious violence?

Dharmasamanvaya, as taught by Sri Ramakrishna and Swami Vivekananda, is based upon a view of reality in which the highest or ultimate reality can be viewed and approached from a wide array of perspectives. According to Sri Ramakrishna, this is an effect, at least in part, of divine grace. The divine reality wants us to achieve realization and thus accommodates our limited perspectives so that we can approach and eventually experience that goal. According to Sri Ramakrishna, the divine reality has become all things, and is ultimately not separable from the self or the world. In describing his own state of realization, or *vijñāna*, Ramakrishna affirms that the realization of the impersonal Brahman of the Advaita Vedānta tradition leads to the insight that nothing other than the infinite

Brahman exists, that Brahman has become all things. Brahman can thus be perceived in and through all things: "That which is realized as Brahman through the eliminating process of 'Not this, not this' is then found to have become the universe and all its living beings. The *vijñānī* sees that the Reality which is *nirguṇa* is also *saguṇa* . . . Those who realize Brahman in *samādhi* . . . find that it is Brahman that has become the universe and its living beings . . . This is known as *vijñāna*" (Ramakrishna; Nikhilananda 1942, 103–104).

Anekāntavāda, as already discussed, is based upon a view of reality as including a vast array of aspects or facets, any of which can form the basis of a valid, if incomplete, perspective on the nature of existence. *Anekāntavāda* thus has the capacity to greatly enrich the scope and the detail of the ontology of the harmony of religions. What are the relations among the various facets of Brahman as these are experienced by the *vijñānī*? What is the logic by which seemingly contrary facets of this reality (such as being simultaneously beyond the realm of time and space and being that of which time and space both consist) can be brought together to form an internally consistent picture of reality?

Similarly, *dharmasamanvaya* introduces to *anekāntavāda* the idea that the various partial views of the world's religions and philosophies, rather than simply being seen as incomplete and in need of fulfillment by a more comprehensive worldview, can anchor spiritual practice in ways that have unique and important impacts upon the consciousness of the practitioner and thus give rise to insights that might not otherwise be available. Interestingly, the *dharmasamanvaya* approach of the Ramakrishna tradition is anticipated by the eighth-century CE Śvetāmbara Jain thinker Haribhadrasūri. In his *Yogadṛṣṭisamuccaya*, or *Collection of Views on Yoga*, Haribhadra argues that the experience of *mokṣa*, or liberation, is essentially one, but is described differently by the great masters of various traditions who have attained it in order to meet the needs of their particular disciples and the times in which they lived. The proper attitude, therefore, to hold toward all the great founders of the various paths to liberation, or *yoga*s—such as Kāpila and the Buddha, whom he refers to as "omniscient ones"—is veneration and respect. Disputation with rival schools is thus to be avoided as non-conducive to the supreme and common goal of *mokṣa* or *nirvāṇa*:

> The ultimate truth transcending all states of worldly existence and called *nirvāṇa* is essentially and necessarily one even if it be designated by different names.
>
> It is this very entity that is designated by words like Sadāśiva, Parabrahman, Siddhātman, Tathatā, etc.—words which have got the same meaning and a proper meaning at that.
>
> For there is no dispute about the definition of this ultimate truth (i.e. of the ultimate state of the soul's existence) inasmuch as it is (unanimously) said to be free from all disturbance, free from all ailment, free from all activity, and that on account of its undergoing no birth, etc.
>
> Having comprehended by means of *asaṃmoha* [calm composure] the essential nature of the truth called *nirvāṇa* it is impossible for thoughtful persons to quarrel as to how to express one's loyalty to this truth.
>
> Since it is a necessary truth that *nirvāṇa* is open to an omniscient person alone, the short path leading from omniscience to *nirvāṇa* ought to be straight. How, then, can there be a difference (of opinion) among those possessing omniscience?
>
> Their teaching exhibits diversity of types parallel to the diversity of levels possessed by the understanding of the disciples concerned; for these great personages are competent physicians in relation to the ailment called worldly existence.
>
> They thus enlightened different types of disciples in different manners, only keeping in mind that in each case the sowing of seed (of religious faith) was possible and the remaining operations were so performed that the plant would go on growing smoothly (and would ultimately bear fruit).
>
> Or we might say that their teaching is really one and the same but that it appears different to the different

> members of the audience owing to the inscrutable capacity of the virtuous acts earlier performed by them (i.e. performed by these members of the audience or by these teachers in their earlier births).
>
> This teaching thus turns out to be beneficial to all—but to each in a way that specially suits him. That again is how this teaching well demonstrates its fruitful character in each and every case.
>
> Or we might say that the teaching in question—though essentially rooted in omniscience—has come forth from the sages themselves in a diversified form due to the diversity of standpoints [*nayas*] (adopted by the various sages) or to the diversity in the periods of time (when the various sages preached) or some other diversity of a kindred type. (*Yogadṛṣṭisamuccaya* 129–138, trans. by Dixit 1970, 66–69)

To be sure, both approaches—*anekāntavāda* and *dharmasamanvaya*—even when each is enriched by the insights of the other, face the challenge of how to translate their insights into practice, to shape the interactions of living human beings. As of this writing, it has been 130 years since Swami Vivekananda proclaimed the harmony of religions in Chicago. Yet the world remains torn by conflict—often violent conflict—and polarization among the adherents of diverse views of reality. It is this pragmatic challenge that remains to be met by those of us who would see humanity evolve beyond its current state of conflict and toward a collective conversation marked by mutual respect and the ability to draw insight from others.

Conclusion

Anekāntavāda promises to give a philosophical grounding to pluralism. It can thus help to cultivate a wider cosmopolitanism that is open to truth in many worldviews and accessible to persons with diverse perspectives on reality, knowledge, and ethics. The project of developing ways from within diverse worldviews for the adherents of those worldviews to arrive at *anekāntavāda* is thus an imperative if *anekāntavāda* is to be applied in a productive way to the project of human coexistence. This chapter has been the merest sketch of how this development might proceed. But it is offered in the hope that it might, one day, bear fruit in the world not only between Jains and Hindus but also between all of those who seem to possess seemingly irreconcilable, though perhaps at least at minimum mutually informing, worldviews.

Notes

1. Bronkhorst (2003) has recently challenged this argument.
2. The story as told here is my paraphrasing of the earliest known extant version found in an early Buddhist source: *Udāna* 6.4:66–69.
3. Author's translation.

References

Bronkhorst, Johannes. 2003. "Jainism's First Heretic and the Origin of Anekānta-vāda." In *Jainism and Early Buddhism: Essays in Honor of Padmanabh S. Jaini*, edited by Olle Qvarnström. Asian Humanities Press.

Clooney, Francis X. 2010. *Comparative Theology: Deep Learning Across Religious Borders*. Wiley-Blackwell.

Cort, John E. 2000. "'Intellectual Ahiṃsa' Revisited: Jain Tolerance and Intolerance of Others." *Philosophy East and West* 50 (3): 324–347.

Gandhi, Mohandas K. 1981 [1926]. *Young India: 1919–1931*. Vol. 8, 1926. Navajivan Publishing House.

Haribhadrasūri. 1970. *Yogadṛṣṭisamuccaya and Yogaviṃśikā*. Translated by Krishna Kumar Dixit. L. D. Institute of Indology.

Matilal, Bimal Krishna. 1981. *Anekāntavāda: The Central Philosophy of Jainism*. L. D. Institute of Indology.

Nikhilananda, Swami, trans. 1942. *The Gospel of Sri Ramakrishna*. Ramakrishna Vivekananda Center.

Vivekananda, Swami. 1979 [1893]. *Complete Works*. Advaita Ashrama.

Contributors

Johannes Beltz has studied theology, Indian studies, and religious studies at the universities of Halle, Strasbourg, Paris, and Lausanne. On numerous occasions throughout the 1990s, he undertook research in India for his PhD thesis. From 1999 to 2002, he worked at the renowned South Asia Institute of the University of Heidelberg before taking up a post at the Museum Rietberg, where he is now curator of the collection of Indian bronzes, sculptures and textiles, and the South East Asian collection. He has chaired the museum's curatorial board since 2009, and was appointed assistant director in 2016. In addition, Johannes Beltz has lectured regularly at the University of Zürich.

Cogen Bohanec is assistant professor in Jain and Sanskrit studies at Arihanta Institute, a visiting assistant professor at Claremont School of Theology (CST), and he has taught numerous classes on South Asian Religions and Sanskrit at the Graduate Theological Union (GTU) in Berkeley. Dr. Bohanec specializes in comparative dharma traditions, philosophy of religion, and Sanskrit language and literature, and he has numerous publications in those areas. He has a PhD in Historical and Cultural Studies of Religion with an emphasis in Hindu studies from GTU, where his research emphasized ancient Indian languages, literature, and philosophical systems. He also holds an MA in Buddhist studies from the Institute of Buddhist Studies at GTU.

Shivani Bothra is assistant professor in the Department of Religious Studies at California State University, Long Beach. She worked earlier as a postdoctoral researcher at Rice University in Houston,

Texas, and was a lecturer in religious studies at the University of California, Santa Barbara. She earned her doctorate from the Victoria University of Wellington in New Zealand. Her focus is South Asian traditions, Jainism, and nonviolence. Shivani's primary research areas are transnational Jainism, emphasizing contemporary Jainism.

Andrew Bridges holds the Bhagwan Shantinath Lectureship at California State University, Fullerton, where he teaches the course "Non-Violence, Animal Rights and Diet in Jainism" and helps to organize the annual Peace and Religion Symposium. He teaches in both the Religious Studies Department and Philosophy Department at Cal State Fullerton. His research interests include comparative epistemology, contemporary applications of *anekānta-vāda*, and ethics.

Christopher Key Chapple is Doshi Professor of Indic and comparative theology and founding director of the Master of Arts in Yoga Studies at Loyola Marymount University in Los Angeles. A specialist in the religions of India, he has published more than twenty books, including the recent *Living Landscapes: Meditations on the Elements in Hindu, Buddhist, and Jain Yogas* (SUNY Press). He serves as advisor to multiple organizations including the Forum on Religion and Ecology (Yale), the Ahimsa Center (Pomona), the Dharma Academy of North America (Berkeley), the Jain Studies Centre (SOAS, London), the South Asian Studies Association, and International School for Jain Studies (New Delhi). He teaches online through the Center for Religion and Spirituality (LMU) and Glo.

Jonathan Dickstein is Tirthankara Shreyansnath Endowed Assistant Professor of Jain and vegan studies at Arihanta Institute and specializes in South Asian religions, religion and ecology, and comparative religious ethics. He received his doctoral degree in religious studies from the University of California, Santa Barbara, where he wrote his dissertation on ancient Indian animal taxonomies and their relevance for religious ritual and dietary practice. Jonathan's current work focuses on Jainism and contemporary ecological issues, and accordingly extends into critical animal studies, food studies, and diaspora studies. Jonathan has published in a wide array of interdisciplinary journals on topics such as veganism and politics, yoga and diet, Jain veganism, and the ethic of nonviolence (*ahiṃsā*). Jonathan considers himself a scholar-practitioner, having spent many years not only in libraries but also in public advocating for justice for both humans and nonhumans alike.

Parveen Jain is the founder, chairman of the board, and chief executive officer of Arihanta Institute. He is a resident of the Silicon Valley, where he enjoys life after an exciting corporate career of over thirty years as a founder and chief executive of multiple technology companies, including a senior executive role at McAfee, the cybersecurity company. Parveen has always cherished philanthropy and has held leadership roles in various nonprofit organizations. He has been a longtime trustee of the International Mahavira Jain Mission, where he has been deeply involved with the growth of Siddhachalam, the first Jain tīrtha outside of India, from its founding. He led the team to build the Jain Temple in the San Francisco Bay Area, has served as chairman and president of Jain Center of Northern California, and continues to be an active advisor. Previously, he was a founding director of the Sunnyvale Hindu Temple, served as a trustee of the American Foundation for the Blind, and was a founding team member of the South Asian Heart Center. Currently, besides other nonprofits, Parveen serves as a founding director of Stanford Center for Asian Health Research and Education (Stanford-CARE). In addition, he enjoys mentoring bright entrepreneurs and serves on the boards of several technology companies. Besides the philanthropic and mentoring activities, Parveen joyously spends time with his grandkids, self-studies, and writes.

Corinna May Lhoir, MA, is a PhD candidate of classical Indology and a contract lecturer for Beginner's Sanskrit and Origins of Yoga at Universität Hamburg as well as an entrepreneur with her own online learning platform with focus on studies of yoga and Sanskrit (yogastudien.de). She holds a BA in Languages and Cultures of India and Tibet with focus on classical Indology from Universität Hamburg and an MA in Traditions of Yoga and Meditation from SOAS, University of London. She also has an MA in Oriental Languages and Cultures India from Ghent University in Belgium, where her studies focused on Jainism.

Jeffery D. Long is the Carl W. Zeigler Professor of Religion, Philosophy, and Asian Studies at Elizabethtown College, in Pennsylvania, where he has taught since receiving his doctoral degree from the University of Chicago Divinity School in the year 2000. He has authored, among other works, *Hinduism in America: A Convergence of Worlds* (2020), *Jainism: An Introduction* (2009), and, with Michael Long, *Nonviolence in the World's Religions: A Concise Introduction* (2021). In 2021, he received the Ranck Award for Research Excellence from Elizabethtown College, and in 2022 he received an Ahimsa Award from the International Ahimsa Foundation for his work to promote nonviolence through his scholarship. In 2022, he also received the Rajinder and Jyoti Gandhi Award for Excellence in Philosophy, Theology, and Critical Reflection from DANAM (the Dharma Academy of North America) for *Hinduism in America*. He has spoken at a variety of prestigious venues, including three talks at the United Nations. He is the editor of the Lexington Books series Explorations in Indic Traditions: Ethical, Philosophical, and Theological.

Christopher Jain Miller is the co-founder, vice president of academic affairs, and professor of Jain and Yoga studies at Arihanta Institute. He is also a visiting researcher at the University of Zürich's Asien-Orient-Institut and visiting professor at Claremont School of Theology where he co-developed and co-directs a remotely available master's degree program and PhD program focusing on engaged Jain studies. He completed his PhD in the study of religion at the University of California, Davis. His current research focuses on modern yoga and engaged Jainism, and he is the author of a number of articles and book chapters concerned with Jainism and the history and practice of modern yoga. He is the author of *Embodying Transnational Yoga: Eating, Singing, and Breathing in Transformation* (2024) and the co-editor of the volume *Beacons of Dharma: Spiritual Exemplars for the Modern Age* (2020).

Alba Rodríguez Juan is a PhD candidate in the Department for the Study of Religion at the University of California, Riverside. She completed a master's degree in yoga studies at Loyola Marymount University, California. Her research focuses on South Asian philosophical and religious traditions, with a main focus on the continuities and discontinuities between traditional and contemporary forms of Jain meditation and ethical practices.

Atul K. Shah has a PhD from the London School of Economics and is author of *Inclusive and Sustainable Finance* (2022), *Jainism and Ethical Finance* (with Aidan Rankin, 2017), *The Politics of Financial Risk, Audit and Regulation* (2018), *Reinventing Accounting and Finance Education* (2018), *Celebrating Diversity* (2007), and *Boardroom Diversity: The Opportunity* (2010). He is passionate about business ethics, education reform, and diversity. Dr. Shah has published a number of papers in international academic journals such as *Accounting, Organizations and Society; Accounting, Auditing and Accountability Journal; European Accounting Review; Journal of Financial Regulation and Compliance; Business Ethics: A European Review*. Between 1995 and 1998, he published a series of papers predicting the global financial crisis, focusing in particular on derivatives and systemic risk, and regulatory arbitrage. His work has been profiled in BBC and *Forbes*, and Dr. Shah is presently working on a series of projects around financial risk management, diverse ethics, and regulation. He has broadcast experience, with credits including BBC Radio 4, BBC World Service, Channel 4, Five Live, BBC Radio 2, Guardian, and BBC Asian Network. Professor Shah also writes and comments for the *Financial Times*. In 2010 Professor Shah embarked on a historic 1,500-mile Masala tour of Britain to showcase the depth and breadth of the diversity in Britain and help the country improve its cultural intelligence — this was featured in the *Guardian*. The tour was also widely covered on BBC radio nationally. He is also founder of the global Young Jains Movement and founding editor of *Jain Spirit Magazine*. Presently he is writing a new book for Routledge on "inclusive" accounting and finance leadership, a theme that is virtually absent from the business literature. He is also a top business ethics writer for *The Conversation* and his research on global accounting won the Best Paper award in 2019.

Joey Tuminello is an assistant professor of philosophy at McNeese State University in Lake Charles, Los Angeles. His research interests include the philosophies of food/animals/environment through the lenses of hermeneutics, pragmatism, and Jainism. Joey's work has appeared in the journals *Food, Culture, and Society;*

Sofia Philosophical Review; and *Humana.Mente: Journal of Philosophical Studies*, as well as several edited volumes including *The Routledge Handbook of Religion and Animal Ethics, Food Justice in U.S. and Global Contexts*, and *The Future of Meat Without Animals*. Joey is also a Fellow of the Oxford Centre for Animal Ethics and a program coordinator for the nonprofit organizations Farm Forward and Better Food Foundation.

Tine Vekemans holds the Ācārya Mahāprajña Chair for Jain Studies at Ghent University. Additionally, she is a postdoctoral research fellow funded by Research Foundation–Flanders (FWO). Her approach to Jain studies combines ethnography with textual study, but always starts from practices and experiences of contemporary Jains. Over the past decade, her research touched upon diverse aspects of modern Jainism, including Jain migration history, changing lay-mendicant relations, Jainism in the digital age, and processes of knowledge transfer within the Jain diaspora.

Steven M. Vose (PhD, South Asia studies, University of Pennsylvania) is a historian of Śvetāmbara Jain communities of western India. His first book, *Reimagining Jainism in Islamic India: Jain Intellectual Culture in the Delhi Sultanate* (forthcoming), focuses on Jain intellectual exchanges with the Delhi Sultanate and the transformations to Jain communities that resulted from these interactions. The book won the Edward C. Dimock Jr. Book Prize in the Indian Humanities from the American Institute of Indian Studies (AIIS). He is currently researching the emergence of transnational Jain communities in post-liberalization India. He is an assistant professor in the Department of History at the University of Colorado-Denver, where he holds the Bhagwan Suparshvanatha Endowed Chair in Jain Studies.

Benjamin Zenk is instructor of management in the College of Business and Economics at the University of Hawaii at Hilo. There, he teaches critical thinking, business ethics, environmental ethics, and introductory business. Dr. Zenk also works with the university's department of philosophy, where he has taught intro to philosophy, ethics, reasoning, symbolic logic, histories of Indian and Buddhist philosophy, and comparative philosophy. He received his PhD in philosophy from the University Hawaii at Manoa in 2018 on the topic of cross-cultural philosophical disagreement. Prior to this, he received an MA in philosophy from the University of Hawaii at Manoa and a bachelor's degree in philosophy from Loyola Marymount University (LMU). Dr. Zenk utilizes a broad array of cross-cultural and interdisciplinary materials in his business and management courses, stemming from his studies of world philosophy, logic, and ethics, as well as both German and Sanskrit language and literature.

Yifan Zhang obtained his PhD in religious studies from Renmin University of China and is a PhD candidate in Indian Languages and Cultures at Ghent University. The title of his doctoral project at Ghent University is "The Jains in Contemporary Southeast Asia (Thailand, Malaysia and Singapore): Their Distinctiveness and Identities," wherein he is currently undertaking ethnographic research in never-before-studied Southeast Asian Jain communities. His research project focuses on diasporic Jain communities, Jain folk religious practices, and South and Southeast Asia using ethnography on Jains in contemporary Southeast Asia, specifically Thailand, Malaysia, and Singapore. The experience of his cross-cultural investigations spans the Asia-Pacific region, encompassing diverse areas, where he has engaged with local communities and villages of different cultural and religious backgrounds. He also explores local discourses of storytelling and narratives in South and Southeast Asia.

Index